Review Special Issue: Recent Advances in Personalized Medicine

Review Special Issue: Recent Advances in Personalized Medicine

Guest Editor

David Alan Rizzieri

MDPI

Basel • Beijing • Wuhan • Barcelona • Belgrade • Novi Sad • Cluj • Manchester

Guest Editor
David Alan Rizzieri
Novant Health Cancer Institute
Winston Salem, NC
USA

Editorial Office
MDPI AG
Grosspeteranlage 5
4052 Basel, Switzerland

This is a reprint of the Special Issue, published open access by the journal *Journal of Personalized Medicine* (ISSN 2075-4426), freely accessible at: https://www.mdpi.com/journal/jpm/special_issues/M996L073B5.

For citation purposes, cite each article independently as indicated on the article page online and as indicated below:

Lastname, A.A.; Lastname, B.B. Article Title. *Journal Name* **Year**, *Volume Number*, Page Range.

ISBN 978-3-7258-8493-3 (Hbk)
ISBN 978-3-7258-8494-0 (PDF)
https://doi.org/10.3390/books978-3-7258-8494-0

Contents

Journal of Personalized Medicine

MDPI

Review

Red-Haired People's Altered Responsiveness to Pain, Analgesics, and Hypnotics: Myth or Fact?—A Narrative Review

Annelie Augustinsson [1,*], Elisabeth Franze [1], Martina Almqvist [1], Margareta Warrén Stomberg [1], Carina Sjöberg [1] and Pether Jildenstål [1,2,3,4,5]

1 Care in High Technological Environments, Department of Health Sciences, Lund University, 221 00 Lund, Sweden
2 Institute of Health and Care Sciences, Sahlgrenska Academy, University of Gothenburg, 405 30 Gothenburg, Sweden
3 Department of Anesthesia and Intensive Care, Institute for Clinical Sciences, Sahlgrenska Academy, University of Gothenburg, 405 30 Gothenburg, Sweden
4 Department of Anesthesiology, Surgery and Intensive Care, Sahlgrenska University Hospital, 405 83 Gothenburg, Sweden
5 Department of Anesthesiology and Intensive Care, Örebro University Hospital and School of Medical Sciences, Örebro University, 701 85 Örebro, Sweden
* Correspondence: annelie.augustinsson@med.lu.se

Abstract: Red hair has been linked to altered sensitivity to pain, analgesics, and hypnotics. This alteration may be impacted by variants in the melanocortin-1 receptor (*MC1R*) gene, which are mainly found in redheads. The aim of this narrative review was to explore and present the current state of knowledge on red hair and its plausible associations with altered responsiveness to pain, analgesics, and hypnotics. Structured searches in the PubMed, CINAHL Complete, and Scopus electronic databases were conducted. Evidence suggests that women with red hair have an increased sensitivity to pain. Conversely, data also indicate a higher pain tolerance in homozygous carriers of *MC1R* variant alleles. Varied responses to analgesia have been reported, with both increased analgesic responsiveness in homozygous carriers of *MC1R* variant alleles and less analgesia in redheads. Data indicate an increased need for hypnotics in redheads. However, failed attempts to find statistical associations between red hair and altered responsiveness to hypnotics are also evident. Even though there seems to be an association between red hair and an altered responsiveness to pain, analgesics, and/or hypnotics, the results of this narrative review are inconclusive. Further research studies with larger populations and *MC1R* testing are needed.

Keywords: melanocortin-1 receptor; MC1R; redheads; pain; analgesics; hypnotics; response

1. Introduction

There is uncertainty regarding redheads' responsiveness to pain, analgesics, and hypnotics. Redheads' plausible altered responsiveness seems to be associated with a dysfunction in the melanocortin-1 receptor (MC1R), a receptor that besides contributing to red hair also contributes to a more sensitive light skin with poor tanning ability, predisposition to sunburn, and increased risk for melanoma [1,2]. MC1R is a seven-transmembrane G-protein-coupled receptor primarily located on the surface of melanocytes and transformed melanoma cells. The receptor is activated by melanocyte-stimulating hormone (MSH) and/or adrenocorticotropic hormone (ACTH), controlling melanogenesis [3]. The receptor plays a crucial role in determining human pigmentation by regulating which type of melanin, i.e., the dark brown/black UV protective eumelanin or the red/blonde pheomelanin pigment, will be produced [3,4]. Individuals with a dysfunctional MC1R may therefore have a decreased synthesis of eumelanin, which leads to fair skin and an increased sensitivity to UV exposure.

Table 1. Key characteristics of the ten included studies, arranged by year of publication.

Authors	Study Design	Sample Size (*n*)		Primary Objective	Intervention	Analysis of *MC1R*	Quality
		Total	Red-Heads				
Mogil et al. (2003) [10]	Experimental case-control study	42	21	To evaluate redheads' and non-redheads' responses to κ-opioids and pain.	Thermal and ischemic pain assessments after administration of κ-opioids or saline.	Yes	High
Chua et al. (2004) [11]	Experimental case-control study	39	20	To evaluate resistance to sedative drugs in redheads and non-redheads.	Pain assessment after experimentally induced pain through application of capsaicin.	No	High
Liem et al. (2004) [12]	Experimental case-control study	20	10	To evaluate whether women with red hair have a greater requirement of volatile anesthesia than women with dark hair.	Measurements of depth of anesthesia through pain stimuli with bilateral intradermal needles in the anterior thighs and end-tidal concentration of inhaled gas.	Yes	High
Liem et al. (2005) [13]	Experimental case-control study	60	30	To evaluate if women with red hair are more sensitive to pain compared to women with dark hair.	Pain assessments through cold and heat stimuli during local anesthesia, both subcutaneous and on the skin.	No	High
Mogil et al. (2005) [14]	Experimental case-control study	47	29	To evaluate redheads' responses to pain and μ-opioid analgesia compared to individuals with other hair colors.	Assessments of electrode-induced acute pain in the legs after administration of μ-opioids.	Yes	High
Andresen at al. (2010) [15]	Experimental case-control study	40	20	To evaluate if pain sensitivity differs between women with red hair compared to women with blond/dark hair.	Pain assessments to different phasic experimental stimulus modalities and capsaicin-induced hyperalgesia.	No	High
Myles et al. (2012) [16]	Prospective, matched cohort study	468	32	To evaluate the effects of hair color on requirements and response to general anesthesia and on postoperative recovery.	Measurements of end-tidal concentration and depth of volatile anesthesia.	No	Moderate
Doufas et al. (2013) [17]	Experimental case-control study	29	13	To evaluate the hypnotic effect of propofol in healthy volunteers with red and dark hair.	Measurements of BIS and drug concentrations before, during, and after anesthesia.	No	High
Gradwohl et al. (2015) [18]	Prospective cohort study	1914	319	To evaluate the risk of awareness, need for anesthesia, and postoperative recovery in redheads.	A secondary analysis where redheads were compared to non-redheads.	No	Moderate
Fontanillas et al. (2022) [19]	Cohort study	PSQ: 25,321 CPT: 6853	PSQ: 693 CPT: 240	To identify genetic factors contributing to individual pain perception.	Self-assessment forms and CPT intervention in the participants' home environments.	Yes	High

Abbreviations: BIS, bispectral index; CPT, cold pressor test; MAC, minimum alveolar concentration; *MC1R*, melanocortin-1 receptor; PSQ, pain sensitivity questionnaire.

Table 2. Reported associations between hair color and responsiveness to pain, analgesics, and/or hypnotics in the ten included studies, arranged by year of publication.

Authors	Response to	Measures	Hair Color or *MC1R* Genotype: Redheads or >1 Variant Alleles	Hair Color or *MC1R* Genotype: Non-Redheads or 0/1 Variant Allele	*p* Value	Comments
Mogil et al. (2003) [10]	Pain and analgesics	IPT:				Significantly greater pentazocine analgesia in women with >1 *MC1R* variant alleles than in women with 0/1 allele, and significantly higher ischemic PT and ratings of intensity and unpleasantness in women with >1 *MC1R* variant alleles than in women with 0/1 allele, but not in men.
		Women	408.0 (284.1)	37.1 (82.9)	<0.05	
		Men	46.4 (149.3)	84.1 (182.8)	>0.05	
		SIPI:				
		Women	84.8 (50.3)	16.9 (41.9)	<0.05	
		Men	18.7 (36.2)	37.8 (38.3)	>0.05	
		SIPU:				
		Women	79.6 (45.7)	9.0 (49.6)	<0.05	
		Men	24.2 (41.0)	33.0 (49.0)	>0.05	
		STPI:				
		Women	28.0 (48.9)	–22.8 (40.1)	<0.05	
		Men	9.2 (51.0)	26.2 (56.5)	>0.05	
Chua et al. (2004) [11]	Hypnotics	OAA/S:				Significantly less sedation and cognitive impairment in volunteers with red hair than in those with blond or brown hair. BIS values did not differ between groups.
		Placebo	5.0 (0.0)	5.0 (0.0)	>0.05	
		Midozolam	5.0 (0.0)	4.0 (2.0)	0.004	
		Drowsiness VAS:				
		Placebo	0 (5)	0 (3)	>0.05	
		Midozolam	42 (54)	67 (47)	0.034	
		BIS:				
		Placebo	97 (3)	97 (4)	>0.05	
		Midazolam	85 (13)	80 (9)	>0.05	
Liem et al. (2004) [12]	Hypnotics	Desfluran requirement (%)	6.2 (5.9–6.5)	5.2 (4.9–5.5)	0.0004	A significant increase in volatile anesthesia requirement in redheads compared with controls.
Liem et al. (2005) [13]	Pain and analgesics	CSPT (°C)	30.7 (30.3–31.0)	30.5 (29.9–31.2)	0.596	Significantly higher sensitivity to cold pain perception and tolerance, as well as lower PT threshold at stimulation after subcutaneous lidocaine in women with red hair than in women with dark hair.
		CPPT (°C)	22.6 (15.1–26.1)	12.6 (0.0–20.0)	0.004	
		CPTT (°C)	6.0 (0.0–9.7)	0.0 (0.0–2.0)	0.001	
		HSPT (°C)	33.8 (33.5–34.0)	33.5 (33.4–33.8)	0.015	
		HPPT (°C)	41.4 (39.7–43.1)	42.4 (41.3–44.6)	0.059	
		HSTT (°C)	46.3 (45.7–47.5)	47.7 (46.6–48.7)	0.009	

Table 2. *Cont.*

Authors	Response to	Measures	Hair Color or *MC1R* Genotype: Redheads or >1 Variant Alleles	Hair Color or *MC1R* Genotype: Non-Redheads or 0/1 Variant Allele	*p* Value	Comments
Liem et al. (2005) [13]	Pain and analgesics	PT thresholds (mA):				Significantly higher sensitivity to cold pain perception and tolerance, as well as lower PT threshold at stimulation after subcutaneous lidocaine in women with red hair than in women with dark hair.
		2000 Hz	11.0 (8.5–16.5)	>20 (14.5–>20)	0.005	
		250 Hz	5.0 (4.0–9.0)	11.6 (8.0–13.0)	0.003	
		5 Hz	6.3 (3.2–10.2)	8.5 (7.0–14.2)	0.013	
Mogil et al. (2005) [14]	Pain and analgesics	PT (mA):				Significantly greater PT and analgesic response in individuals with *MC1R* variants than in controls.
		Baseline	20.9 (1.7)	15.8 (1.2)	0.018	
		Ischemic	1.18 (0.04)	1.49 (0.09)	0.003	
Andresen at al. (2010) [15]	Pain	PTT (kPa/s)	713.6 (403.8)	673.5 (226.1)	0.80	No differences in PTT or HTT between redheads and controls.
		HTT (°C)	47.4 (2.8)	47.8 (1.7)	1.0	
		aaMAC	1.28 (0.27)	1.31 (0.34)	0.46	
Myles et al. (2012) [16]	Hypnotics	Equivalents (mg × kg^{-1}):				No evidence of increased anesthetic requirements in redheads compared with patients with black hair.
		Midazolam	0.028 (9.026)	0.028 (0.026)		
		Morphine	0.80 (1.15)	0.75 (0.85)		
		Propofol	2.11 (2.00)	2.22 (1.75)		
		Vecuronium	0.12 (0.11)	0.12 (0.09)		
Doufas et al. (2013) [17]	Hypnotics	$Ce_{50\ BIS}$ (μg/mL)	2.57 (1.68–3.60)	2.71 (2.28–3.36)	>0.05	No difference in the hypnotic effect of propofol between volunteers with red and dark hair.
Gradwohl et al. (2015) [18]	Hypnotics	aaMAC	0.92 (1.18)	0.91 (0.18)	0.476	No difference in the anesthetic management between redheads and matched controls without red hair.
Fontanillas et al. (2022) [20]	Pain	Redhead × sex *	0.2597 (0.1300)		0.046	Significantly higher sensitivity to pain in red-haired women and self-perceived pain in individuals with >1 *MC1R* variant alleles.
		CPT: *				
		>1 alleles	0.1253 (0.0515)		0.015	
		0/1 allele	0.0517 (0.0191)		0.0068	

* Linear models on PSQ score. Abbreviations: aaMAC, age-adjusted minimum alveolar concentration; BIS, bispectral index; CPPT, cold pain perception threshold; CPT, cold pressor test; CPTT, cold pain tolerance threshold; CSPT, cold sensory perception threshold; HPPT, heat pain perception threshold; HPTT; heat pain tolerance threshold; HSPT, heat sensory perception threshold; HTT, heat tolerance threshold; Hz, Hertz; IPT, ischemic pain tolerance; MC1R, melanocortin-1 receptor; OAA/S, observer's assessment of alertness/sedation; PSQ, pain sensitivity questionnaire; PT, pain tolerance; PTT, pressure tolerance threshold; SIPI, sum ischemic pain intensity; SIPU, sum ischemic pain unpleasantness; STPI, sum thermal pain intensity; VAS, visual analog scale.

3. Results

3.1. Altered Responsiveness to Pain

Evidence suggests that women with red hair have an increased sensitivity to pain. In a study by Fontanillas et al. [19], the relationship between the human genome and pain sensitivity, specifically regarding hair color and the *MC1R* gene, was evaluated. Here, a total of 25,321 participants answered a pain sensitivity questionnaire (PSQ) and 6853 participants performed a cold pressure test (CPT). The results showed that red-haired women had higher PSQ scores compared to women with other hair colors and men ($p = 0.046$). However, no significant difference could be detected between red-haired men and men with other hair colors.

Based on the hypothesis that red-haired women are more sensitive to pain, Liem et al. [13] evaluated differences between redheads ($n = 30$) and non-redheads ($n = 30$). In this study, participants' responsiveness to pain was tested with the Neurometer® CPT/C and the TSA-II NeuroSensory Analyzer device. Results showed that women with red hair were more sensitive to both cold and heat stimuli ($p = 0.001$ and $p = 0.009$, respectively) compared to non-redheads. Conversely, no significant differences regarding responses to pressure- and heat-induced pain between red-haired women ($n = 20$) and women with other hair colors ($n = 20$) were reported in a study by Andresen et al. [15], where responses to pain through heat and pressure stimulations and topical application of capsaicin were evaluated. However, this study indicated that redheads were significantly less sensitive to capsaicin-induced hyperalgesia compared to non-redheads ($p = 0.014$).

Both Liem et al. [13] and Andresen et al. [15] examined pain response to heat. The studies were conducted in a similar way and on similar populations. Even though Liem et al. showed a significant difference in the response to thermal stimuli in red-haired women compared to women with other hair colors [13], Andresen et al. reported no difference between the groups [15]. These results could possibly be explained by the use of different temperatures in the studies, which may have resulted in varied nociceptive responses [21].

In addition, studies on individuals who were genotyped for *MC1R* variants showed varied results on pain responsiveness between *MC1R* variant carriers and non-carriers. In the study by Fontanillas et al. [19], significantly higher PSQ scores were reported by carriers of one ($p = 0.0068$) or two or more ($p = 0.015$) *MC1R* SNPs compared to carriers of wild-type alleles. Conversely, they did not observe an association between being a carrier of *MC1R* variants and CPT duration. However, the tests in this study were conducted in the participants' home environments without the presence of a researcher. Therefore, it is challenging to ascertain whether they were performed correctly. This could have led to compromised reliability of the investigation and, consequently, varied validity of the results. In contrast, in a study by Mogil et al. [14], individuals with *MC1R* variants exhibited significantly higher pain tolerance compared to controls when acute pain was induced through electrodes placed on the skin over the tibial bone of the left leg ($p = 0.018$).

3.2. Altered Responsiveness to Analgesics

In another study by Mogil et al. [10], the responsiveness to analgesics after being given ischemic and thermal pain stimuli was evaluated in 42 participants who underwent genotyping for *MC1R* variants. *MC1R* variants were shown to significantly influence the response to analgesia, however, only in red-haired women and not in red-haired men. When using the κ-opioid Pentazocine, women with two *MC1R* variant alleles were the only ones that had a clear effect of, and response to, the given analgesics. In the more recent study published by the same authors [14], it was further investigated whether the difference in response to analgesics depended on the received type of opioid. The results indicated that *MC1R* variant carriers had an increased response to μ-opioid (morphine) induced analgesia compared to the control group ($p = 0.003$). Whereas the first study by Mogil et al. [10] showed a difference in the responsiveness to analgesics between women and men, which is consistent with results from other previous studies, i.e., that gender has an association with perceived pain [22,23], no significant difference between sexes could be demonstrated in the more recent study [14]. Further investigation is needed to determine whether the observed difference in response is attributable to gender in general or if it is directly linked to μ- and κ-opioids.

The responsiveness to analgesia in redheads and non-redheads was also evaluated in the study by Liem et al. [13]. When the effect of the subcutaneously administered lidocaine was evaluated, a lower effect was shown in redheads compared to dark-haired participants, where redheads showed significantly lower pain tolerance thresholds at 2000 Hz, 250 Hz, and 5 Hz stimulation ($p = 0.005$, $p = 0.03$, and $p = 0.013$, respectively). However, no significant difference was observed between the two groups in response to cutaneous administered lidocaine when evaluating the effect of local anesthetics ($p = 0.46$). While both studies by Mogil et al. [10,14] showed an increased response to opioids in *MC1R* SNP carriers compared to the controls, Liem et al. [13] showed that red-haired women had a weaker response to analgesics. This may be explained by the variation in pain character, the use of different types of analgesics, and different ways of administering the drug [24]. Another possibility is that the individual's own experience of pain could have affected the outcome, i.e., perceived pain, in both tests, even though participants who had been part of earlier pain studies were excluded [14]. It is difficult to draw any conclusion from the studies by Mogil et al. [10,14] and Liem et al. [13]. These studies included small populations and the researchers were not blinded to participants' hair color. In addition, it must be considered that the researchers could have influenced the results by observational bias, and participants could have modified their behavior knowing that they were part of a study, the so-called Hawthorne effect [20]. The participants had, however, not been informed of the hypotheses of the studies, which may strengthen the results.

3.3. Altered Responsiveness to Hypnotics

Redheads may require more sedation compared to non-redheads. Studies regarding a possible increased need for hypnotics in redheads measured the used amount of volatile anesthetic agent and hypnotic depth, e.g., using the bispectral index (BIS) and end-tidal inhalation concentration, i.e., minimal alveolar concentration (MAC). In an experimental study by Liem et al. [12], all participants ($n = 20$) underwent genotyping for *MC1R* variants. Study participants were anesthetized by sevoflurane and subsequently transitioned to desflurane, maintaining anesthesia with an end-tidal concentration of 5.5–7.5%. The response to anesthesia was measured by bilateral electrical stimuli on the front of the thighs for ten seconds using transdermal needles. If the person moved their legs in response to the stimuli, the amount of volatile agent was increased by 0.5%. In contrast, if there was no response, the amount was decreased by 0.5%. The study showed a significant difference in the need for volatile agents between red-haired women and the control group, with redheads requiring 19% more ($p = 0.0004$). Additionally, Chua et al. [11] conducted a blinded randomized study on redheads' responsiveness to hypnotics, in which the participants ($n = 39$) received either intravenous midazolam or saline. The study showed significant differences between the groups regarding the observer's assessment of alertness/sedation (OAA/S) and the drowsiness visual analog scale (VAS), where the redheads required more sedation compared to non-redheads ($p = 0.004$ and $p = 0.034$, respectively). BIS values were not different between the groups [12]. No significant differences between redheads and non-redheads in terms of anesthetic requirements were reported in the three studies by Myles et al. [16], Gradwohl et al. [18], and Doufas et al. [17], where none of the participants were genotyped for *MC1R* variants. The study by Gradwohl et al. [18] was conducted on a large population. However, it included patients at higher risk of intraoperative awareness, resulting in them receiving larger doses of both volatile and intravenous anesthesia as well as muscle relaxants. Because they were given higher doses of medication, it may have affected the result [25].

To measure responses to hypnotics, most of the studies used the BIS tool [11,16–18]. Only Chua et al. [11] used several different validated measuring tools. It is interesting, though, that the only objective measuring tool where one can imagine that the evidence is more reliable, no significant differences were shown, neither in the study by Chua et al. [11] nor in any of the other studies [16–18]. This raises the question of whether the results would have been different if other objective measuring tools had been used. Even Gradwohl et al. [18] question the use of BIS to assess the depth of anesthesia as it is a surrogate measure and does not fully reflect the neurobiological depth of anesthesia. Hence, it is possible that redheads may have needed more volatile anesthesia than indicated. To obtain more valid results, consideration should have been given to the type of anesthesia each patient received. The measurement shown by electroencephalogram (EEG) monitoring varies according to the type of anesthesia the patient receives and the patient's age can also affect the results [26]. The studies that evaluated the response of hypnotics took place between 2004 and 2015. It is possible that the outcome would have been different if the studies had been implemented in the present due to the progress of medical techniques. In addition, there is a possibility that the results could have been different if another measuring tool, e.g., spectral edge frequency (SEF), had been used as well since it shows more individualized EEGs with higher precision [26].

Only one of the studies where the participants were genotyped for *MC1R* variants evaluated the responsiveness to hypnotics. In this study, by Liem et al. [12], a significant increase in the requirement of volatile anesthesia in redheads compared to the controls was reported. However, the MAC value was lower than what is usually needed for surgical stimuli in this study. This was expected though since the depth of anesthesia should always be adjusted according to the patient's age and the anticipated stimuli [27]. In the more recent study by Liem et al. [13], one could also assume that all red-haired participants had two *MC1R* variant alleles since the genetic analysis from the earlier study had evidence for this [20]. This also coheres with other studies that have examined genetic *MC1R* SNPs associated with red hair [28,29]. However, Mogil et al. [10] reported that individuals with red hair can have a functioning MC1R and that the red hair color could be caused by something else than a non-functioning MC1R. With regard to the hypothesis that variants in *MC1R* affect the responsiveness to pain, analgesics, and hypnotics, it is possible that the outcome could have been different in the studies where the participants were not genotyped. In addition, it is difficult to know if any exclusion criteria were made with regard to the patients' habits, e.g., use of drugs and/or alcohol, which could have increased the need for hypnotics [30].

Variants in the *MC1R* gene are mostly known for their regulation of pigmentation of skin and hair color [6] but may also be associated with pain sensitivity and altered responsiveness to analgesics and hypnotics. This could indicate that genetic variations in *MC1R* result in altered responsiveness and would therefore be of clinical relevance [1,31].

4. Conclusions

The largest challenge for people with red hair seems to be an altered responsiveness to pain and analgesics. It is important to implement multimodal pain management since redheads have shown varied sensitivity to opioids. In addition, redheads seem to have a certain tolerance toward volatile anesthesia, which leads to total intravenous anesthesia being preferred. EEG-based depth of anesthesia monitoring should be used to increase patient safety. One consideration for future preoperative routines regarding this population of individuals might be to enhance the possibility of genetic testing of *MC1R*. It seems that studies regarding the responsiveness to pain, analgesics, or hypnotics in red-haired people are limited. The results of this narrative review indicate a need for more randomized intervention studies. Few studies have been made, and mostly on relatively small populations, with a scarcity of studies incorporating *MC1R* genotyping. Due to population heterogeneity, certain genotypes may hold importance in determining the effects of medication. Hence, pharmacogenomic associations need validation for each therapeutic indication, particularly with the advent of new drugs and in diverse subgroups. Recognizing these limitations is crucial for accurately interpreting genetic factors influencing drug response and for effectively translating pharmacogenomic findings into clinical practice. Because the studies had different designs and populations, it was difficult to draw any general conclusions. However, this narrative review shows some associations between red hair, including people with genetic variants in *MC1R*, and altered responsiveness to pain, analgesics, and hypnotics. Further studies on this subject are, however, needed, including larger populations and *MC1R* genotyping.

Author Contributions: Conceptualization, A.A. and P.J.; methodology, A.A., E.F., M.A. and P.J.; software, A.A.; validation, E.F., M.A., C.S., M.W.S. and P.J.; formal analysis, A.A., E.F. and M.A.; writing—original draft preparation, A.A., E.F., M.A. and P.J.; writing—review and editing, A.A., E.F., M.A., C.S., M.W.S. and P.J; visualization, A.A.; supervision, P.J. All authors have read and agreed to the published version of the manuscript.

Funding: This research received no external funding.

Institutional Review Board Statement: The study did not require ethical approval.

Informed Consent Statement: Not applicable.

Data Availability Statement: No new data were created.

Conflicts of Interest: The authors declare no conflicts of interest.

References

1. Zorina-Lichtenwalter, K.; Maixner, W.; Diatchenko, L. Detangling red hair from pain: Phenotype-specific contributions from different genetic variants in melanocortin-1 receptor. *Pain* **2020**, *161*, 938–948. [CrossRef]
2. Garcia-Borron, J.C.; Abdel-Malek, Z.; Jimenez-Cervantes, C. MC1R, the cAMP pathway, and the response to solar UV: Extending the horizon beyond pigmentation. *Pigment. Cell Melanoma Res.* **2014**, *27*, 699–720. [CrossRef]
3. Wolf Horrell, E.M.; Boulanger, M.C.; D'orazio, J.A. Melanocortin 1 Receptor: Structure, Function, and Regulation. *Front. Genet.* **2016**, *7*, 95. [CrossRef] [PubMed]
4. Zorina-Lichtenwalter, K.; Lichtenwalter, R.N.; Zaykin, D.V.; Parisien, M.; Gravel, S.; Bortsov, A.; Diatchenko, L. A study in scarlet: MC1R as the main predictor of red hair and exemplar of the flip-flop effect. *Hum. Mol. Genet.* **2019**, *28*, 2093–2106. [CrossRef] [PubMed]
5. Sherry, S.T.; Ward, M.; Sirotkin, K. dbSNP-database for single nucleotide polymorphisms and other classes of minor genetic variation. *Genome Res.* **1999**, *9*, 677–679. [CrossRef] [PubMed]
6. Morgan, M.D.; Pairo-Castineira, E.; Rawlik, K.; Canela-Xandri, O.; Rees, J.; Sims, D.; Tenesa, A.; Jackson, I.J. Genome-wide study of hair colour in UK Biobank explains most of the SNP heritability. *Nat. Commun.* **2018**, *9*, 5271. [CrossRef] [PubMed]
7. Rees, J.L. The melanocortin 1 receptor (MC1R): More than just red hair. *Pigment. Cell Res.* **2000**, *13*, 135–140. [CrossRef] [PubMed]
8. Guyatt, G.; Oxman, A.D.; Akl, E.A.; Kunz, R.; Vist, G.; Brozek, J.; Norris, S.; Falck-Ytter, Y.; Glasziou, P.; DeBeer, H.; et al. GRADE guidelines: 1. Introduction—GRADE evidence profiles and summary of findings tables. *J. Clin. Epidemiol.* **2011**, *64*, 383–394. [CrossRef] [PubMed]
9. Critical Appraisal Skills Programme. CASP Checklists. Available online: https://casp-uk.net/casp-tools-checklists/ (accessed on 15 February 2023).
10. Mogil, J.S.; Wilson, S.G.; Chesler, E.J.; Rankin, A.L.; Nemmani, K.V.S.; Lariviere, W.R.; Groce, M.K.; Wallace, M.R.; Kaplan, L.; Staud, R.; et al. The melanocortin-1 receptor gene mediates female-specific mechanisms of analgesia in mice and humans. *Proc. Natl. Acad. Sci. USA* **2003**, *100*, 4867–4872. [CrossRef]
11. Chua, M.V.; Tsueda, K.; Doufas, A.G. Midazolam causes less sedation in volunteers with red hair. *Can. J. Anaesth.* **2004**, *51*, 25–30. [CrossRef]
12. Liem, E.B.; Lin, C.-M.; Suleman, M.-I.; Doufas, A.G.; Gregg, R.G.; Veauthier, J.M.; Loyd, G.; Sessler, D.I. Anesthetic requirement is increased in redheads. *Anesthesiology* **2004**, *101*, 279–283. [CrossRef] [PubMed]
13. Liem, E.B.; Joiner, T.V.; Tsueda, K.; Sessler, D.I. Increased sensitivity to thermal pain and reduced subcutaneous lidocaine efficacy in redheads. *Anesthesiology* **2005**, *102*, 509–514. [CrossRef]
14. Mogil, J.S.; Ritchie, J.; Smith, S.B.; Strasburg, K.; Kaplan, L.; Wallace, M.R.; Romberg, R.R.; Bijl, H.; Sarton, E.Y.; Fillingim, R.B.; et al. Melanocortin-1 receptor gene variants affect pain and -opioid analgesia in mice and humans. *J. Med. Genet.* **2005**, *42*, 583–587. [CrossRef]
15. Andresen, T.; Lunden, D.; Drewes, A.M.; Arendt-Nielsen, L. Pain sensitivity and experimentally induced sensitisation in red haired females. *Scand. J. Pain* **2011**, *2*, 3–6. [CrossRef]
16. Myles, P.S.; Buchanan, F.F.; Bain, C.R. The effect of hair colour on anaesthetic requirements and recovery time after surgery. *Anaesth. Intensiv. Care* **2012**, *40*, 683–689. [CrossRef]
17. Doufas, A.G.; Orhan-Sungur, M.; Komatsu, R.; Lauber, R.; Akca, O.; Shafer, S.L.; Sessler, D.I. Bispectral index dynamics during propofol hypnosis is similar in red-haired and dark-haired subjects. *Anesth. Analg.* **2013**, *116*, 319–326. [CrossRef] [PubMed]

18. Gradwohl, S.C.; Aranake, A.; Ben Abdallah, A.; McNair, P.; Lin, N.; Fritz, B.A.; Villafranca, A.; Glick, D.; Jacobsohn, E.; Mashour, G.A.; et al. Intraoperative awareness risk, anesthetic sensitivity, and anesthetic management for patients with natural red hair: A matched cohort study. *Can. J. Anaesth.* **2015**, *62*, 345–355. [CrossRef]
19. Fontanillas, P.; Kless, A.; Bothmer, J.; Tung, J.Y. Genome-wide association study of pain sensitivity assessed by questionnaire and the cold pressor test. *Pain* **2022**, *163*, 1763–1776. [CrossRef] [PubMed]
20. Wickström, G.; Bendix, T. The "Hawthorne effect"—What did the original Hawthorne studies actually show? *Scand. J. Work Environ. Health* **2000**, *26*, 363–367. [CrossRef]
21. Yucel, A.; Andersen, O.K.; Nielsen, J.; Arendt-Nielsen, L. Heat hyperalgesia in humans: Assessed by different stimulus temperature profiles. *Eur. J. Pain* **2002**, *6*, 357–364. [CrossRef]
22. Morin, C.; Lund, J.P.; Villarroel, T.; Clokie, C.M.; Feine, J.S. Differences between the sexes in post-surgical pain. *Pain* **2000**, *85*, 79–85. [CrossRef] [PubMed]
23. Zheng, H.; Schnabel, A.; Yahiaoui-Doktor, M.; Meissner, W.; Van Aken, H.; Zahn, P.; Pogatzki-Zahn, E. Age and preoperative pain are major confounders for sex differences in postoperative pain outcome: A prospective database analysis. *PLoS ONE* **2017**, *12*, e0178659. [CrossRef] [PubMed]
24. Argoff, C.E.; Silvershein, D.I. A comparison of long- and short-acting opioids for the treatment of chronic noncancer pain: Tailoring therapy to meet patient needs. *Mayo Clin. Proc.* **2009**, *84*, 602–612. [CrossRef] [PubMed]
25. Avidan, M.S.; Jacobsohn, E.; Glick, D.; Burnside, B.A.; Zhang, L.; Villafranca, A.; Karl, L.; Kamal, S.; Torres, B.; O'Connor, M.; et al. Prevention of intraoperative awareness in a high-risk surgical population. *N. Engl. J. Med.* **2011**, *365*, 591–600. [CrossRef] [PubMed]
26. Jildenstål, P.; Bäckström, A.; Hedman, K.; Warrén-Stomberg, M. Spectral edge frequency during general anaesthesia: A narrative literature review. *J. Int. Med. Res.* **2022**, *50*, 3000605221118682. [CrossRef] [PubMed]
27. Ni, K.; Cooter, M.; Gupta, D.K.; Thomas, J.; Hopkins, T.J.; Miller, T.E.; James, M.L.; Kertai, M.D.; Berger, M. Paradox of age: Older patients receive higher age-adjusted minimum alveolar concentration fractions of volatile anaesthetics yet display higher bispectral index values. *Br. J. Anaesth.* **2019**, *123*, 288–297. [CrossRef] [PubMed]
28. Valverde, P.; Healy, E.; Jackson, I.; Rees, J.L.; Thody, A.J. Variants of the melanocyte–stimulating hormone receptor gene are associated with red hair and fair skin in humans. *Nat. Genet.* **1995**, *11*, 328–330. [CrossRef] [PubMed]
29. Rees, J.L. Genetics of hair and skin color. *Annu. Rev. Genet.* **2003**, *37*, 67–90. [CrossRef]
30. Beaulieu, P. Anesthetic implications of recreational drug use. *Can. J. Anaesth.* **2017**, *64*, 1236–1264. [CrossRef]
31. Trescot, A.M.; Faynboym, S. A review of the role of genetic testing in pain medicine. *Pain Physician* **2014**, *17*, 425–445. [CrossRef]

Journal of
*Personalized
Medicine*

MDPI

Review

A Critical Review of the Impact of *SMARCA4* Mutations on Survival Outcomes in Non-Small Cell Lung Cancer

Peter Manolakos *, Luigi Boccuto and Diana S. Ivankovic

Healthcare Genetics and Genomics PhD Program, Clemson University, Clemson, SC 29634, USA; lboccut@clemson.edu (L.B.); divanko@clemson.edu (D.S.I.)
* Correspondence: pmanola@clemson.edu

Abstract: This critical review investigates the impact of SWI/SNF-related, matrix-associated, actin-dependent regulator of chromatin, subfamily A, member 4 (*SMARCA4*) mutations on survival outcomes in non-small cell lung cancer (NSCLC) through an analysis of 21 peer-reviewed articles. Survival analyses across this review demonstrated consistently worse outcomes for *SMARCA4*-mutated vs. *SMARCA4* wild-type NSCLC patients, specifically emphasizing class 1 truncating mutations as an independent factor for poor overall survival. In addition, this review explores the clinicopathologic characteristics of *SMARCA4* mutations and their impact on various treatment modalities, including immune checkpoint inhibitors (ICIs) both with and without Kirsten rat sarcoma viral oncogene homolog (*KRAS*) co-mutations. The potential ineffectiveness of ICI treatment in NSCLC is explored through the impact of *SMARCA4/KRAS* co-mutations on the tumor microenvironment. Moreover, this NSCLC review consistently reported statistically worse overall survival outcomes for *SMARCA4/KRAS* co-mutations than *SMARCA4* wild-type/*KRAS*-mutated cohorts, extending across ICIs, chemo-immunotherapy (CIT), and *KRAS* G12C inhibitors. Designing prospective clinical *SMARCA4*-mutated or *SMARCA4/KRAS* co-mutated NSCLC trials to evaluate targeted therapies and immunotherapy may lead to a better understanding of how to improve cancer patients' outcomes and survival rates.

Keywords: *SMARCA4*; mutation; *KRAS*; co-mutation; *KRAS/SMARCA4*; NSCLC; non-small cell lung cancer; survival; treatment outcome; immunotherapy

1. Introduction

Over the past twenty years, the Food and Drug Administration (FDA) has approved a minimum of 20 new molecular entities that target oncogenic driver mutations in non-small cell lung cancer (NSCLC) [1]. These targeted therapies have led to some NSCLC studies reporting a median overall survival (OS) over three years in the metastatic setting [2]. While more than fifty percent of non-squamous NSCLC patients may have a mutation with an FDA-approved therapy, there remains a distinct unmet medical need for those with epigenetic dysregulation that may be more challenging to target [1,3]. This need is particularly vital given that the five-year survival rate for Stage IV NSCLC patients in 2020 was only 8.2% [4].

This critical review analyzes the current literature on the impact of mutations in the SWI/SNF-related, matrix-associated, actin-dependent regulator of chromatin, subfamily A, member 4 (*SMARCA4*) gene, focusing on the survival outcomes for patients with NSCLC. Typically, patients with *SMARCA4*-deficient NSCLC clinically present with adenocarcinoma, larger invasive tumor size, a smoking history, and fewer epidermal growth factor receptor (EGFR) mutations ($p < 0.05$) [5,6]. In addition, *SMARCA4*-mutated NSCLCs are associated with a higher likelihood of negative or low programmed cell death ligand-1 (PD-L1) expression ($p = 0.03$) and higher tumor mutational burden (TMB) as compared to wild-type (WT) cases ($p < 0.001$) [7,8].

SMARCA4 mutations occur in approximately 5–7% of all human cancers and 7–11% of NSCLC cases [6,9–11]. Two classes of *SMARCA4* alterations are linked to epigenetic dysregulation [12]. Class 1 mutations encompass truncating mutations, fusions, and homozygous deletions, typically associated with protein loss and loss of function. Class 2 mutations involve missense mutations, which are suggested to employ dominant-negative or gain-of-function effects. Some reports indicate a loss of function leading to reduced accessibility and diminished chromatin remodeling activity, mainly observed in lung cancer [11]. In a comprehensive study of 4813 tumors from NSCLC patients, Schoenfeld et al. discovered that 212 patients (4% of the total population) exhibited class 1 *SMARCA4* alterations (52% of the *SMARCA4* variants) [8]. In contrast, 195 patients (4% of the total population) had tumors with class 2 *SMARCA4* alterations (48% of the *SMARCA4* variants) [8]. Of particular interest, *SMARCA4* mutations are associated with altered MYC gene expression, which is essential in regulating cell growth and proliferation [13].

SMARCA4 is a tumor suppressor gene located on chromosome 19p13.2 that encodes the Brahma-Related Gene 1 (BRG1) protein, which is one of two mutually exclusive critical DNA-dependent ATPases (Brahma is the other) that regulates gene expression by altering the chromatin structure [14]. In addition, the BRG1 protein contains a bromodomain that plays a critical role in gene transcription and is essential in recognizing acetylated lysine residues on N-terminal tails of histones [14].

BRG1 is part of the mammalian-type switch/sucrose non-fermenting (mSWI/SNF) chromatin-regulatory complex (CRC) [15]. The mSWI/SNF remodeling complex is essential in regulating chromatin structures and contains approximately 10–12 subunits [16]. Utilizing energy obtained through ATP hydrolysis, the catalytic subunits of human mSWI/SNF change nucleosome positioning. This alteration modulates the accessibility of transcriptional machinery to DNA, ultimately impacting the activation or repression of specific genes. The mSWI/SNF CRC protein subunits of interest are AT-Rich Interaction Domain 1A (ARID1A), SWI/SNF Related, Matrix-Associated, Actin-Dependent Regulator of Chromatin, Subfamily B, Member 1 (SMARCB1), and BRG1. They are among the most studied CRCs and have higher rates of mutations in human cancers than other CRC subunits [17].

The most frequent co-mutations found in the Massachusetts General Hospital analysis of 29 *SMARCA4* patients that lacked BRG1 protein expression affected *TP53* (N = 17, 59%), *STK11* (N = 15, 52%), *KEAP1* (N = 12, 41%), and *KRAS* (N = 10, 34%) [6]. These co-mutation frequencies were validated in a more extensive Foundation Medicine data set with *SMARCA4* co-mutations in *TP53* (74%), *CDKN2A* (38%), *STK11* (34%), *KRAS* (26%), and *KEAP1* (15%) [6].

Further research is needed to unravel the intricate interplay between *SMARCA4*, chromatin remodeling, and tumorigenesis in non-small cell lung cancer. A comprehensive understanding of the nuanced interplay between *SMARCA4* and *KRAS* co-occurring mutations in the context of NSCLC is paramount, as *KRAS* mutations commonly co-occur with various mutations and have been found to have a poor prognosis across several NSCLC studies [18]. This review aims to summarize the clinical studies that have elucidated the potential implications of *SMARCA4* mutations and *SMARCA4/KRAS* co-mutations on survival outcomes when treating metastatic NSCLC patients across various treatments (i.e., chemotherapy and immune checkpoint inhibitors).

2. Materials and Methods

PubMed and the Web of Science were searched using the following keywords: "SMAR CA4" and "NSCLC". Boolean operators were used to connect specific search keywords. Peer-reviewed articles published in English between 2018 and 2023 were included, and duplicate records were removed. Articles were included if they contained any of the following concerning NSCLC patients with *SMARCA4* mutations vs. *SMARCA4* WT: OS hazard ratio (HR), progression-free survival (PFS) HR, median OS, or median PFS. Articles were excluded if they were solely pre-clinical or diagnostic. Articles were also excluded if the majority of *SMARCA4* lung cancer patients were diagnosed with non-NSCLC (i.e., small-cell), an undifferentiated tumor, or sarcomatoid *SMARCA4* NSCLC. Articles were loaded into Raayan [19] and reviewed by all authors. Discrepancies were discussed until a consensus was reached on included vs. excluded articles.

The search strategy was as follows: (smarca4 [Title/Abstract]) AND (nsclc [Title/Abstract]) Filters: Full text, Humans, from 2018–2023. The study selection process is outlined in the PRISMA flow diagram (Figure 1) [20].

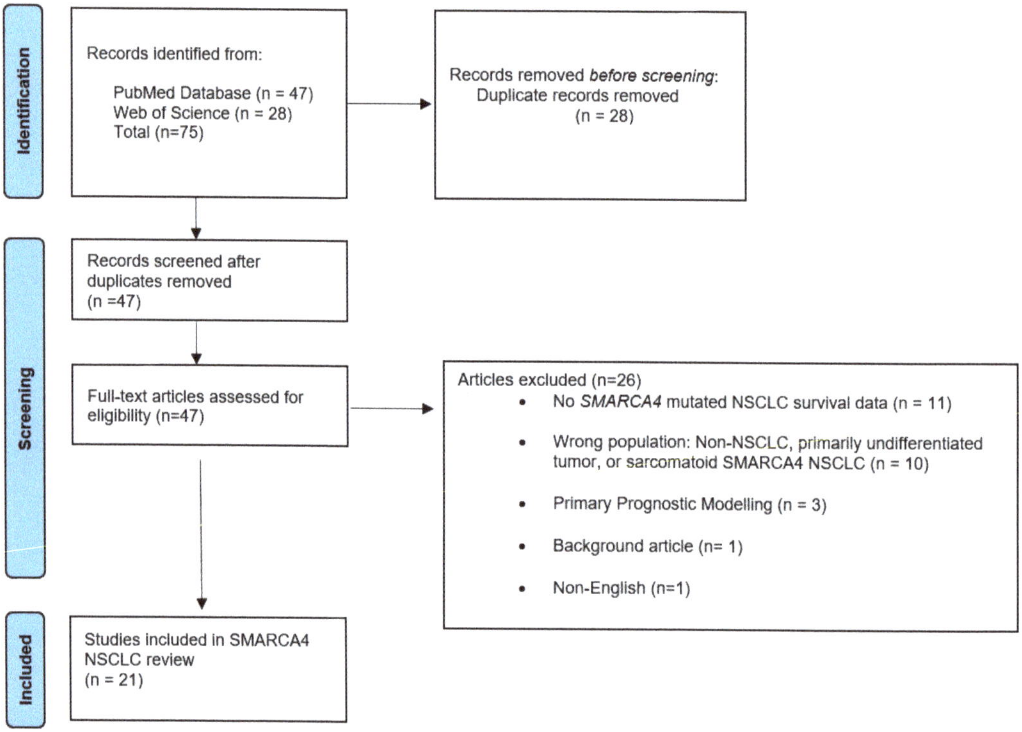

Figure 1. PRISMA flow diagram illustrating the study selection process.

3. Results

3.1. Results and Description of Studies

In this critical review, 75 articles were identified by applying the search strategy. Twenty-eight articles were excluded and removed as duplicate records, and 47 articles were fully reviewed. Twenty-six articles were excluded due to the lack of *SMARCA4*-mutation NSCLC survival outcomes, primary prognostic modeling, lack of incorrect patient population (i.e., sarcomatoid histology), review articles, and being written in non-English.

Twenty-one studies were included and reviewed in this critical review of *SMARCA4* NSCLC. The included articles focus on survival outcomes across various patient categories, clinicopathologic characteristics, and immune checkpoint inhibitors (ICIs) cancer treatment. Moreover, a separate subheading focusing on *SMARCA4* and *KRAS* co-mutation survival outcomes in patients with NSCLC is included, as this has recently become a medically relevant topic in the lung cancer community. Table 1 summarizes the NSCLC mutation analyzed, treatment, outcome, and relevance of each study in this review.

Table 1. Summary of articles included in this critical review. (A) *SMARCA4* Mutations. (B) *SMARCA4/KRAS* Co-mutations.

(A)					
Author	**Publication Year**	**Treatment**	**NSCLC Mutation Analyzed**	**Number of NSCLC Patients with Mutation Analyzed**	**Outcomes/Relevance**
Schoenfeld	2020	Various SOC	*SMARCA4*	N = 292 mut [class 1 mut (N = 149) and class 2 (N = 143)]	In a multivariate analysis, both *SMARCA4* mut class 1 and 2 had worse OS ($p < 0.001$) vs. WT. Class 1 mut had worse OS compared to class 2 mut or WT ($p < 0.001$).
		ICI cohort	*SMARCA4*	N = 87 mut	OS improvement for *SMARCA4* mut with ICI treatment vs. without ICI treatment regardless of class 1 or class 2 mut status ($p = 0.01$). The unadjusted ICI analysis showed no difference in PFS ($p = 0.74$) or OS ($p = 0.35$) with class 1 mut vs. class 2 mut.
Alessi	2023	CIT	*SMARCA4*	114 mut	In multivariate analysis: worse OS for *SMARCA4* mut vs. WT (8.1 versus 15.0 months, HR: 1.70; $p < 0.001$) and worse PFS: (2.7 versus 6.1 months, HR: 1.62; $p < 0.001$).
Alessi	2021	Various SOC	*SMARCA4*	163 mut	*SMARCA4* mut had worse OS (15.6 months) vs. *SMARCA4* WT (25 months) (HR: 0.64; $p < 0.001$).
		ICI or ICI/CTLA4 cohort	*SMARCA4*	57 mut class 1 non-sense, frameshift, and splice site mut (N = 26) and class 2 missense mut (N = 31)	There were no significant differences in *SMARCA4* WT vs. mut: PFS (3.1 vs. 2.1 months; HR = 0.93, $p = 0.62$) or OS (12.4 vs. 11 months; HR = 0.83, $p = 0.25$ months). There was no OS difference in outcomes after receiving ICI therapy when comparing class 1 nonsense, frameshift, and splice site mut (6.7 months; $p = 0.11$) vs. WT patients (12.4 months) vs. class 2 missense mut (11.9 months, HR = 1.03, $p = 0.87$).
Fernando	2020	Various SOC	*SMARCA4*	*SMARCA4* mut in four categories: (1) homozygous truncated (N = 102), (2) homozygous nontruncated (N = 101), (3) heterozygous truncated (N = 16), (4) heterozygous nontruncated (N = 49)	There was a significant OS difference when comparing *SMARCA4* homozygous truncated mut vs. *SMARCA4* WT (7.9 vs. 16.3 months, HR: 1.85; $p < 0.0001$), but no significant differences when comparing the other *SMARCA4* mut categories with WT.
		ICI cohort		*SMARCA4* mut four categories: (1) homozygous truncated (N = 38), (2) homozygous nontruncated (N = 41), (3) heterozygous truncated (N = 5), (4) heterozygous nontruncated (N = 23)	There was a significant OS difference when comparing *SMARCA4* mut homozygous truncated vs. *SMARCA4* WT (9.9 vs. 19.5 months, HR: 1.62; $p = 0.01$), but no significant differences when comparing the other *SMARCA4* mut categories with WT.
Dagogo-Jack	2020	Chemo or CIT	*SMARCA4*	16 mut	Extremely short PFS for chemo and CIT treatment (38 and 35 days), respectively.

Table 1. *Cont.*

(A)					
Author	**Publication Year**	**Treatment**	**NSCLC Mutation Analyzed**	**Number of NSCLC Patients with Mutation Analyzed**	**Outcomes/Relevance**
Liang	2023	Various SOC	*SMARCA4* *SMARCA4*	Stage III mut (N = 21), Stage IV mut (N = 69) 221 mut women (N = 88), men (N = 25)	Median OS survival for *SMARCA4* mut vs. *SMARCA4* WT patients was notably lower in Stage III (23.73 vs. 29.43 months, p = <0.01) and Stage IV (11.93 vs. 28.23 months, p = <0.01). Multivariate analysis resulted in statistically worse OS for women vs. men (HR = 4.1, p = 0.04).
Talvitie	2022	Various SOC	*SMARCA4* *SMARCA4*	135 mut Stage III mut (N = 31)	*SMARCA4* mut patients had a worse OS than *SMARCA4* WT (HR: 3.522; p < 0.002). Stage III multivariate analysis *SMARCA4* mut patients had a worse OS vs. WT patients (HR:1.93; p = 0.04).
Xu	2023	Various SOC	*SMARCA4*	Four Arms: (1) *SMARCA4* WT, TMB Low (N = 761), (2) *SMARCA4* WT, TMB High (N = 722), (3) *SMARCA4* mut, TMB Low (N = 26), and (4) *SMARCA4* mut, TMB High (N = 69).	Statistically better OS for *SMARCA4* WT/TMB High (p = 0.00019).
Miao	2023	Alectinib (ALK)	*SMARCA4/ALK*	3 mut	In a multivariate analysis, *SMARCA4* mut patients with brain metastasis were the only co-mut with *ALK* with worse outcomes (HR: 8.76; p = 0.009).
Pan	2023	Various SOC	*SMARCA4*	44 mut: women (N = 19), men (N = 25)	Multivariate analysis with *SMARCA4* mut: men had a significantly worse OS than women (2.75 months vs. un-estimable, HR:14.2; p = 0.02).
Wang	2021	Atezo (ICI) or docetaxel	*SMARCA4* *SMARCA4*	100 mut 39 mut	OAK analysis: there is no statistical difference in OS when comparing atezolizumab vs. docetaxel in *SMARCA4* mut, whether PDL-1 high or negative (HR = 0.67; p = 0.256). No difference in OS with PDL-1 high vs. low when treated with atezo (HR = 1.185, p = 0.513)
Marinelli	2020	Atezo (ICI)	*SMARCA4*	18 mut	OAK uni-variate analysis: *SMARCA4*-mutated patients receiving atezo did not fare worse than *SMARCA4* WT patients (HR: 1.70; p = 0.064).
Velut	2022	Nivolumab or pembro	*SMARCA4*	7 mut	SD-NSCLC patients had a shorter OS than patients with non-SD-NSCLC, considering either from the date of diagnosis (p = 0.01, HR: 2.9) or from the date of immunotherapy (p = 0.006, HR: 3.2). OS rates at 1 year were not significantly different between *SMARCA4* mut and WT patients but dropped significantly at 2 (58% vs. 74%) and 5 years (37% vs. 53%).

Table 1. *Cont.*

(A)					
Author	**Publication Year**	**Treatment**	**NSCLC Mutation Analyzed**	**Number of NSCLC Patients with Mutation Analyzed**	**Outcomes/Relevance**
Chang	2022	ICI (87% of patients)	*SMARCA4*	16 mut	No significant PFS difference in *SMARCA4* WT vs. mut (6.3 vs. 3.9 months, HR: 0.64; $p = 0.15$).
Yang	2023	Various SOC	*SMARCA4*	5 mut	*SMARCA4* mut patients had a worse OS compared to WT patients (4.5 months vs. 13.3 months; HR: 2.86; $p = 0.031$). Significantly worse PFS for *SMARCA4* mut vs. WT (2.3 months vs. 8.1 months, HR: 2.80; $p = 0.035$).
Wang	2021	SOC	*SMARCA4*	4 mut	In multivariate analysis, *SMARCA4* mut patients fared worse than *SMARCA4* WT (HR = 3.098, $p = 0.038$) and had worse PFS (3 vs. 8 months, $p = 0.007$).
Le Fleur	2019	Various SOC	*SMARCA4*	21 mut	In a multivariate all-cause mortality analysis, *SMARCA4* mut were independently associated with a worse OS prognosis (HR: 2.06, $p = 0.003$).
(B)					
Author	**Publication Year**	**Treatment**	**NSCLC Mutations Analyzed**	**Number of NSCLC Patients with Mutations Analyzed**	**Outcomes/Relevance**
Cooper	2022	Various SOC	*SMARCA4/KRAS* G12D co-mut *SMARCA4* WT/*KRAS* G12D mut	8 co-mut 49 mut	Significantly worse PFS for co-mut patients; PFS: *SMARCA4/KRAS* G12D mut vs. *SMARCA4* WT/*KRAS* G12D mut (1.5 vs. 4.0 months; $p = 0.0039$). No significant difference in OS: *SMARCA4/KRAS* G12D co-mut vs. *SMARCA4* WT/*KRAS* G12D mut (6.1 vs. 17.3 months; $p = 0.4202$).
Negrao	2023	Sotorasib or adagrasib	*SMARCA4/KRAS* G12C co-mut *SMARCA4* WT/*KRAS* G12C	20 co-mut 214 mut	*SMARCA4/KRAS* co-mut patients had significantly worse PFS than *SMARCA4* WT/*KRAS* mut (1.6 months vs. 5.4, HR: 3.04; $p < 0.001$) and had a significantly worse OS (4.9 months vs. 11.8 months, HR: 3.07; $p < 0.001$).
Boiarsky	2023	Various SOC	*SMARCA4/KRAS* co-mut *SMARCA4* WT/*KRAS* mut	33 co-mut 231 mut	OS was significantly worse for *SMARCA4/KRAS* co-mut patients with brain metastasis vs. *SMARCA4* WT/*KRAS*-mutated (7.4 months vs. 15.0 months, HR: 2.1; $p = 0.0003$). Liver metastasis: *SMARCA4/KRAS* co-mut had worse outcomes vs. *SMARCA4* WT/*KRAS*-mutated (5.2 months vs. 13.2 months, HR: 2.1; $p = 0.00015$).

Table 1. *Cont.*

(B)					
Author	**Publication Year**	**Treatment**	**NSCLC Mutations Analyzed**	**Number of NSCLC Patients with Mutations Analyzed**	**Outcomes/Relevance**
Alessi	2021	CIT	*SMARCA4/KRAS* co-mut *SMARCA4* WT/*KRAS* mut	44 co-mut 232 mut	Significantly worse OS (6.6 vs. 14.6 months; HR: 2.52, $p < 0.001$) and PFS (2.2 vs. 6.2 months; HR: 2.39, $p < 0.001$) in *SMARCA4/KRAS* co-mut vs. *SMARCA4* WT/*KRAS* mut patients.
Alessi	2023	Single-agent ICI or ICI combined with CTLA-4	*SMARCA4/KRAS* co-mut *SMARCA4* WT/*KRAS* mut	17 co-mut 159 mut	*SMARCA4/KRAS* co-mut had significantly shorter PFS (1.4 vs. 4.1 months, HR: 0.25; $p < 0.001$) and OS (3 vs. 15.1 months, HR: 0.29; $p < 0.001$) compared with *SMARCA4* WT/*KRAS* mut patients. The presence of a *SMARCA4/KRAS* co-mut may confer a worse outcome to ICIs.
Schoenfeld	2020	Various SOC	*SMARCA4/KRAS* co-mut	110 co-mut 58 co-mut (class 1 *SMARCA4*) 52 co-mut (class 2 *SMARCA4*)	Multivariate *SMARCA4/KRAS* co-mut analysis resulted in worse statistical OS regardless of class 1 or 2 alterations. [Class 1: HR: 1.59, and class 2: HR: 2.75] vs. WT ($p < 0.001$).
Liu	2021	Various SOC	*SMARCA4/KRAS* co-mut *SMARCA4* WT/*KRAS* mut	Cohort A: *SMARCA4/KRAS* co-mut (N = 9) vs. *SMARCA4* WT/*KRAS* mut (N = 146) Cohort B: *SMARCA4/KRAS* co-mut (N = 34) vs. *SMARCA4* WT/*KRAS* mut (N = 280) Cohort C: *SMARCA4/KRAS* co-mut (N = 9) vs. *SMARCA4* WT/*KRAS* mut (N = 68) Cohort D: *SMARCA4/KRAS* co-mut (N = 2) vs. *SMARCA4* WT/*KRAS* mut (N = 16)	Cohort A: *SMARCA4/KRAS* co-mut vs. *SMARCA4* WT/*KRAS* mut had worse OS (15.73 vs. 19.73 months) in non-immunotherapy cohort in The Cancer Genome Atlas (TCGA) (HR: 2.32, $p = 0.047$). Cohort B: *SMARCA4/KRAS* co-mut vs. *SMARCA4* WT/*KRAS* mut had worse OS (5.2 vs. 6.5 months) in non-immunotherapy MSK-CT cohort (HR: 1.95, $p = 0.015$). Cohort C: *SMARCA4/KRAS* co-mut vs. *SMARCA4* WT/*KRAS* mut (1.73 vs. 4.22 months) had worse PFS in immunotherapy MSK-IO cohort (HR: 2.15; $p = 0.048$). Cohort D: *SMARCA4/KRAS* co-mut vs. *SMARCA4* WT/*KRAS* mut had worse OS in immunotherapy Wake Forest cohort (HR: 11.98, $p = 0.0018$).

Atezo, atezolizumab; chemo, chemotherapy; co-mut, co-mutation; CTLA-4, Cytotoxic T-Lymphocyte Antigen 4; ICI, Immune Checkpoint Inhibitor; HR, Hazard Ratio; mets, metastasis; mut, mutation; OS, Overall Survival; PD1, Programmed Cell Death protein 1; PDL-1, Programmed Cell Death Ligand-1; pembro, pembrolizumab; PFS, Progression Free Survival; SOC, Standard of Care; WT, Wild-type.

3.2. *SMARCA4* Mutations

Schoenfeld et al. examined the clinicopathologic characteristics in a multivariate NSCLC analysis and determined that both *SMARCA4*-mutated class 1 (N = 149) and class 2 (N = 143) had worse OS vs. WT ($p < 0.001$) using Kaplan–Meir methods [8]. In addition, class 1 *SMARCA4*-mutated patients had the worst OS compared to class 2 mutated or WT patients (N = 996) via a log-rank test analysis [8]. Furthermore, an ICI survival treatment analysis (N = 87) showed an OS improvement for *SMARCA4*-mutated patients receiving ICI treatment vs. without ICI treatment regardless of class 1 or class 2 mutation status ($p = 0.01$). However, there was no significant difference in PFS ($p = 0.74$) or OS ($p = 0.35$) for *SMARCA4*-mutated patients receiving ICIs when comparing class 1 vs. class 2 alterations in an unadjusted analysis [8].

Both studies from Alessi et al. further support *SMARCA4* mutations as an independent factor that leads to worse outcomes for NSCLC patients [21,22]. In one of the most extensive NSCLC studies of patients with *SMARCA4* mutations who received chemo-immunotherapy (CIT), Alessi et al. reported that patients with non-squamous histology who had *SMARCA4* mutations (N = 114) vs. WT (N = 593) had significantly worse survival: PFS (2.7 versus 6.1 months, HR: 1.62; $p < 0.001$), and OS (8.1 versus 15.0 months, HR: 1.70; $p < 0.001$) from the start of CIT [22]. A multivariable analysis using inverse probability weighting was conducted to address potential selection bias due to the absence of Programmed Death Ligand-1 (PDL-1) reporting. The analysis revealed that confirmed *SMARCA4* mutations independently correlated with reduced survival: PFS (*SMARCA4*-mutated HR: 1.61; $p < 0.001$), OS (*SMARCA4*-mutated HR: 1.66; $p < 0.001$) to CIT [22].

A separate Alessi et al. study reported better OS in NSCLC patients with *SMARCA4* WT (N = 1327) vs. *SMARCA4*-mutated patients (N = 163): *SMARCA4* WT 25.0 months vs. *SMARCA4*-mutated 15.6 months (HR: 0.064; $p < 0.001$) [21]. However, in the immunotherapy-treated cohort of *SMARCA4*-mutated (N = 57) and WT patients (N = 475), which included single-agent checkpoint therapy or ICI in combination with a Cytotoxic T-Lymphocyte Antigen 4 (CTLA-4) inhibitor, there were no significant differences in *SMARCA4* WT vs. *SMARCA4*-mutated patients: PFS (3.1 vs. 2.1 months, HR: 0.93; $p = 0.62$) or OS (12.4 months vs. 11 months, HR: 0.83; $p = 0.25$) [21]. When getting more granular and looking at different types of *SMARCA4* mutations class 1 (N = 26) vs. class 2 (N = 31), there was no statistical OS difference in outcomes after receiving PDL-1 therapy when comparing *SMARCA4*-mutated class 1 [nonsense, frameshift, and splice site] (6.7 months; $p = 0.11$) vs. WT patients (N = 275, 12.4 months) vs. *SMARCA4*-mutated class 2 missense mutations (11.9 months, HR: 1.03; $p = 0.87$) [21].

When examining class 1 or class 2 mutations regardless of the type of treatment, Fernando et al. compared patients with *SMARCA4* WT (N = 2194) vs. *SMARCA4* NSCLC mutations in four categories: (a) homozygous truncated (N = 102), (b) homozygous nontruncated (N = 101), (c) heterozygous truncated (N = 16), and (d) heterozygous nontruncated (N = 49] [11]. There was a significant OS difference when comparing *SMARCA4*-mutated homozygous truncated vs. WT (7.9 vs. 16.3 months, HR: 1.85; $p < 0.0001$) but no significant differences when comparing other *SMARCA4*-mutated categories vs. *SMARCA4* WT [11].

Fernando et al. conducted a separate analysis when looking at the same four *SMARCA4* mutation categories but for patients who received immunotherapy (nivolumab, pembrolizumab, atezolizumab, or durvalumab) at any time during their cancer treatment [11]. This ICI treatment analysis compared patients with *SMARCA4* WT (N = 1069) vs. *SMARCA4* NSCLC mutations in four categories: (a) homozygous truncated (N = 38), (b) homozygous nontruncated (N = 41), (c) heterozygous truncated (N = 5), and (d) heterozygous nontruncated (N = 23). Similar to the non-treatment-specific OS analysis, there was a significant OS difference when comparing *SMARCA4*-mutated homozygous truncated vs. *SMARCA4*-WT (9.9 vs. 19.5 months, HR: 1.62; $p = 0.01$), but no significant differences when comparing WT with the other *SMARCA4*-mutated categories in the ICI-treated patients [11].

In a different study with the largest number of *SMARCA4* mutations in this review (N = 3305), the authors focused on clinicopathologic characteristics of patients with *SMARCA4* mutations and BRG1-deficient NSCLC [6]. Even though this study had a large number of *SMARCA4* patients, they only performed a *SMARCA4* mutation PFS analysis (N = 16) with 11 patients on chemotherapy and five on CIT. These patients had extremely short PFS of only 38 and 35 days, respectively [6].

Several studies included OS multivariate analysis across stages to address the outcomes of patients with *SMARCA4* mutations in the context of Stage III vs. Stage IV disease. One study conducted by Liang et al. revealed that individuals with *SMARCA4* mutations experienced significantly poorer survival in both locally advanced (Stage III) (N = 21) and metastatic (Stage IV) (N = 69) scenarios when compared to those with WT status [5]. The median survival for *SMARCA4*-mutated vs. WT patients was notably lower in Stage III (23.73 vs. 29.43 months, $p < 0.01$) and Stage IV (11.93 vs. 28.23 months, $p < 0.01$) [5]. To support this finding in Stage III patients, Talvitie et al.'s multivariate analysis on *SMARCA4*-mutated patients (N = 31) also revealed worse OS vs. WT patients (HR:1.93; $p = 0.04$) [23]. Regardless of stage, both authors conducted a multivariate analysis showing that *SMARCA4* WT (N = 221) patients had a better OS than mutated patients [(N = 105),

28.23 months vs. 12.17 months; $p < 0.001$] and *SMARCA4*-mutated patients had a worse OS than WT (HR: 3.522; $p < 0.002$) [5,23].

In association with *SMARCA4* mutations and clinico-genomic biomarkers across two different studies, tumor mutational burden (TMB) and brain metastasis in Anaplastic Lymphoma Kinase (ALK)-positive NSCLC were evaluated [24,25]. In exploring the relevance of TMB, Xu et al. conducted an NSCLC adenocarcinoma multivariate analysis [24]. The four arms were as follows: (a) *SMARCA4* WT, TMB Low (N = 761), (b) *SMARCA4* WT, TMB High (N = 722), (c) *SMARCA4*-mutated, TMB Low (N = 26), and (d) *SMARCA4*-mutated, TMB High (N = 69) [24]. The results showed a statistically better overall survival for *SMARCA4* WT, TMB High ($p = 0.00019$) [24]. In the context of brain metastasis, one study examined clinico-genomic outcomes in patients with (ALK)-positive NSCLC treated with alectinib [25]. They determined that *SMARCA4*-mutated patients (N = 3) with brain metastasis were the only group with co-mutations (*SMARCA4*/*ALK*) to do statistically worse across a multivariate analysis (HR: 8.76; $p = 0.009$).

When addressing *SMARCA4* mutation OS differences in a multivariate analysis of biological sex, two OS results were mixed between the sexes [5,26]. Pan et al. conducted a retrospective multivariate analysis, which included a cohort across 21 medical centers. There were 44 NSCLC patients with *SMARCA4* mutations, and men (N = 25) had a significantly worse OS than women (N = 19) (2.75 months vs. inestimable, HR:14.2; $p = 0.02$) [26]. The authors shared that one reason for the inestimable survival may be the low sample size of *SMARCA4* NSCLC patients. In the second study, the authors conducted a multivariate analysis, which resulted in statistically worse OS for women (N = 88) vs. men (N = 25) (HR: 4.1; $p = 0.04$) [5].

There were two NSCLC analyses of the OAK study involving atezolizumab. In the first OAK study analysis, Wang et al. discovered that *SMARCA4* was more likely to be seen in the negative PDL-1 expression group, but there was no statistical difference in OS when comparing atezolizumab vs. docetaxel in *SMARCA4*-mutated (N = 100) whether the patients were PDL-1 high or negative (HR = 0.67; $p = 0.256$) [27]. In addition, there was no difference in OS in *SMARCA4*-mutated NSCLC patients (N = 39) vs. *SMARCA4* WT (N = 491) whether the patients were PDL-1 high or negative when treated with atezolizumab (HR = 1.185, $p = 0.513$) [27]. In a second OAK uni-variate analysis, *SMARCA4*-mutated patients (N = 18) receiving atezolizumab did not fare worse than *SMARCA4* WT patients (N = 181) (HR: 1.70; $p = 0.064$) [28].

In the analysis by Velut et al., NSCLC patients with *SMARCA4* mutations (N = 7) did worse than WT (N = 70), independent of whether they received ICI therapy or not (HR: 3.2; $p = 0.006$) [29]. Interestingly, OS rates at 1 year were not significantly different between *SMARCA4*-mutated and WT patients but dropped significantly at 2 (58% vs. 74%) and 5 years (37% vs. 53%). In addition, patients were significantly younger upon diagnosis with *SMARCA4* mutation vs. without (61.9 years vs. 66.6 years; $p = 0.01$) [29]. A second single-institution analysis demonstrated a numerical, but not statistical, PFS benefit (6.3 vs. 3.9 months, HR: 0.64; $p = 0.15$) in *SMARCA4* WT (N = 130) vs. *SMARCA4*-mutated (N = 16) patients receiving ICIs (87% received combination ICI-chemotherapy) [30].

Three additional studies demonstrated significantly worse OS outcomes for NSCLC patients with *SMARCA4* mutations than wild-type patients across a multivariate analysis. In the first study, Yang et al.'s analysis resulted in worse OS for mutated (N = 5) vs. WT (N = 32) patients (4.5 months vs. 13.3 months, HR: 2.86; $p = 0.031$) [31]. The second multivariate analysis obtained a worse PFS (3 vs. 8 months; $p = 0.007$) for *SMARCA4*-mutated (N = 4) vs. WT patients (N = 99), and the results concluded that *SMARCA4* mutations were independently associated with a worse OS (HR: 3.098; $p = 0.038$) [32]. The last *SMARCA4* mutation analysis highlighted that the differences in all-cause mortality remained significant between the adenocarcinoma NSCLC patients that were mutated (N = 21) vs. wild-type (N = 204) (HR: 2.06; $p = 0.003$) [33].

3.3. *SMARCA4/KRAS* Co-Mutations

Seven NSCLC publications contained *SMARCA4/KRAS* co-mutation survival outcomes [8,21,22,33–36]. Two of these studies had specific *SMARCA4/KRAS* point mutation outcomes (i.e., *KRAS* G12C and G12D), and one analyzed survival with co-mutations in patients across clinical characteristics (i.e., brain and liver mets) [34–36]. Moreover, two different co-mutated analyses were performed by Alessi et al., highlighting robust results across many types and combinations of ICIs and chemotherapy [21,22]. Across various treatments, Schoenfeld et al.'s multivariate *SMARCA4/KRAS* co-mutation analysis resulted in worse statistical OS regardless of class 1 (N = 58) or 2 alterations (N = 52) (class 1: HR: 1.59 and class 2: HR: 2.75 vs. WT; $p < 0.001$) [8].

Negrao et al. produced the only publication focusing on NSCLC patients with co-mutations and *KRAS* G12C inhibitors (sotorasib or adagrasib). All NSCLC patients in their study had *KRAS* G12C mutations [35]. *SMARCA4/KRAS* G12C co-mutated patients (N = 18) had significantly worse PFS than *SMARCA4* WT/*KRAS* G12C-mutated patients (N = 213) (1.6 vs. 5.4 months, HR: 3.04; $p < 0.001$) and had a significantly worse OS (4.9 months vs. 11.8 months, HR: 3.07; $p < 0.001$) [35]. In relation to these survival outcomes, *SMARCA4* was one of the three tumor suppressor genes significantly enriched in the early progressing subgroup ($p = 0.001$) [35].

The second study that contained granular co-mutation outcomes (*KRAS* G12D) demonstrated statistically worse PFS for NSCLC patients; PFS: *SMARCA4/KRAS* G12D-co-mutated (N = 8) vs. *SMARCA4* WT/*KRAS* G12D-mutated (N = 49) (1.5 vs. 4.0 months; $p = 0.0039$) [34]. However, OS was only numerically worse but not statistically significant: *SMARCA4/KRAS* G12D-co-mutated vs. *SMARCA4* WT/*KRAS* G12D-mutated (6.1 vs. 17.3 months; $p = 0.4202$) [34].

Boiarsky et al. demonstrated that more than two times the number of patients had co-mutated *SMARCA4/KRAS* NSCLC Stage IV disease upon diagnosis (14%, N = 214) vs. Stage I (5%, N = 83) ($p = 0.038$), and these co-mutated patients had worse outcomes across patterns of metastatic spread (i.e., the brain) [36]. For example, OS was significantly worse for *SMARCA4/KRAS*-co-mutated (N = 33) patients with brain metastasis vs. *SMARCA4* WT/*KRAS*-mutated (N = 231) patients (7.4 months vs. 15.0 months, HR: 2.1; $p = 0.0003$) [36]. This HR was similar to *SMARCA4/KRAS*-co-mutated (N = 25) patients with liver metastasis vs. *SMARCA4* WT/*KRAS*-mutated (N = 155) patients (5.2 months vs. 13.2 months, HR: 2.1; $p = 0.00015$) [36].

SMARCA4-mutated patients had worse CIT treatment outcomes than *SMARCA4* WT patients in both *KRAS* WT and *KRAS*-mutated non-squamous NSCLC [22]. In reference to how co-mutated *SMARCA4/KRAS* non-squamous patients (N = 44) fared vs. *SMARCA4* WT/*KRAS*-mutated patients (N = 232), they fared even worse: PFS: *SMARCA4/KRAS*-mutated vs. *SMARCA4* WT/*KRAS*-mutated (2.2 vs. 6.2 months, HR: 2.39; $p < 0.001$), OS: *SMARCA4/KRAS*-mutated vs. *SMARCA4* WT/*KRAS*-mutated (6.6 vs. 14.6 months, HR: 2.52; $p < 0.001$) [22]. In the second Alessi et al. analysis with single-agent ICI or ICI-combination with CTLA-4, *KRAS*-mutant NSCLC was the most common co-mutation in the *SMARCA4* mutant subset (N = 17) [21]. The *SMARCA4/KRAS*-co-mutated patients had significantly shorter PFS (1.4 versus 4.1 months, HR: 0.25; $p < 0.001$) and OS (3 versus 15.1 months, HR: 0.29; $p < 0.001$) compared with NSCLC patients with *SMARCA4* WT/*KRAS* mutations (N = 159). Thus, the presence of a *SMARCA4/KRAS* co-mutation may confer a worse outcome to ICIs [21].

The last analysis from Liu et al. demonstrated significantly worse OS for all four *SMARCA4/KRAS*-mutated adenocarcinoma NSCLC cohorts across ICI-treated and non-ICI-treated NSCLC patients [37]. In Cohort A, *SMARCA4/KRAS*-co-mutated vs. *SMARCA4* WT/*KRAS*-mutated patients had worse OS (15.73 vs. 19.73 months) in a non-immunotherapy cohort in The Cancer Genome Atlas (TCGA) (HR: 2.32, $p = 0.047$). In Cohort B, *SMARCA4/KRAS*-co-mutated vs. *SMARCA4* WT/*KRAS*-mutated patients had worse OS (5.2 vs. 6.5 months) in a non-immunotherapy MSK-CT cohort (HR: 1.95, $p = 0.015$). In Cohort C, *SMARCA4/KRAS* co-mutated vs. *SMARCA4* WT/*KRAS*-mutated patients (1.73 vs.

4.22 months) had worse PFS in an immunotherapy MSK-IO cohort (HR: 2.15; $p = 0.048$). In Cohort D, *SMARCA4/KRAS*-co-mutated vs. *SMARCA4* WT/*KRAS*-mutated patients had worse OS in the immunotherapy Wake Forest cohort (HR: 11.98, $p = 0.0018$) [37].

4. Discussion

This *SMARCA4* NSCLC critical review focuses on survival outcomes across clinicopathological characteristics, *KRAS* co-mutations, and treatment with ICIs within twenty-one peer-reviewed articles. Eleven of thirteen (85%) *SMARCA4* mutation survival analyses in this review demonstrated significantly worse overall survival for *SMARCA4*-mutated NSCLC patients regardless of cancer treatment type. There were somewhat mixed results across *SMARCA4*-mutated treatment analysis for patients receiving ICIs and ICIs in combination with chemotherapy or CTLA-4 treatment. Three of the seven ICI analyses had worse OS for *SMARCA4*-mutated patients, three had no OS differences, and one outlier study highlighted that the patients with *SMARCA4* mutations did better on ICIs regardless of the class of *SMARCA4* mutation. Regarding *SMARCA4/KRAS* co-mutations, all seven treatment analyses (four with ICIs, two with non-ICIs, and one with *KRAS* G12C inhibitors) indicated that co-mutated *SMARCA4/KRAS* NSCLC patients consistently had significantly worse OS than *SMARCA4* WT/*KRAS*-mutated cohorts [8,21,22,34–37].

4.1. SMARCA4 Molecular Sub-Types and Genomic Features

In the largest *SMARCA4*-mutated survival analysis in this review (N = 407), the authors determined that class 1 truncating mutations were the strongest independent factor for significantly worse OS for NSCLC patients [8]. Class 1 mutations are typically associated with BRG1 protein loss compared to class 2 mutations, not losing any BRG1 protein expression (81% vs. 0%, $p < 0.001$) [8]. This lack of protein expression was also seen in an analysis completed at Massachusetts General Hospital (MGH), where 84% of patients with class 1 truncating mutations lacked BRG1 protein expression [6]. However, class 2 mutations (missense, nontruncating) also had worse OS, indicating that protein function could be impacted even though protein expression was evident [8].

As the only outlier in this review, *SMARCA4*-mutated NSCLC patients treated with ICI therapy had a longer OS ($p = 0.01$) [8]. In contrast, this ICI treatment OS benefit is not seen as appreciable when looking at *SMARCA4* WT vs. class 1 or 2 *SMARCA4* mutations. Alessi et al. point out that Schoenfeld's results may differ from their extensive *SMARCA4* ICI therapy analysis due to imbalances in unreported baseline clinicopathological characteristics in the Schoenfeld publication, which could have altered the OS [21].

As further support, both Alessi et al. studies highlight *SMARCA4* mutations as an independent factor in a significantly worse outcome for NSCLC patients [21,22]. However, different conclusions arose in their two separate publication analyses of ICI treatment: (1) based on whether it was used in the first line with chemotherapy (CIT), or (2) in pretreated patients as a single agent (ICI) or ICI/CTLA4 combination therapy. In the first-line setting, *SMARCA4* mutations were associated with significantly worse OS to first-line CIT treatment in non-squamous NSCLC (*SMARCA4*-mutated 8.1 months vs. *SMARCA4* WT 15.0 months ($p < 0.001$) [22]. In the pre-treatment setting, the authors did not find an association between *SMARCA4* mutational status and ICI treatment on PFS or OS, or whether the patient had a class 1 or 2 *SMARCA4* mutation [21].

When looking more granularly at truncated vs. nontruncated *SMARCA4* mutations or homozygous vs. heterozygous, there was a significantly worse OS when comparing *SMARCA4* homozygous truncated vs. WT (7.9 vs. 16.3 months, HR: 1.85; $p < 0.0001$) but no significant differences when comparing other *SMARCA4*-mutated categories vs. WT [11]. This significant OS difference was also demonstrated when looking specifically at ICI treatment when comparing homozygous truncated vs. WT (9.9 vs. 19.5 months, HR: 1.62; $p = 0.01$), but no significant differences were obtained when comparing WT with the other *SMARCA4*-mutated categories in the ICI-treated patients [11].

TMB is a genomic feature being analyzed in NSCLC across various ICI studies [38]. It is being reviewed as a possible biomarker for the use of ICIs in *SMARCA4*-mutated NSCLC [21]. Xu et al. showed a worse OS for NSCLC patients that are *SMARCA4*-mutated (TMB Low or TMB High) as compared to *SMARCA4* WT/TMB High ($p = 0.00019$) [24].

4.2. Clinicopathological Features

Multiple studies, including Liang et al. and Talvitie et al., conducted OS multivariate analyses across different stages, revealing consistently poorer survival for patients with *SMARCA4* mutations [5,23]. Liang et al.'s study demonstrated significantly worse OS in both locally advanced (Stage III) and metastatic (Stage IV) *SMARCA4*-mutated scenarios compared to WT status (Stage III (23.73 vs. 29.43 months, $p < 0.01$) and Stage IV (12.17 vs. 28.23 months, $p < 0.01$) [5]. Talvitie et al.'s analysis in Stage III patients further supported worse OS for *SMARCA4*-mutated patients [23]. Regardless of which stage, multivariate analyses consistently showed worse OS for *SMARCA4*-mutated patients, highlighting the impact of these mutations on survival outcomes.

This *SMARCA4* review illustrated statistically significant OS differences based on brain metastasis and mixed results based on biological sex [5,25,26]. In the context of brain metastases, Miao et al. investigated clinicogenomic outcomes in *ALK*-positive NSCLC patients treated with alectinib, finding that *SMARCA4*-mutated patients with brain metastases were the only group with co-mutations to exhibit statistically worse outcomes in a multivariate analysis (HR: 8.76; $p = 0.009$) [25]. In two multivariate analyses of the impact of biological sex on *SMARCA4* mutation OS differences, one analysis demonstrated significantly worse survival for men, and the other demonstrated worse survival for women [5,26]. Pan et al. reported that male NSCLC patients with *SMARCA4* mutations had a markedly worse OS than females (HR: 12.64; $p = 0.002$), while Liang et al.'s study highlighted a worse OS for women across a cohort of Stage IV *SMARCA4*-mutated patients (HR:14.2; $p = 0.02$) [5,26]. Although women had a statistically significant worse OS in the multivariate analysis, the authors share that one of the reasons for the possible large female survival discrepancy was due to lower numbers of females than males in the study (88 vs. 133) [5].

In the context of *SMARCA4* NSCLC patients treated with immune checkpoint inhibitors (ICIs), one study found that those with *SMARCA4* mutations had worse outcomes than WT patients regardless of ICI treatment or not (HR = 3.2; $p = 0.006$), and two separate OAK trial NSCLC analyses showed no OS differences with atezolizumab (ICI) vs. docetaxel in pre-treated NSCLC *SMARCA4*-mutated patients [27–29]. Three additional studies demonstrated significantly worse OS outcomes for NSCLC patients with *SMARCA4* mutations vs. WT patients across a multivariate analysis and various standards of care treatments [30–32].

4.3. *SMARCA4/KRAS* Co-Mutations

All seven *SMARCA4/KRAS* co-mutation NSCLC publications in this review showed either a significantly worse PFS or OS as compared to *SMARCA4* WT/*KRAS* mutation analyses across standard-of-care cancer treatments or within a specific treatment analysis (i.e., *KRAS* G12C inhibitor, ICIs, or non-ICIs) [8,21,22,34–37]. Two of these studies presented granular survival outcomes specific to two *KRAS* isoforms (G12C and G12D) [34,35]. Finally, one analysis demonstrated significantly worse survival for *SMARCA4/KRAS*-co-mutated patients as they presented at a higher rate of Stage IV NSCLC with a significantly higher propensity of brain or liver metastasis [36]. These higher rates of metastatic spread led to significantly worse survival for co-mutated *SMARCA4/KRAS* vs. *SMARCA4* WT/*KRAS*-mutated patients who either had brain or liver metastasis (i.e., brain metastasis 7.4 months vs. 15.0 months, HR: 2.1; $p = 0.0003$) [36].

SMARCA4/KRAS co-mutations are among the most common co-mutations within this review. Among the largest co-mutation analyses within the review, *SMARCA4/KRAS* was co-mutated at a rate of 36% in NSCLC [8]. Within this multi-variate analysis and across various treatments, the *SMARCA4/KRAS* co-mutation analysis by Schoenfeld et al.

resulted in worse OS regardless of class 1 or 2 alteration [class 1: HR: 1.59, and class 2: HR: 2.75] vs. WT ($p < 0.001$) [8]. Cooper et al.'s PFS co-mutation *SMARCA4/KRAS* G12D analysis demonstrated significantly worse outcomes for co-mutated patients vs. *SMARCA4* WT/*KRAS* G12D-mutated patients (1.5 vs. 4.0 months; $p = 0.0039$) [34]. However, as the outlier in this critical review focusing on *KRAS* G12D, the *SMARCA4/KRAS* G12C co-mutation OS analysis did not result in a significant difference as compared to *SMARCA4* WT/*KRAS*-mutated NSCLC patients (6.1 vs. 17.3 months; $p = 0.42$) [34].

4.4. *SMARCA4/KRAS* Co-Mutation Treatment Analysis

Four studies reported six *SMARCA4/KRAS* co-mutation OS survival treatment analyses [21,22,35,37]. All six treatment analyses across various treatment types (i.e., ICI, non-ICI, or *KRAS* G12C inhibitor) resulted in a significantly worse OS ($p < 0.05$) for *SMARCA4/KRAS*-co-mutated NSCLC patients. Negrao et al. had the only publication focusing on *KRAS* G12C NSCLC patients with co-mutations and *KRAS* G12C inhibitors (sotorasib or adagrasib) [35]. NSCLC patients with *SMARCA4/KRAS* G12C co-mutations vs. *SMARCA4* WT/*KRAS* G12C mutations had significantly worse OS (4.9 months vs. 11.8 months, HR: 3.07; $p < 0.001$). In relation to these survival outcomes, *SMARCA4* was one of the three tumor suppressor genes significantly enriched in the early progressing subgroup ($p = 0.001$) [35].

Across two publications by Alessi et al., whether the co-mutated NSCLC patients were treated in the first line with CIT or in $\geq$ 2nd line with single-agent ICI in combination with CTLA-4, the patients had statistically worse OS [21,22]. Co-mutated *SMARCA4/KRAS* non-squamous CIT-treated patients had worse OS compared to *SMARCA4* WT/*KRAS*-mutated OS (6.6 vs. 14.6; $p < 0.001$) [22]. In the second Alessi et al. analysis with single-agent ICIs or an ICI combination with CTLA-4, co-mutated NSCLC patients had significantly worse OS compared with NSCLC patients with *SMARCA4* WT/*KRAS* mutations (3 months versus 15.1 months, HR: 0.29; $p < 0.001$) [21]. Thus, the authors concluded that *SMARCA4/KRAS* co-mutation may confer worse NSCLC survival outcomes to ICIs [21].

Liu et al.'s ICIs and non-ICIs treatment adenocarcinoma NSCLC analysis was associated with significantly worse OS or PFS across all four *SMARCA4/KRAS* co-mutated vs. *SMARCA4* WT/*KRAS*-mutated cohorts [37]. Cohort A and B *SMARCA4KRAS*-mutated patients were associated with worse OS when treated with non-ICIs ($p = 0.047$ and $p = 0.015$). In Cohort C and Cohort D, *SMARCA4KRAS*-mutated patients treated with immunotherapy had worse PFS and OS (Cohort C (PFS): $p = 0.048$ and Cohort D (OS): $p = 0.0018$) [37].

There are potential reasons why current treatments are not highly effective in treating *SMARCA4/KRAS* NSCLC co-mutations, as the tumor microenvironment (TME) plays an important role in metastatic NSCLC [39]. Regarding ICI therapy, Liu et al. used a signature gene panel to evaluate the level of immune cell type across each NSCLC individual [37]. They found that *SMARCA4/KRAS*-co-mutated patients had a significantly lower estimated proportion of Cluster of Differentiation 8 (CD8+) T-cells ($p = 0.015$) and activated CD4+ memory T cells ($p = 0.0035$) than *SMARCA4* WT/*KRAS*-mutated subjects [37]. This suggests that CD8+ T-cell function may be impacted by regulatory T cells (Tregs), which can lead to a more immunosuppressive tumor microenvironment landscape [39]. Beyond ICI monotherapy and looking at CIT, *SMARCA4* mutations can activate Nuclear Factor Erythroid 2-Related Factor 2 (NRF2) signaling, leading to the up-regulation of cytoprotective genes and enabling platinum therapy resistance [40].

5. Future Direction

The majority of *SMARCA4*-mutated NSCLC patient analyses within this review demonstrated a worse overall survival as compared to *SMARCA4* wild-type patients. Mutations in this gene should be explored as a prospective biomarker across ICI, CIT, and *KRAS* G12C inhibitor clinical trials. As each *SMARCA4/KRAS* co-mutated treatment analysis in this review showed a statistically worse OS or PFS than *SMARCA4* WT/*KRAS*-mutated patients, a prospective comprehensive immune cell analysis could be considered for *SMARCA4*-mutated and co-mutated *SMARCA4/KRAS* patients to understand better how these mutations and co-mutations impact the tumor microenvironment. Utilization of this prospective biomarker approach and immune cell data analysis could inform the design of future NSCLC clinical trials.

6. Limitations

The vast majority of mutation and treatment analyses (i.e., single agent and combination approaches) in this review are retrospective and vary in *SMARCA4* mutation sample size. The scope of the publications was limited to those in the English language published from 2018 through 2023. *KRAS* was the primary co-mutated gene included, rather than analyzing other possible co-mutations with *SMARCA4* (e.g., *KEAP1/STK11*). Given these limitations, this review's strength is that it is one of the largest *SMARCA4* overall survival NSCLC reviews completed to date.

7. Conclusions

In one of the largest reviews to date of *SMARCA4*-mutated overall survival data in NSCLC, two consistent trends emerged from the twenty-one publications in scope: First, *SMARCA4* NSCLC mutated patients had statistically worse OS than *SMARCA4* WT patients. Secondly, NSCLC patients with *SMARCA4/KRAS* co-mutations tended to have significantly worse overall survival than *SMARCA4* WT/*KRAS*-mutated patients, regardless of treatment type, within each treatment analysis. Moreover, designing prospective clinical *SMARCA4*-mutated or *SMARCA4/KRAS*-co-mutated NSCLC trials to evaluate targeted therapies and immunotherapy may lead to a better understanding of how to improve cancer patients' outcomes and survival rates. These findings may have implications for future research and clinical practice.

Author Contributions: Conceptualization, P.M.; methodology, P.M.; validation, P.M.; formal analysis, P.M.; investigation, P.M.; resources, P.M. and D.S.I.; data curation, P.M. and L.B.; writing—original draft preparation, P.M.; writing—review and editing, P.M., L.B. and D.S.I.; supervision, L.B. and D.S.I.; project administration, L.B. All authors have read and agreed to the published version of the manuscript.

Funding: This research received no external funding.

Institutional Review Board Statement: Ethical review and approval was not sought for this literature review.

Informed Consent Statement: Not applicable.

Data Availability Statement: No new data were created or analyzed in this study. Data sharing is not applicable to this article.

Acknowledgments: A special thank you to A.M. for all her support. Also, thank you to Janice Withycombe for her help in the initial editing of the manuscript.

Conflicts of Interest: P.M. is an employee of and a stockholder in Novartis®. L.B. and D.I. declare no conflicts of interest.

References

1. Compilation of CDER-NME-New Biologic Approvals from 1985–2022. Available online: https://www.fda.gov/media/135308/download (accessed on 1 February 2024).
2. Ramalingam, S.S.; Vansteenkiste, J.; Planchard, D.; Cho, B.C.; Gray, J.E.; Ohe, Y.; Zhou, C.; Reungwetwattana, T.; Cheng, Y.; Chewaskulyong, B.; et al. FLAURA Investigators Overall Survival with Osimertinib in Untreated, EGFR-Mutated Advanced NSCLC. *N. Engl. J. Med.* **2020**, *382*, 41–50. [CrossRef] [PubMed]
3. Skoulidis, F.; Heymach, J.V. Co-occurring genomic alterations in non-small-cell lung cancer biology and therapy. *Nat. Rev. Cancer* **2019**, *19*, 495–509. [CrossRef] [PubMed]
4. Surveillance Epidemiology and End Results (SEER). Cancer Stat Facts: Lung and Bronchus Cancer. Available online: https://seer.cancer.gov/statfacts/html/lungb.html (accessed on 1 March 2024).

Journal of
Personalized Medicine

MDPI

Review

Management of Severe Bilateral Symptomatic Internal Carotid Artery Stenosis: Case Report and Literature Review

Mircea Robu [1], Bogdan Radulescu [1,*], Irina-Maria Margarint [1,*], Anca Dragan [2], Ovidiu Stiru [1], Gabriel-Petre Gorecki [3], Cristian Voica [4], Vlad Anton Iliescu [1] and Horatiu Moldovan [1,5]

[1] Faculty of Medicine, Carol Davila University of Medicine and Pharmacy, 050474 Bucharest, Romania; mircea.robu@drd.umfcd.ro (M.R.); ovidiu.stiru@umfcd.ro (O.S.); vladanton.iliescu@gmail.com (V.A.I.); horatiu.moldovan@umfcd.ro (H.M.)
[2] 1st Department of Cardiovascular Anesthesiology and Intensive Care, Prof. Dr. C. C. Iliescu Emergency Institute for Cardiovascular Diseases, 022328 Bucharest, Romania; anca.dragan1978.14@gmail.com
[3] Faculty of Medicine, Titu Maiorescu University, 031593 Bucharest, Romania; gabriel.gorecki@prof.utm.ro
[4] Department of Cardiovascular Surgery, Emergency Clinical Hospital Bucharest, 014461 Bucharest, Romania; cristian.voica@drd.umfcd.ro
[5] Academy of Romanian Scientists, 50711 Bucharest, Romania
* Correspondence: bogdan.radulescu@umfcd.ro (B.R.); irina-maria.margarint@drd.umfcd.ro (I.-M.M.)

Abstract: Multiple strategies for tandem severe carotid artery stenosis are reported: bilateral carotid artery endarterectomy (CEA), bilateral carotid artery stenting (CAS), and hybrid procedures (CEA and CAS). The management is controversial, considering the reported high risk of periprocedural stroke, hemodynamic distress, and cerebral hyperperfusion syndrome. We present the case of a 64-year-old patient with severe symptomatic bilateral internal carotid artery stenosis (95% stenosis on the left internal carotid artery with recent ipsilateral watershed anterior cerebral artery–medial cerebral artery (ACA-MCA) and medial cerebral artery–posterior cerebral artery (MCA-PCA) ischemic strokes and 90% stenosis on the right internal carotid artery with chronic ipsilateral frontal ischemic stroke) managed successfully with staged CEA within a 3-day interval. The patient had a history of coronary angioplasty and stenting. Strategies for brain protection included shunt placement after the evaluation of carotid stump pressure, internal carotid backflow, and near-infrared spectroscopy. A collagen and silver-coated polyester patch was used to complete the endarterectomy using a 6.0 polypropylene continuous suture in both instances. Management also included neurological consults after extubation, dual antiplatelet therapy, head CT between the two surgeries, myocardial ischemia monitoring, and general anesthesia. Staged CEA with a small time interval between surgeries can be an option to treat tandem symptomatic carotid artery stenosis in highly selected patients. The decision should be tailored according to the patient's characteristics and should also be made by a cardiology specialist, a neurology specialist, and an anesthesia and intensive care physician.

Keywords: staged carotid artery endarterectomy; severe bilateral carotid artery stenosis; ischemic stroke

1. Introduction

Carotid artery stenosis is responsible for 10% of ischemic strokes, one of the main causes of long-term disability. The prevalence of bilateral carotid artery stenosis is nearly 8–39% among patients with stroke [1,2]. The management of this situation is controversial and carries a high risk of periprocedural stroke, hemodynamic distress, and cerebral hyperperfusion syndrome [3]. Multiple strategies for tandem severe carotid artery stenosis are reported: bilateral carotid artery endarterectomy (CEA), bilateral carotid artery stenting (CAS), and hybrid procedures with CEA and CAS. However, there are no guidelines for the exact timing and order of these options. CEA and CAS can be performed simultaneously or staged. When considering the staged strategy, the optimal time interval between procedures is not well determined. With the hybrid approach, there is no consensus regarding which technique should be used first regardless of the staged or simultaneous strategy. Staged CEA was the first technique to emerge for tandem severe carotid artery stenosis and was considered for obvious reasons to be safer than simultaneous bilateral CEA [4,5]. Carotid artery stenting began as an alternative to this initial strategy, with the development of carotid artery stents, initially as an adjuvant to CEA, but also for high-risk patients [6] and patients with CEA restenosis [7]. We review different strategies and present the management of a 64-year-old male with severe bilateral symptomatic carotid artery stenosis, successfully managed with staged CEA with a 3-day interval.

2. Case Report

We present the case of a 64-year-old male patient with a recent history (one month) of left ACA-MCA and MCA-PCA ischemic strokes with right hemiparesis, documented on cerebral CT. A chronic frontal right ischemic lesion was also documented. Neurological examination on admission revealed right minor central facial palsy, 3/5 MRC right hemiparesis, and mild right hemihypoesthesia, consistent with an NIHSS score of 4. Past medical history revealed ischemic heart disease, with severe stenosis at the proximal level of the anterior descending artery, treated with balloon angioplasty and two drug-eluting stents 6 months before admission. Also, the patient was diagnosed with hypertension, type II diabetes, and obesity. The patient was on dual antiplatelet therapy with Aspirin and Clopidogrel. At admission, he was stable, with a 110–120 mmHg systolic blood pressure, a 95 bpm regular pulse, and a 98% peripheral oxygen saturation. He had almost complete resolution of the right hemiparesis with the rest of the clinical examination within normal limits. The blood test revealed hyperlipidemia. The EKG showed normal sinus rhythm, without any ST-T changes, and the chest XR was without any pathological findings. Transthoracic echocardiography showed normal biventricular function, no significant valvular pathology, and no pericardial effusion. Arterial Doppler ultrasound of the carotid arteries revealed 90–95% stenosis at the level of the left common carotid artery bifurcation, extending to the internal carotid artery, and 85–90% stenosis at the level of the right common carotid artery bifurcation, extending at the level of the internal carotid artery. The atheromatous plaques responsible for the severe bilateral stenosis were both of mixt echogenicity (Figure 1).

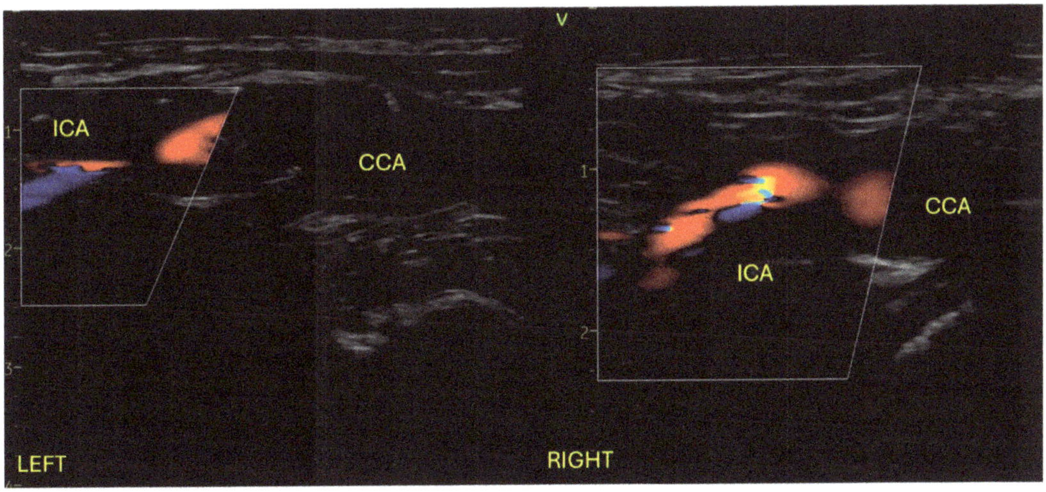

Figure 1. Arterial Doppler ultrasound of the carotid system showing bilateral severe stenosis at the level of common carotid artery bifurcation extending at the level of the internal carotid artery. ICA: internal carotid artery; CCA: common carotid artery.

Cervical CT angiography confirmed the severe lesions at the level of the carotid arteries (Figure 2A–C). Additionally, considering the history of ischemic heart disease, coronary angiography was obtained, and carotid angiography was performed in the same setting. Figure 3 shows severe suboclusive stenosis at the level of the left common and internal carotid artery. Unfortunately, the cannulation of the right carotid artery was not possible. Coronary arteries were without any significant stenosis, and the stents at the level of the anterior descending artery were patent.

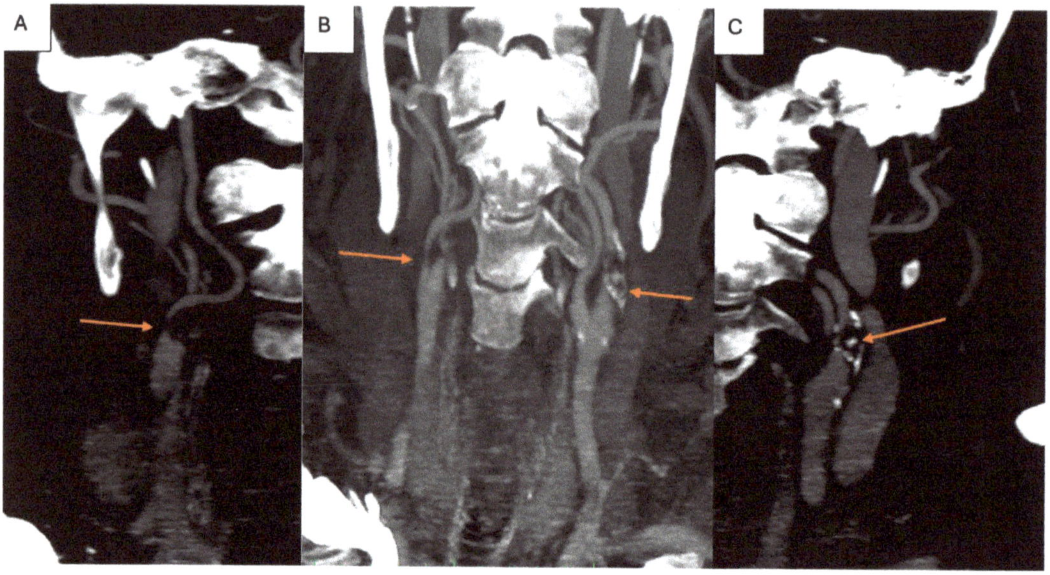

Figure 2. Cervical CT angiography showing right severe internal carotid artery stenosis ((**A**), arrow), left severe internal carotid artery stenosis ((**C**), arrow), and bilateral severe internal carotid artery stenosis ((**B**), arrows).

The management strategy used was determined by a team that included a cardiology specialist, a neurology specialist, a vascular surgeon, an anesthesia specialist, and an intensive care physician. The decision was made to perform the left CEA first due to the recent ipsilateral ischemic stroke, and then as soon as possible afterwards the right CEA was performed. The reason for the relative short interval between surgeries included high-grade stenosis on the right internal carotid artery, with a history of ischemic stroke. Also, the mixed echogenicity aspect of the plaque at the echocardiography suggested a high risk of cerebral embolization. Stenting of the right carotid lesion as an alternative for right CEA was not an option for several reasons. First, our center's experience with carotid stenting is low, with fewer than 10 cases per year, and second, from a technical point of view, we did not have stents with an embolic prevention system at that time. A head CT and a neurologic consultation were planned after the first intervention in order to identify hemorrhagic lesions that would contraindicate the second intervention. Also, the dual antiplatelet therapy was continued during the entire hospitalization, considering the high risk of cerebral thromboembolism. The patient signed both the informed consent and the publication consent form for the case and was scheduled for surgery the next day.

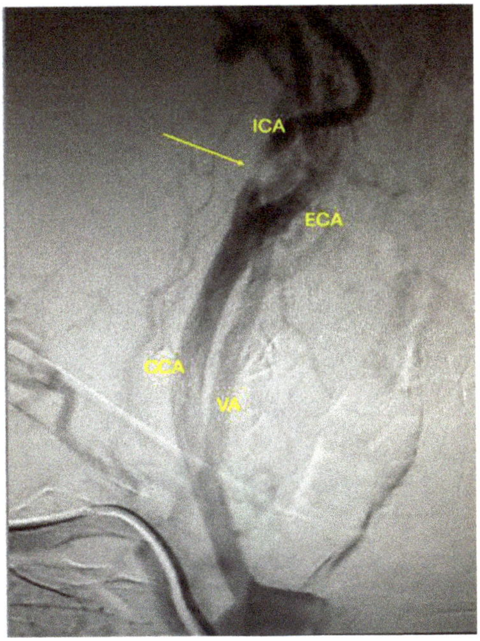

Figure 3. Carotid artery angiography showing suboclusive stenosis at the level of the left common and internal carotid artery with patent left vertebral artery. CCA: common carotid artery; ICA: internal carotid artery; ECA: external carotid artery; VA: vertebral artery.

2.1. Surgical Technique

After the provision of general anesthesia, an incision was made along the left medial border of the sternocleidomastoid muscle. After the dissection of subcutaneous fat tissue and a platysma muscle incision, the sternocleidomastoid muscle was retracted laterally, the internal jugular vein was also retracted, and the carotid sheath was incised. The common, internal, and external carotid arteries were isolated carefully, so as not to injure the vagus and hypoglossal nerves. We administrated 3500 units of unfractionated heparin, and after 2 min, the carotid arteries could be clamped. The systolic blood pressure was maintained over 140 mmHg in order to augment cerebral blood flow during carotid artery clamping. Retrograde pressure at the level of the internal carotid artery was measured (24 mmHg) and was below 40 mmHg. A longitudinal incision was made, beginning at the level of the common carotid artery, moving over the carotid artery bifurcation, and extending to the level of the internal carotid artery 1 cm distal to the end of the plaque felt at palpation. The clamp at the level of the ICA was removed, and backflow was evaluated and deemed unsatisfactory. We used near-infrared spectroscopy (NIRS) to monitor cerebral oxygenation, and the values dropped on the left side after carotid clamping from 65% to 45%. All of the above (reduced backflow, reduced retrograde blood pressure, drop in NIRS) led us to insert a shunt in order to augment cerebral perfusion during carotid clamping (Figure 4A). After the shunt insertion, NIRS values returned to normal. Continuous transcranial Doppler ultrasonography and EEG monitoring were not available in our institution. The plaque was excised down to the level of the intima, and two 7.0 polypropylene sutures were used to fix the layers at the distal end of the endarterectomy. Macroscopic examination of the plaque confirmed the mixed heterogenicity shown on the Doppler ultrasound with thrombotic material attached to the inner surface (Figure 4B). Figure 4C shows the plaque extracted at the time of the right CEA. A collagen and silver-coated polyester patch was used to complete the endarterectomy using a 6.0 polypropylene continuous suture. After the shunt was extracted, the arteries were deaired, the suture was finished, and then all arteries were declamped in the reverse order of clamping: the external carotid artery, common carotid arteries, and internal carotid artery. The carotid artery clamp time was 24 min. The final result is shown in Figure 4D. A surgical drain was inserted via contra incision. Both CEAs were performed with the same surgical technique. The second CEA had a 21 min period of carotid artery clamping. For the second CEA, shunt insertion was not necessary.

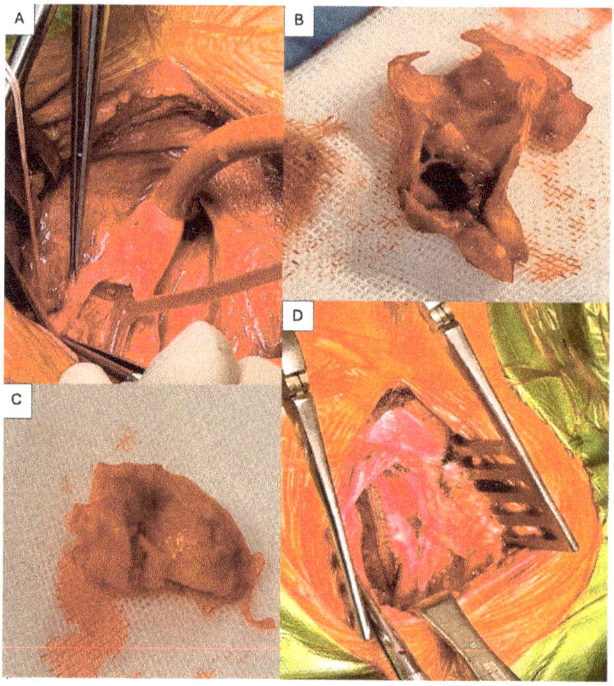

Figure 4. (**A**) A shunt inserted in the left common and internal carotid arteries. (**B**) Plaque extracted from the left carotid artery. (**C**) Plaque extracted from the right carotid artery. (**D**) Final result of left CEA with collagen and silver-coated polyester.

2.2. Postoperative Evolution

After the left CEA, the patient was extubated after 3 h. He had no new neurological deficits according to the neurological consult. Myocardial enzymes, serial EKG, and transthoracic echocardiography showed no signs of myocardial ischemia in the immediate postoperative period. The only postoperative complication was postoperative arterial hypertension. Regarding blood pressure values, the highest value was for systolic blood pressure between 170 and 190 mmHg when the sedation was stopped. It was rapidly managed with intravenous calcium channel blockers (Nicardipine) and continued the whole stay in intensive care with normal values for the blood pressure. The patient was transferred to the surgical ward the following day with oral medication for hypertension. The surgical drain was extracted on the same day. On the second day, we obtained a head CT and a neurological consult. Because there were not any clinical or imaging signs of new cerebral ischemia or cerebral hemorrhage, the neurologist cleared the patient for the second CEA. On the third postoperative day, the patient was transferred to the operating room, and a right CEA was performed using the same technique described above. Postoperative evolution was uneventful, the patient was extubated after 5 h, no neurological complications were documented, transthoracic echocardiography was performed within normal limits, and myocardial enzymes and serial EKG showed no signs of myocardial ischemia. He was transferred to the surgical ward the following day. The surgical drain was extracted on the second day after the right CEA, and no cervical hematoma was observed at daily evaluations. After another neurological consultation and a final cardiological examination, the patient was discharged on the seventh day after the initial left CEA. At discharge, hypoesthesia and hemiparesis were almost completely reversed with mild deficit persistence on right upper limb, consistent with an NIHSS score of 2 (minor facial palsy and mild deficit on the right upper limb). Follow-up at 1, 3, and 6 months and 1 year were uneventful.

3. Review

Stroke is the second most common cause of death worldwide and is characterized by high morbidity. Furthermore, half of stroke survivors have severe disability, and subsequently, these patients are a heavy burden on public health [8]. Recurrent ischemic stroke contributes massively to this burden and inflicts potentially debilitating sequelae on a group of already fragile patients. Thus, preventive measures should be developed and implemented. While the control of risk factors is beneficial for secondary prevention, the identification of the specific mechanism, such as internal carotid artery stenosis ipsilateral to ischemic stroke or transitory ischemic accident (TIA), will guide decision-making for further prevention [9].

Reported for the first time in 1954 by Eastcott et al. [10], carotid endarterectomy (CE) has proven to have a beneficial effect on stroke prevention in patients with internal carotid artery stenosis. In 1991, the North American Symptomatic Carotid Endarterectomy Trial (NASCET) and the European Carotid Surgery Trail (ECST) reported a beneficial effect of CE in patients with angiographic evidence of symptomatic stenosis with comparable rates of periprocedural rates of stroke and death. They concluded that CE was highly beneficial for symptomatic stenosis, ranging from 70% to 99%, and moderately beneficial for symptomatic carotid stenosis, ranging from 50 to 69% [11,12].

Since then, numerous societies have elaborated guidelines for the management of extracranial carotid stenosis. The 2021 American Heart Association Guidelines for the Prevention of Stroke in Patients with Stroke and Transient Ischemic Attack (TIA) recommend CE for both 70% to 99% and 50% to 69% carotid artery stenosis and ipsilateral TIA or nondisabling ischemic stroke occurring within the past 6 months if the perioperative morbidity and mortality risk is below 6%. For the 50% to 69% group of patients age, sex and comorbidities should be considered before surgery. CE is also the preferred method for stroke prevention over carotid artery stenting (CAS) in patients over 70 years old, while CAS is recommended in severe carotid artery stenosis (over 70%) with a high risk of surgery [13]. The European Society for Vascular Surgery Clinical Practice Guidelines on the Management of Atherosclerotic Carotid and Vertebral Artery Disease have recommendations for both symptomatic and asymptomatic patients [14]. For 60% to 99% asymptomatic carotid stenosis cases, CE is recommended in the presence of one or more imaging or clinical characteristics that may be associated with increased risk of stroke, provided that 30-day stroke/death rates are below 3% and patient life expectancy exceeds five years. CAS is recommended if surgery is deemed high risk in the same conditions. Symptomatic patients treated within the preceding six months with a 70–99% carotid artery stenosis have a class I indication for CE provided that the risk of 30-day risk of death/stroke is below 6%. Patients with 50–69% carotid artery stenosis have a class IIa indication. CAS is the preferred method for treatment in patients over 70 years old in accordance with the American Heart Association Guidelines. CE should be performed within 14 days from the onset of symptoms to increase the likelihood of a stroke-free outcome, a recommendation stated in both of the societies' guidelines. The European Stroke Organization recommends CE for patients with more than 60% asymptomatic carotid artery stenosis with an increased risk of stroke with medical therapy alone, and this is also a recommendation for patients over 75 years old with a life expectancy of more than 5 years. Patients with symptomatic 70–99% carotid artery stenosis have a strong recommendation for CE, while CE is suggested for symptomatic 50–69% stenosis. Early CE within 2 weeks of the first neurological event also has a strong recommendation [15].

While it is clear that symptomatic severe carotid artery stenosis has strong recommendation for CE, the guidelines do not specify the management for severe bilateral carotid artery stenosis, especially in the presence of symptoms and or ulcerous high-risk embolism plaques. The frequency of bilateral carotid stenosis varies and is reported to be between 3.2% and 39% in the literature [2,16,17]. In this group of patients, impaired cerebral hemodynamics may contribute to cognitive dysfunction, neurological symptoms, and even stroke, even in the absence of symptoms, and it is believed that this group of patients could benefit from the more aggressive management of carotid revascularization [18]. The management of this situation carries a high risk of periprocedural stroke, besides hemodynamic complications and hyperperfusion syndrome [17]. Strategies for the treatment of these patients include bilateral CEA, bilateral carotid artery stenting (CAS), and a hybrid approach with CEA and CAS. However, the optimal sequence that is simultaneous or staged has not been determined.

3.1. Bilateral Carotid Endarterectomy (BCAE)

Bilateral CEA can be performed simultaneously (sbCEA) or staged (SCEA) with a variable interval between the two surgeries. Advocates of SCAE consider that leaving an interval of time between the two interventions reduces the risk of brain injury, but the optimal interval between the first and second surgery has not been defined [19,20]. Kim et al. performed SCAE in 43 patients within 30 days or less (the mean time interval was 12 days). Compared with the group of patients with unilateral CEA, there were no differences with regard to nerve cranial nerve palsy and non-neurological CEA-related complications. Age was the only risk factor associated with ipsilateral stroke in multivariate analysis, while SCEA was not associated with stroke. The two groups did not differ significantly with regard to stroke, myocardial infarction, or death during the periprocedural period or ipsilateral stroke within 3 years after CEA. Also, similar rates of survival were communicated [20]. Rodrigues et al. performed SCEA with a main interval of 4 days in 154 patients and reported no increase in immediate and 30-day morbidity and mortality when compared to unilateral CEA [21]. Darling et al. report 102 cases with a mean interval between surgeries of 2 days with no operative mortality and only one permanent neurological deficit. They communicate a stroke mortality rate of 1% and a 1.5% rate of transient neurological deficits comparable with those undergoing unilateral CEA [22]. Schroeder et al. reported in a series of 56 patients that postendarterectomy hypertension was significantly higher following the second procedure when the procedures were performed less than 3 weeks apart and was linked with the occurrence of new neurological symptoms. The author advises at least a three-week interval between the first and the second CEA and a conservative attitude towards the contralateral asymptomatic lesion [5]. In accordance with Schroeder, several other reports describe the association between postoperative hypertension and new-onset neurological symptoms, supporting the idea that the second CEA should be performed after more than 3 weeks [23–25]. A short interval time between CEA and the occurrence of postoperative hypertension was also reported by Maxwell et al. He communicated a 5.6% death and stroke rate in 161 patients with SCEA [26]. The most recent study to this date investigating changes in blood pressure after CEA identified hypertension as an independent predictor of perioperative stroke following bilateral CEA irrespective of the interval between surgeries. Also, bilateral CEA was associated with postoperative hypertension together with gender, emergency admissions, and plaque morphology [27].

Those in favor of SBCEA advocate that repeated anesthesia, repeated surgical stress, prolonged intensive care and hospitalization times, and increased risk of cranial hemorrhage because of second heparinization increase the risk of SBCEA [28]. Although neither SCEA nor SBCEA have been proven to be the correct strategy for bilateral severe carotid artery stenosis, particular lesions like patients with bilateral stenosis of more than 90%

and those with ulcerous, calcified, and high-risk embolism plague SBCEA seem to be a rationale choice [28–30].

Ketonen et al. reported, in 1979, a series of 18 patients with SBCEA. He communicated a 3.8% hospital mortality, 5% rate of transient neurological deficits, and 5% rate of permanent neurological deficit [4]. While the results of the above study do not favor SBCEA, multiple studies comparing SCEA with SBCEA report no significant differences between the two aspects. Farask et al. compared 6 patients with SBCEA with 20 patients with SCEA and found no differences regarding mortality, myocardial infarction, respiratory problems, or permanent neurological damage of the central nervous system. The only complication reported in the SBCEA was transient hypoglossal paresis [29]. Dimakakos et al. report their initial experience, comparing 11 BSCEA with 12 SCEA and 155 cases of unilateral CEA regarding death, myocardial infarction, or permanent neurological dysfunction. No differences were found, and reports in the SBCEA group included a case of transient ischemic attack and transient vocal cord paresis [31]. The same author reported the same results, with no significant differences between 17 BSCEA and 17 SCEA with a zero mortality rate. The conclusion favors SCEA, with SBCEA being reserved for strictly selected patients [29].

Besides an experienced surgical team, the type of anesthesia appears to play an important role when considering SBCEA. Regional anesthesia offers the advantage of monitoring the neurological status and determining the shunt indication, while general anesthesia seems to have a protective effect for cerebral hypoxia [32]. Regional anesthesia also decreases the need for shunt placement from 43% to 14%, a significant advantage considering that shunt placement has a 1% to 3% risk of embolism and dissection [30,31]. Also, general anesthesia is linked to a study with a higher incidence of myocardial infarction [33]. Despite the fact that regional anesthesia does not appear to influence the postoperative results of CEA and has the advantage of increasing patient comfort, no need for recovery like general anesthesia and reducing hospitalization costs and complications like phrenic nerve, vagus nerve, and stellate ganglion lesions can be observed [28].

3.2. *Hybrid Procedures and Bilateral Carotid Artery Stenting*

Another strategy for bilateral severe carotid artery stenosis is a hybrid approach with carotid artery stenting (CAS) and either staged or simultaneous CEA.

Xu et al. report a series of eight patients with severe bilateral carotid stenosis with simultaneous CAS and CEA. Three patients had CAS before CEA and five patients had CEA as the first intervention. There were no deaths, and only one patient developed hyperperfusion syndrome [34]. Hokari et al. discuss two patients with severe bilateral carotid artery stenosis with CEA performed first for the symptomatic side and CAS performed for the contralateral side after three weeks. There were no deaths, one of the patients developed hyperperfusion syndrome after CEA with full recovery and the second patient developed severe hypotension requiring catecholamines but also with good evolution [34]. Beach et al. also report 22 patients with staged CEA and CAS. CEA was performed first with a 4.5% rate of perioperative stroke and myocardial infarction and a 9.1% rate of cranial nerve injuries [35].

Shchehlov et al. report 10 years of experience with bilateral simultaneous CAS in 39 patients. In all cases, stenting was performed with success, with two periprocedural neurological complications, one TIA, and one minor stroke, as well as with no deaths or myocardial infarction recorded [1]. Chen et al. also report 10 patients with simultaneous bilateral CAS deemed high risk for surgery, and Mubarak et al. report 5 cases treated for CEA restenosis, with no periprocedural complications [6,7]. Lai et al. performed a meta-analysis to evaluate the safety of bilateral simultaneous CAS. Based on 333 cases reported in the literature, they conclude that besides hyperperfusion syndrome, other periprocedural complications including hemodynamic depression, stroke, and myocardial infarction are comparable with unilateral CAS [3]. Oshita et al. compare simultaneous with staged bilateral CAS, and their conclusion is that bilateral CAS performed simultaneously was not inferior to staged CAS, with an obvious advantage when considering the length of hospital stay [36]. Based on the current data, simultaneous bilateral CAS might increase the risk of intra- or postoperative bradycardia and/or hypotension due to bilateral baroreceptor stimulation or hyperperfusion syndrome resulting from an increase in bilateral intracranial blood flow. On the other hand, simultaneous BCAS has the advantage of being less expensive and more convenient for patients than staged BCAS.

All authors (Table 1) conclude that patients with tandem severe carotid artery stenosis should be carefully examined and the best treatment strategy should be assessed using a multidisciplinary approach.

Table 1. Studies that report the management of severe bilateral carotid artery stenosis. CEA: carotid artery endarterectomy; CAS: carotid artery stenting.

Autor	Year	Management	Complications
Xu et al. [34]	2016	8 simultaneous CEA and CAS	Hyperperfusion syndrome
Kim et al. [21]	2015	43 staged CEA within 30 days	No association with ipsilateral stroke
Farask et al. [30]	2001	12 bilateral simultaneous CEA com pared to 20 stagedCEA	No major neurological complications; no difference in the gropus
Dimakakos et al. [31]	1996	12 bilateral simultaneous CEA and 22 staged CEA	No differences between gropus; one case of TIA and another case of transient vocal cord paresis in the bilateral simultaneous CEA group
Darling et al. [23]	1996	102 staged CEA within 2 days	Combined stroke mortality rate of 1%
Hokari et al. [3]	2014	Hybrid procedure: 2 CEA (symptomatic side) and CAS after 2 months	Severe hypotension after CAS
Schroeder et al. [5]	1986	56 staged CEA within 3 weeks	Postendarterectomy hypertension was significantly higher following the second procedure, when operations were staged less than 3 weeks apart
Maxwell et al. [27]	1992	161 staged CEA	5.6% stroke and death rate; death was associated with postoperative hypertension and a short intersurgical interval
Kavakli et al. [29]	2015	1 bilateral simultaneous CEA with regional anesthesia	No complications
Ketonen et al. [4]	1979	18 bilateral simultaneous CEA	3.8% mortality, 5% permanent neurological deficits
Mubarak et al. [7]	1998	5 bilateral CAS	No complications
Chen et al. [6]	2004	10 bilateral CAS	No complications
Sultan et al. [28]	2024	91 staged CEA	Postoperative hypertension as a crucial independent predictor of perioperative stroke
Jumpei et al. [37]	2019	8 bilateral simultaneous CAS and 4 staged bilateral CAS	Bilateral simultaneous CAS is not inferior to staged CAS
Beach et al. [36]	2019	22 hybrid procedures: staged CEA and CAS	One perioperative stroke (4.5%), one patient with postoperative myocardial infarction (4.5%), and two patients (9.1%) with cranial nerve injuries
Shchehlov et al. [1]	2022	39 bilateral simultaneous CAS	Two periprocedural neurological complications, one transient ischemic attack, and one minor stroke

Table 1. *Cont.*

Autor	Year	Management	Complications
Lai et al. [3]	2019	333 bilateral simultaneous CAS	Except for hyperperfusion syndrome, all other periprocedural complications including hemodynamic depression, stroke, and MI were comparable with the literature reports on unilateral carotid artery stenting
Rodriguez et al. [22]	2001	154 staged CEA (4 days)	No increase in immediate and 30-day morbidity and mortality when compared to unilateral CEA

4. Discussion

We presented a case of a 64-year-old male patient with severe bilateral symptomatic carotid artery stenosis. He was successfully managed with staged CEA with a 3-day interval between surgeries. While many strategies are reported for this condition (staged CEA, simultaneous bilateral CEA, hybrid procedure), there are no guidelines and no strategy has been proven superior. We consider that a patient-tailored strategy should be planned considering patient comorbidities and the risk of cerebral thromboembolism. In our case, the presence of severe symptomatic bilateral carotid artery stenosis (recent left ischemic stroke with right hemiparesis and chronic ischemic frontal lesion on the right side), with mixed echogenicity and high risk of cerebral embolism, led us to perform carotid endarterectomy first on the left side and then right carotid endarterectomy within a three-day interval. This strategy is supported by data from the literature. Both Farsk et al. [30] and Dimakakos et al. [31] reported no difference between simultaneous and staged CEA. Rodriguez et al. [22] observed no increase in immediate and 30-day morbidity and mortality when they compared 154 staged CEA cases with a mean interval of 4 days with unilateral CEA. Also, Darling et al. [23] reported a low (1%) combined stroke and mortality rate after analyzing 102 staged CEA with a mean interval of 2 days between surgeries, while Kim et al. [21] did not find any association with ipsilateral stroke in 43 staged CEA cases. However, Maxwell et al. [27] reported a higher rate of stroke and death (5.6%) than Darling et al. A possible explication for this difference could be the evolution of brain protection strategies. We did not proceed with simultaneous bilateral CEA because of the risk of hyperperfusion syndrome associated with severe bilateral stenosis especially in our case with more than 90% bilateral stenosis. The patient developed postoperative hypertension after the first left CEA in accordance with several reports that link this complication to a less than 3-week interval between surgeries [5,28]. This complication was rapidly managed with intravenous calcium channel blockers and did not affect the evolution of the patient. Also, considering the history of ischemic cardiomyopathy with stent implantation, we considered that longer operation times associated with simultaneous bilateral CEA could increase the risk of myocardial ischemia complications. Also, another reason in favor of staged CEA was the high risk of bleeding and cervical hematoma occurrence associated with the dual antiplatelet therapy if not discontinued.

While bilateral CAS is reported to be a safe alternative for CEA with studies that report no complications [6,7,27], it was not an option in our case even if we consider only CAS of the right internal carotid artery. The reason was both the lack of experience and materials (embolic prevention system) needed for a safe procedure.

The planned management also included the following: dual antiplatelet therapy not discontinued because of the risk of thromboembolism; a neurological consultation immediately after each extubation; myocardial ischemia monitoring with serial EKG, myocardial enzymes, transthoracic echocardiography and a coronary angiography performed in the preoperative setting to evaluate the stents implanted and other possible coronary stenosis; a neurological consultation and a head CT before the second CEA in order to evaluate the safety of performing surgery (we looked for new imaging or clinical signs of cerebral hemorrhage that would contraindicate the second CEA); and general anesthesia, with a neurological and cardiological consultation before discharge.

Considering the surgical technique used, strategies for brain protection during carotid artery clamping are essential in this case of severe bilateral carotid artery stenosis. While continuous transcranial Doppler ultrasonography and EEG monitoring were not available at our institution, we measured the pressure in the internal carotid artery after clamping (carotid stump pressure), and we evaluated the backflow in the internal carotid artery. Also, NIRS was used to monitor cerebral oxygenation. A carotid pressure stump pressure below 40 mmHg [38,39], an unsatisfactory backflow, and a more than 20% reduction from baseline in cerebral oxygenation led us to proceed with shunt insertion. Also, careful hemostasis and surgical drains were essential for reducing the risk of cervical hematoma.

General anesthesia was used because studies report a protective effect for cerebral hypoxia. Also, the type of anesthesia does not seem to influence the postoperative results of CEA. Even though regional anesthesia reduces the need for shunt placement, in our case, it was obvious that shunt placement would be very likely. We also wanted to avoid specific neurological complications associated with this type of anesthesia like phrenic nerve, vagus nerve, and stellate ganglion lesions. To reduce the risk of myocardial infarction associated with general anesthesia, we chose to do a staged procedure to minimize the operative times, and dual antiplatelet therapy was not discontinued considering the history of coronary artery stenting 6 months prior.

5. Conclusions

The management of tandem severe symptomatic carotid artery stenosis can be challenging considering the high risk of periprocedural stroke and the lack of consensus regarding this situation. Staged CEA with a small time interval between CEAs can be an option in patients with a high risk of cerebral thromboembolism when postponing the second CEA for another hospital admission. Although simultaneous bilateral CEA is reported, the choice of surgical and anesthesia strategy should be tailored to each patient. Considering the favodrable evolution of this case, we consider staged CEA for bilateral severe symptomatic (more than 90%) carotid artery stenosis to be a safe strategy in very selected cases.

Author Contributions: Conceptualization, M.R., I.-M.M., B.R., O.S., H.M. and V.A.I.; methodology, M.R., O.S., I.-M.M., C.V., G.-P.G. and H.M.; software M.R. and A.D.; validation, M.R., V.A.I., C.V., H.M. and A.D.; formal analysis, M.R., O.S., B.R., H.M. and V.A.I.; investigation, M.R., B.R., I.-M.M. and O.S.; resources, M.R., A.D., G.-P.G., O.S. and H.M.; data curation, M.R., I.-M.M., C.V., A.D., H.M. and V.A.I.; writing—original draft preparation, M.R., B.R. and V.A.I.; writing—review and editing, M.R., I.-M.M., G.-P.G., O.S. and H.M.; visualization, M.R., H.M., C.V., G.-P.G. and V.A.I.; supervision, M.R., H.M., C.V., B.R. and V.A.I.; project administration, B.R., O.S., G.-P.G. and V.A.I.; funding acquisition, H.M. All authors have read and agreed to the published version of the manuscript.

Funding: The publication of this paper was supported by the University of Medicine and Pharmacy Carol Davila through the institutional program "Publish not Perish".

Institutional Review Board Statement: This study was conducted in accordance with the Declaration of Helsinki and approved by the Romanian National Ethics Committee (Approval Code: 167; Approval Date: 24 January 2022).

Informed Consent Statement: Informed consent was obtained from the patient.

Data Availability Statement: Data available on request.

Conflicts of Interest: The authors declare no conflicts of interest.

References

1. Shchehlov, D.V.; Svyrydiuk, O.Y.; Vyval, M.B.; Sydorenko, O.F.; Nosenko, N.M.; Gudym, M.S. Simultaneous bilateral angioplasty and stenting for carotid stenosis—A single center experience. *J. Med. Life* **2022**, *15*, 252–257. [CrossRef] [PubMed] [PubMed Central]
2. Diehm, N.; Katzen, B.T.; Iyer, S.S.; White, C.J.; Hopkins, L.N.; Kelley, L.; BEACH Investigators. Staged bilateral carotid stenting, an effective strategy in high-risk patients—Insights from a prospective multicenter trial. *J. Vasc. Surg.* **2008**, *47*, 1227–1234. [CrossRef] [PubMed]
3. Lai, Z.; Guo, Z.; Shao, J.; Chen, Y.; Liu, X.; Liu, B.; Qiu, C. A systematic review and meta-analysis of results of simultaneous bilateral carotid artery stenting. *J. Vasc. Surg.* **2019**, *69*, 1633–1642. [CrossRef] [PubMed]
4. Ketonen, P.; Luosto, R.; Mattila, S.; Nemes, A.; Ketonen, L. Surgical experience with simultaneous bilateral carotid endarterectomies. *Scand. J. Thorac. Cardiovasc. Surg.* **1979**, *13*, 321–326. [CrossRef] [PubMed]
5. Schroeder, T.; Sillesen, H.; Engell, H.C. Staged bilateral carotid endarterectomy. *J. Vasc. Surg.* **1986**, *3*, 355–359. [CrossRef] [PubMed]
6. Chen, M.S.; Bhatt, D.L.; Mukherjee, D.; Chan, A.W.; Roffi, M.; Kapadia, S.R.; Ziada, K.M.; Chew, D.P.; Bajzer, C.T.; Yadav, J.S. Feasibility of simultaneous bilateral carotid artery stenting. *Catheter. Cardiovasc. Interv.* **2004**, *61*, 437–442. [CrossRef] [PubMed]
7. Al-Mubarak, N.; Roubin, G.S.; Vitek, J.J.; Gomez, C.R. Simultaneous bilateral carotid stenting for restenosis after endarterectomy. *Cathet Cardiovasc. Diagn.* **1998**, *45*, 11–15. [CrossRef] [PubMed]
8. Bangad, A.; Abbasi, M.; de Havenon, A. Secondary Ischemic Stroke Prevention. *Neurotherapeutics* **2023**, *20*, 721–731. [CrossRef] [PubMed] [PubMed Central]
9. Wolf, P.A.; Clagett, G.P.; Easton, J.D.; Goldstein, L.B.; Gorelick, P.B.; Kelly-Hayes, M.; Sacco, R.L.; Whisnant, J.P. Preventing ischemic stroke in patients with prior stroke and transient ischemic attack: A statement for healthcare professionals from the Stroke Council of the American Heart Association. *Stroke* **1999**, *30*, 1991–1994. [CrossRef] [PubMed]
10. Eastcott, H.H.; Pickering, G.W.; Rob, C.G. Reconstruction of internal carotid artery in a patient with intermittent attacks of hemiplegia. *Lancet* **1954**, *267*, 994–996. [CrossRef] [PubMed]
11. North American Symptomatic Carotid Endarterectomy Trial Collaborators; Barnett, H.J.M.; Taylor, D.W.; Haynes, R.B.; Sackett, D.L.; Peerless, S.J.; Ferguson, G.G.; Fox, A.J.; Rankin, R.N.; Hachinski, V.C.; et al. Beneficial effect of carotid endarterectomy in symptomatic patients with high-grade carotid stenosis. *N. Engl. J. Med.* **1991**, *325*, 445–453. [CrossRef] [PubMed]
12. Moore, W.S.; Barnett, H.J.; Beebe, H.G.; Bernstein, E.F.; Brener, B.J.; Brott, T.; Caplan, L.R.; Day, A.; Goldstone, J.; Hobson, R.W., 2nd; et al. Guidelines for carotid endarterectomy. A multidisciplinary consensus statement from the ad hoc Committee, American Heart Association. *Stroke* **1995**, *26*, 188–201. [CrossRef] [PubMed]
13. European Carotid Surgery Trialists' Collaborative Group. Randomised trial of endarterectomy for recently symptomatic carotid stenosis: Final results of the MRC European Carotid Surgery Trial (ECST). *Lancet* **1998**, *351*, 1379–1387. [CrossRef] [PubMed]
14. Kleindorfer, D.O.; Towfighi, A.; Chaturvedi, S.; Cockroft, K.M.; Gutierrez, J.; Lombardi-Hill, D.; Kamel, H.; Kernan, W.N.; Kittner, S.J.; Leira, E.C.; et al. 2021 Guideline for the Prevention of Stroke in Patients with Stroke and Transient Ischemic Attack: A Guideline from the American Heart Association/American Stroke Association. *Stroke* **2021**, *52*, e364–e467. [CrossRef] [PubMed]
15. Naylor, R.; Rantner, B.; Ancetti, S.; de Borst, G.J.; De Carlo, M.; Halliday, A.; Kakkos, S.K.; Markus, H.S.; McCabe, D.J.H.; Sillesen, H.; et al. Editor's Choice–European Society for Vascular Surgery (ESVS) 2023 Clinical Practice Guidelines on the Management of Atherosclerotic Carotid and Vertebral Artery Disease. *Eur. J. Vasc. Endovasc. Surg.* **2023**, *65*, 7–111. [CrossRef] [PubMed]
16. Bulbulia, R.; Halliday, A.; van Herzeele, I.; Koncar, I.; McCabe, D.J.; Lal, A.; Ricco, J.B.; Ringleb, P.; Taylor-Rowan, M.; Eckstein, H.H. European Stroke Organisation guideline on endarterectomy and stenting for carotid artery stenosis. *Eur. Stroke J.* **2021**, *6*, I–XLVII. [CrossRef] [PubMed] [PubMed Central]
17. Li, Y.; Sun, W.; Yin, Q.; Wang, Y.; Cai, Q.; Sun, W.; Huang, Z.; Liu, W.; Xiong, Y.; Xu, G.; et al. Safety and efficacy of simultaneous bilateral carotid angioplasty and stenting. *J. Thromb. Thrombolysis.* **2014**, *37*, 202–209. [CrossRef] [PubMed]
18. Liu, B.; Wei, W.; Wang, Y.; Yang, X.; Yue, S.; Zhang, J. Treatment Strategy for Bilateral Severe Carotid Artery Stenosis: One Center's Experience. *World Neurosurg.* **2015**, *84*, 820–825. [CrossRef] [PubMed]
19. Buratti, L.; Balucani, C.; Viticchi, G.; Falsetti, L.; Altamura, C.; Avitabile, E.; Provinciali, L.; Vernieri, F.; Silvestrini, M. Cognitive deterioration in bilateral asymptomatic severe carotid stenosis. *Stroke* **2014**, *45*, 2072–2077. [CrossRef] [PubMed]
20. Brott, T.G.; Halperin, J.L.; Abbara, S.; Bacharach, J.M.; Barr, J.D.; Bush, R.L.; Cates, C.U.; Creager, M.A.; Fowler, S.B.; Friday, G.; et al. 2011 ASA/ACCF/AHA/AANN/AANS/ACR/ASNR/CNS/SAIP/SCAI/SIR/SNIS/SVM/SVS guideline on the management of patients with extracranial carotid and vertebral artery disease: Executive summary. A report of the American College of Cardiology Foundation/American Heart Association Task Force on Practice Guidelines, and the American Stroke Association, American Association of Neuroscience Nurses, American Association of Neurological Surgeons, American College of Radiology, American Society of Neuroradiology, Congress of Neurological Surgeons, Society of Atherosclerosis Imaging and Prevention, Society for Cardiovascular Angiography and Interventions, Society of Interventional Radiology, Society of NeuroInterventional Surgery, Society for Vascular Medicine, and Society for Vascular Surgery. *Circulation* **2011**, *124*, 489–532, Erratum in *Circulation* **2011**, *124*, e145. [CrossRef] [PubMed]
21. Kim, A.; Kwon, T.W.; Han, Y.; Kwon, S.U.; Kwon, H.; Noh, M.; Cho, Y.P. Clinical outcomes of staged bilateral carotid endarterectomy for bilateral carotid artery stenosis. *Ann. Surg. Treat. Res.* **2015**, *89*, 261–267. [CrossRef] [PubMed] [PubMed Central]

22. Rodriguez-Lopez, J.A.; Diethrich, E.B.; Olsen, D.M. Postoperative morbidity of closely staged bilateral carotid endarterectomies: An intersurgical interval of 4 days or less. *Ann. Vasc. Surg.* **2001**, *15*, 457–464. [CrossRef] [PubMed]
23. Darling, R.C., 3rd; Kubaska, S.; Shah, D.M.; Paty, P.S.; Chang, B.B.; Lloyd, W.E.; Leather, R.P. Bilateral carotid endarterectomy during the same hospital admission. *Cardiovasc. Surg.* **1996**, *4*, 759–762. [CrossRef] [PubMed]
24. Lehv, M.S.; Salzman, E.W.; Silen, W. Hypertension complicating carotid endarterectomy. *Stroke* **1970**, *1*, 307–313. [CrossRef] [PubMed]
25. Satiani, B.; Vasko, J.S.; Evans, W.E. Hypertension following carotid endarterectomy. *Surg. Neurol.* **1979**, *11*, 357–359. [PubMed]
26. Towne, J.B.; Bernhard, V.M. The relationship of postoperative hypertension to complications following carotid endarterectomy. *Surgery* **1980**, *88*, 575–580. [CrossRef] [PubMed]
27. Maxwell, J.G.; Covington, D.L.; Churchill, M.P.; Rutherford, E.J.; Clancy, T.V.; Tackett, A.D. Results of staged bilateral carotid endarterectomy. *Arch. Surg.* **1992**, *127*, 793–798. [CrossRef] [PubMed]
28. Sultan, S.; Acharya, Y.; Dulai, M.; Tawfick, W.; Hynes, N.; Wijns, W.; Soliman, O. Redefining postoperative hypertension management in carotid surgery: A comprehensive analysis of blood pressure homeostasis and hyperperfusion syndrome in unilateral vs. bilateral carotid surgeries and implications for clinical practice. *Front. Surg.* **2024**, *11*, 1361963. [CrossRef] [PubMed] [PubMed Central]
29. Kavaklı, A.S.; Ayoğlu, R.U.; Öztürk, N.K.; Sağdıç, K.; Yılmaz, M.; İnanoğlu, K.; Emmiler, M. Simultaneous Bilateral Carotid Endarterectomy under Cervical Plexus Blockade. *Turk. J. Anaesthesiol. Reanim.* **2015**, *43*, 367–370. [CrossRef] [PubMed] [PubMed Central]
30. Farsak, B.; Oç, M.; Boke, E. Simultaneous bilateral carotid endarterectomy: Our first experience. *Ann. Thorac. Cardiovasc. Surg.* **2001**, *7*, 292–296. [PubMed]
31. Dimakakos, P.B.; Arapoglou, B.; Papasava, M.; Papadimitriou, J. Our first experience applying simultaneous bilateral carotid endarterectomy. *Int. Angiol.* **1996**, *15*, 9–13. [PubMed]
32. Yoshida, K.; Kurosaki, Y.; Funaki, T.; Kikuchi, T.; Ishii, A.; Takahashi, J.C.; Takagi, Y.; Yamagata, S.; Miyamoto, S. Surgical dissection of the internal carotid artery under flow control by proximal vessel clamping reduces embolic infarcts during carotid endarterectomy. *World Neurosurg.* **2014**, *82*, e229–e234. [CrossRef] [PubMed]
33. Leichtle, S.W.; Mouawad, N.J.; Welch, K.; Lampman, R.; Whitehouse, W.M., Jr.; Heidenreich, M. Outcomes of carotid endarterectomy under general and regional anesthesia from the American College of Surgeons' National Surgical Quality Improvement Program. *J. Vasc. Surg.* **2012**, *56*, 81–88.e3. [CrossRef] [PubMed]
34. Xu, R.W.; Liu, P.; Fan, X.Q.; Wang, Q.; Zhang, J.B.; Ye, Z.D. Feasibility and Safety of Simultaneous Carotid Endarterectomy and Carotid Stenting for Bilateral Carotid Stenosis: A Single-Center Experience using a Hybrid Procedure. *Ann. Vasc. Surg.* **2016**, *33*, 138–143. [CrossRef] [PubMed]
35. Hokari, M.; Isobe, M.; Asano, T.; Itou, Y.; Yamazaki, K.; Chiba, Y.; Iwamoto, N.; Isu, T. Treatment strategy for bilateral carotid stenosis: 2 cases of carotid endarterectomy for the symptomatic side followed by carotid stenting. *J. Stroke Cerebrovasc. Dis.* **2014**, *23*, 2851–2856. [CrossRef] [PubMed]
36. Beach, J.M.; Sharma, S.; Bena, J.; Kang, J.; Clair, D.G.; Smolock, C.J. Concomitant ipsilateral carotid endarterectomy and stenting is an effective treatment for tandem carotid artery lesions. *J. Vasc. Surg.* **2020**, *71*, 1579–1586. [CrossRef] [PubMed]
37. Oshita, J.; Sakamoto, S.; Okazaki, T.; Ishii, D.; Kurisu, K. Safety of simultaneous bilateral carotid artery stenting for bilateral carotid artery stenosis. *Interv. Neuroradiol.* **2020**, *26*, 19–25. [CrossRef] [PubMed] [PubMed Central]
38. Crawford, E.S.; De Bakey, M.E.; Morris, G.C., Jr.; Fields, W.S. Arterial reconstructive operation for occlusive disease of the innominate, carotid, subclavian, and vertebral arteries. *Prog. Cardiovasc. Dis.* **1960**, *3*, 145–161. [CrossRef] [PubMed]
39. Kordzadeh, A.; Abbassi, O.A.; Prionidis, I.; Shawish, E. The Role of Carotid Stump Pressure in Carotid Endarterectomy: A Systematic Review and Meta-Analysis. *Ann. Vasc. Dis.* **2020**, *13*, 28–37. [CrossRef] [PubMed] [PubMed Central]

Journal of
Personalized Medicine

MDPI

Review

CITED Proteins in Cardiac Development and Lifelong Heart Function

José Bragança [1,2,3,*], Rute Luísa Cabrita Pinto [1,2], Igor Ventura [1], Silvana Ferreira [1] and António Marreiros [1]

[1] Faculty of Medicine and Biomedical Sciences (FMCB), Campus Gambelas, University of Algarve, 8005-139 Faro, Portugal; ruteluisapinto@gmail.com (R.L.C.P.); a70941@ualg.pt (I.V.); a74779@ualg.pt (S.F.); a87786@ualg.pt (A.M.)
[2] Algarve Biomedical Center-Research Institute (ABC-RI), Campus Gambelas, University of Algarve, 8005-139 Faro, Portugal
[3] Centre for Health Technology and Services Research, Health Research Network (CINTESIS@RISE), University of Algarve, 8005-139 Faro, Portugal
* Correspondence: jebraganca@ualg.pt; Tel.: +351-289-800-900 (ext. 302317)

Abstract

The CITED proteins function as transcriptional modulators that are essential for vertebrate development. These proteins interact with numerous partners, notably transcription factors and co-activators. The hallmark of the CITED family is their conserved carboxy-terminal domain, which interacts strongly with the CBP/p300 co-activators. The expression of CITED genes is detected early during embryogenesis within embryonic and foetal regions critical for cardiac morphogenesis, among other developmental processes. Notably, CITED2 loss of function is strongly associated with congenital heart malformations in mice and zebrafish embryos, as well as congenital heart disease (CHD) in humans, whereas other CITED family members are not critical for cardiogenesis. Emerging evidence implicates CITED2 and CITED4 in regulating heart physiological adaptations and protective responses to pathological stress. This review provides a detailed analysis of CITED proteins and their interactors, focusing on CITED-target genes relevant for cardiogenesis and heart disease. We also highlight recent findings indicating that CITED2 and CITED4 may be instrumental for the development of novel therapeutic strategies to mitigate CHD and preserve adult cardiac function.

Keywords: CITED1; CITED2; CITED4; heart development; heart diseases; congenital heart disease

1. Introduction

Congenital heart diseases (CHDs) are structural and functional anomalies resulting from improper foetal development present in nearly 1% of live births, with an estimated 2–5% risk of familial recurrence. As infant mortality rates decrease, more adults with complex CHDs are surviving and are at risk for severe cardiovascular complications [1]. Many children and adults with CHDs require surgeries and lifelong medical care, but inequalities in access to quality CHD care persist worldwide [2,3]. Mutations in genes encoding for transcriptional and epigenetic/chromatin remodelling factor, cell signalling, adhesion and structural sarcomere proteins, as well as chromosomal abnormalities can disrupt heart development, leading to CHDs [1]. Additionally, inadequate placental function, sporadic developmental errors, and/or maternal environmental stressors, such as diabetes, some medications and drugs abuse, infections, tobacco smoke, alcohol, and harmful chemicals, increase the risk of CHDs [1]. Despite scientific and clinical advancements, CHDs remain a significant global health and economic burden. Non-congenital heart conditions, collectively termed acquired cardiovascular diseases (ACDs), represent a spectrum of common heart disorders that develop after birth, which include coronary artery disease and rheumatic heart disease, among others. ACDs are the accountable cause for more than 30% of deaths worldwide annually. Ischemic (coronary) heart disease remains the dominant cause among cardiovascular deaths, and the burden is significant across all countries and economical levels, although over three quarters of these deaths are recorded in countries with emerging economies. The continuing evolution of ACD epidemiology highlights the need for prevention, screening, and intervention strategies adapted to regional risk profiles and health system capacities [4].

The CBP/p300-interacting transactivator with ED-rich tail (CITED) family includes transcriptional regulators present only in vertebrates that interact strongly with the acetyltransferases and transcriptional co-activators CBP and p300 [5–8]. During mouse embryogenesis, CITED proteins display diverse functions and are crucial for multiple developmental and morphological processes. Among the CITED members, Cited2 is currently the most extensively studied and has been demonstrated to be indispensable for mouse embryonic survival and growth during gestation, as well as for the correct development of the heart, placenta, and other organs [5,9–17]. In humans, abnormal regulation and mutations of *CITED2* have been correlated to CHDs [1]. On the other hand, despite *Cited1* being expressed in key cardiogenic structures and present in embryonic mouse hearts, its role in cardiac development is less critical compared to *Cited2*. *Cited4* is not essential for mouse embryo development, but in adult rodent hearts, its expression is linked to physiological cardiac hypertrophy induced by exercise training [18,19]. *Cited3* is the last member of the *CITED* genes, being expressed exclusively in birds and fish, where it also plays a role in their normal developmental processes [20,21].

Strong evidence suggests that the self-renewal and differentiation defects observed in *Cited2*-deficient mouse embryonic stem cells (ESCs), along with the lethality and multiple organ malformations in *Cited2*-null mouse embryos, can be rescued through supplementation or ectopic expression of human CITED2 protein or other Cited2-regulated proteins, including Wnt5a and Wnt11 [22–25]. Like in mice, *Cited2* depletion from the one-cell stage in zebrafish embryos increased early embryonic death and cardiovascular defects, which were substantially rescued following microinjection of recombinant human CITED2 or Wnt5a/Wnt11 proteins [24]. Therefore, the human CITED2 protein exhibits functional equivalence with the endogenous Cited2 proteins of mice and zebrafish, supporting the notion that CITED2 activity is evolutionarily conserved among vertebrates. In the adult heart, *Cited2* and *Cited4* fulfil distinct yet critical functions for cardiac homeostasis, supporting exercise-induced adaptation and conferring protection against cardiovascular stress and pathology, while *Cited1* plays a minimal role in these mechanisms [6,18,26–28].

In this review, we discuss the roles of CITED family members in cardiogenesis and adult cardiac function, as well as their associations with heart disease. We report advances in understanding the molecular and cellular functions of *Cited* genes, which are essential for elucidating their contributions to normal heart development, homeostasis, and pathology. We also highlight recent research methods and techniques employed to extend the understanding of CITED functions, which could contribute to the development of novel therapeutic strategies to prevent or manage cardiac dysfunction.

2. Heart Development

In vertebrates, the heart is a complex organ composed of multiple diverse cell types, including cardiomyocytes, conduction system cells, endothelial cells, vascular smooth muscle cells, and cardiac fibroblasts [29,30]. The proper organization and localization of those cells within the heart are orchestrated by complex differentiation and patterning processes during embryogenesis. In this section, we will focus on the major steps of heart development taking place from embryonic day (E)16 to E60 in humans and E7.5–E15 in mice [31,32]. All resident cells of the heart are derived from distinct cardiac progenitor cells (CPCs) that are spatially and temporally segregated in the developing embryo [1,33]. The majority of cardiac cells arise from the mesodermal layer, which is initially characterized by the expression of the transcription factor Brachyury/T [34]. Some of these mesoderm cells are further specified into early cardiac mesoderm precursor cells expressing the transcription factor Mesp1 (Figure 1).

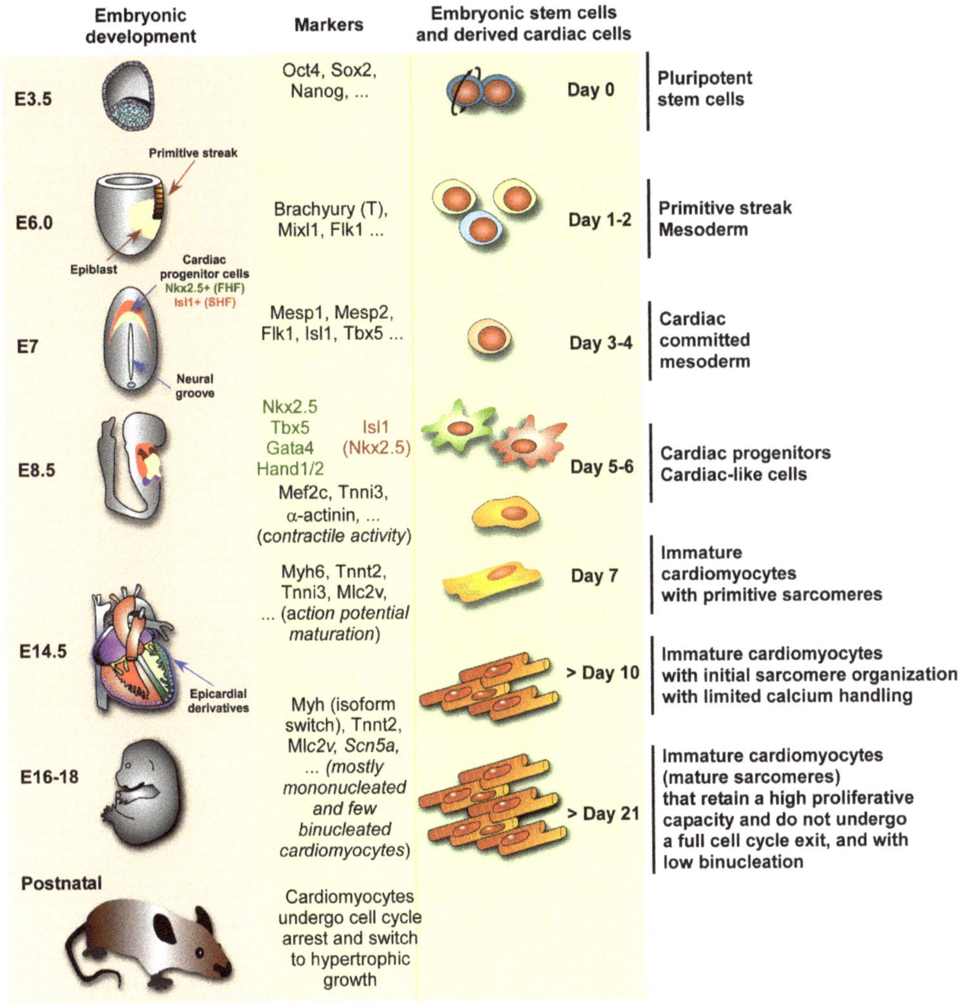

Figure 1. Mouse embryonic development compared to embryonic stem cell cardiac differentiation. Left panel: cardiac structures and timings in embryonic days (E) of mouse embryonic development until birth. Middle panel: some markers specific to each step of heart development and cardiac

differentiation. Right panel: steps and timings of cardiac differentiation from mouse embryonic stem cells (pluripotent stem cells). Note that the cardiac differentiation from ESCs and heart embryonic development follow similar steps and share similar molecular markers. At E3.5, the blastocyst has an inner cell mass (blue cells) from which embryonic pluripotent stem cells are derived, which are characterized by the expression of Nanog, Oct4, and Sox2, among other genes. At E6.0, the formation of the primitive streak initiates, which initiates gastrulation and the generation of the mesoderm. At E7.0, the cardiac crescent is formed, composed of cardiac progenitor cells of the first heart field (FHF) marked by the expression of Nkx2.5 (green field) and the secondary heart field (SHF) marked by the expression of Isl1 (red field), after specification of some cells of the mesoderm into the cardiac mesoderm marked by Mesp1 expression. At 8.5, the linear heart tube is formed, and cardiac contractile activity is detected. By E14.5, the heart is formed by 4 chambers with cells of the FHF contributing to the left ventricle and atrium, and cells of the SHF contributing to the right ventricle and atrium. Epicardial cells will derive from the epicardium. After birth, many cardiomyocytes undergo one final nuclear mitosis without complete cell division, leading to multinucleation (cells with two or more nuclei), which is a hallmark of the switch from a proliferative state (hyperplasia) to hypertrophic growth (cells increase in size rather than number). The information about ESCs and differentiation stages was adapted from [35–38].

Around mouse E6.5–7.0 (human E21–28), Mesp1-positive cells exit the primitive streak and rapidly originate two distinct populations of CPCs called the first heart field (FHF) and second heart field (SHF). The FHF is marked by the expression of the transcription factors Nkx2.5 and Tbx5, whereas the transcription factor Isl1 is specifically expressed in a subset of Mesp1-derived cells contributing to the SHF [39]. By mouse E8.5 and around human E20, cells of the FHF form the cardiac crescent and next migrate and fuse at the midline of the embryo to form the primitive linear heart tube. This structure is composed of an outer (myocardium) and an inner cell layer (endocardium), separated by an extracellular matrix (ECM) called the cardiac jelly. The linear heart tube contributes to the formation of the future left ventricle and atrial chambers [34,40]. By mouse E8.0 and human E21–22, the heart tube initiates rhythmic contractions due to cardiomyocyte activity and undergoes a rightward looping at around mouse E9.0 and human E24–28 [34,40–42]. The SHF progenitors, on the other hand, which are initially present medially and posteriorly to the cardiac crescent (Figure 1), migrate into the linear heart tube, extend into the pharyngeal mesoderm, and participate in the looping heart tube. CPCs of the SHF also contribute to the formation and elongation of the outflow tract (OFT), right ventricle, atrium, venous pole of the heart, and the primary atrial septum [34,40–42]. At this stage, another type of progenitor, the proepicardium cardiac progenitors, migrates onto the outer cardiac surface to produce the cells of the epicardium which cover the myocardium [43]. The sinus venosus comprising the sinoatrial node and the sinus horns derives from a distinct population of cardiac precursors expressing Tbx18 [34,44]. Some epicardial cells undergo an epithelial-to-mesenchymal (EMT) transition and originate epicardium-derived progenitor cells, which migrate into the heart and differentiate into smooth muscle cells, cardiac fibroblasts, and endothelial cells, which contribute to the coronary vasculature [43].

By E9.5 in mice and E34 in humans, endocardial cushions form in the atrioventricular canal (AVC) and OFT through migration of endocardial cells between the endocardium and myocardium [45]. These structures are predominantly composed of mesenchymal cells generated via endocardial EMT [46]. The muscular interventricular septum develops from the myocardium at the caudal end of the forming ventricle, starting around mouse E10.5 and human E52, and will separate the right and left ventricles [32,34]. Atrial septation begins at approximately mouse E10.5–E11.5 and human E32–34 [32]. During this process, the septum primum and septum secundum (membranous structures growing from the roof of the primitive atrium) extend toward the developing endocardial cushions. These structures partially divide the common atrium and leave an opening, the foramen ovale, which allows oxygenated foetal blood to flow from the right atrium to the left atrium. Normally, the foramen ovale closes soon after birth, and failure of this closure results in an atrial septal defect (ASD). At the same time, the common OFT is divided into the aorta and pulmonary artery, a process requiring contributions from cardiac neural crest cell progenitors, which migrate from the neural tube by mouse E9.5 and also participate in remodelling the pharyngeal arch arteries, valvulogenesis, and the development of the cardiac conduction system [34,47]. Atrioventricular valvulogenesis occurs around E14.5–E17.5 in mice and E44–E60 in humans [31,47].

Thus, the intricate orchestration of cardiac development involves the precise timing and coordination of multiple cell lineages, including mesodermal progenitors, neural crest cells, and epicardium-derived cells, to form the heart's chambers, valves, and great vessels. Disruptions in the coordinated cellular and molecular events of heart development may lead to CHDs, highlighting the importance of these processes for proper cardiac function.

3. Tracing the Role of CITED in Heart Development

Cited1 protein expression was detected in early mouse embryos from the two-cell to the blastocyst stage and primarily localized in the cytoplasm [48]. At later stages, *Cited1* is expressed in cultured trophoblast lineages and in the trophectoderm (TE) of early mouse embryos at higher levels than in the inner cell mass (ICM) cells [48]. *Cited1* depletion in mouse ESCs led to a compromised trophoblast differentiation induced by Bmp4, while its overexpression in those cells induces a trophoblast-like state through activation of the BMP signalling pathway. Additionally, Cited1 overexpression upregulated trophoblast signature genes while downregulating pluripotency-related genes, indicating that Cited1 promotes trophectodermal differentiation rather than ICM identity [48]. *Cited2* is expressed in both trophectoderm- and mesoderm-derived placental cells, with particularly high expression levels in the junctional zone of the placenta and invasive trophoblast cells that migrate from this zone into the uterine parenchyma in rodents [14,16,17]. Similarly, in humans and rats, CITED2 is present in extravillous trophoblasts, where it plays a critical role in placental development and function [16]. In addition, in mice, *Cited2* disruption leads to smaller, poorly vascularized placentas with reduced numbers of differentiated trophoblast cell types, resulting in placental insufficiency and embryonic lethality [14,17].

Prior to gastrulation at mouse E5.5 (Figure 2), *Cited2* is expressed in the anterior visceral endoderm (AVE), while *Cited1* is detected in the embryonic visceral endoderm and the visceral yolk sac endoderm [49]. The AVE derives from the visceral endoderm and produces secreted factors to signal the epiblast and orchestrate the correct primitive streak formation, anterior patterning of the embryo, and cardiac development. Later during gastrulation, *Cited2* expression is observed in the anterior mesoderm located next to the AVE (Figure 2B). At mouse E7.0–E7.5, in the cells that derive from the epiblast, *Cited1* transcripts are first detected in the nascent mesoderm adjacent to the primitive streak, while *Cited2* is concurrently expressed in the ventral node and cardiogenic mesoderm [13, 49]. Next, *Cited1* and *Cited2* expression is maintained throughout the cardiac crescent and in the myocardium (Figure 2B). At E8.5, *Cited2* is broadly expressed throughout the myocardium of the primitive heart tube of mouse embryos and is essential for early cardiac morphogenesis. In contrast, *Cited1* is present in the developing heart at this stage but exhibits a more restricted and lower expression pattern than *Cited2* [13,49]. The precise localization of *Cited1* expression within the heart tube is less characterized than the expression of *Cited2*, and its role in cardiac development appears to be less critical than that of *Cited2* [13,49]. Between E8.5 and E9.5, *Cited2* expression is detected in the presumptive septum transversum and the first and second branchial arches [13,49]. *Cited2* expression is also high in CPCs of embryonic hearts at E9.5, particularly cardiac progenitors of the SHF [22]. The function of *Cited2* in CPCs remains to be elucidated.

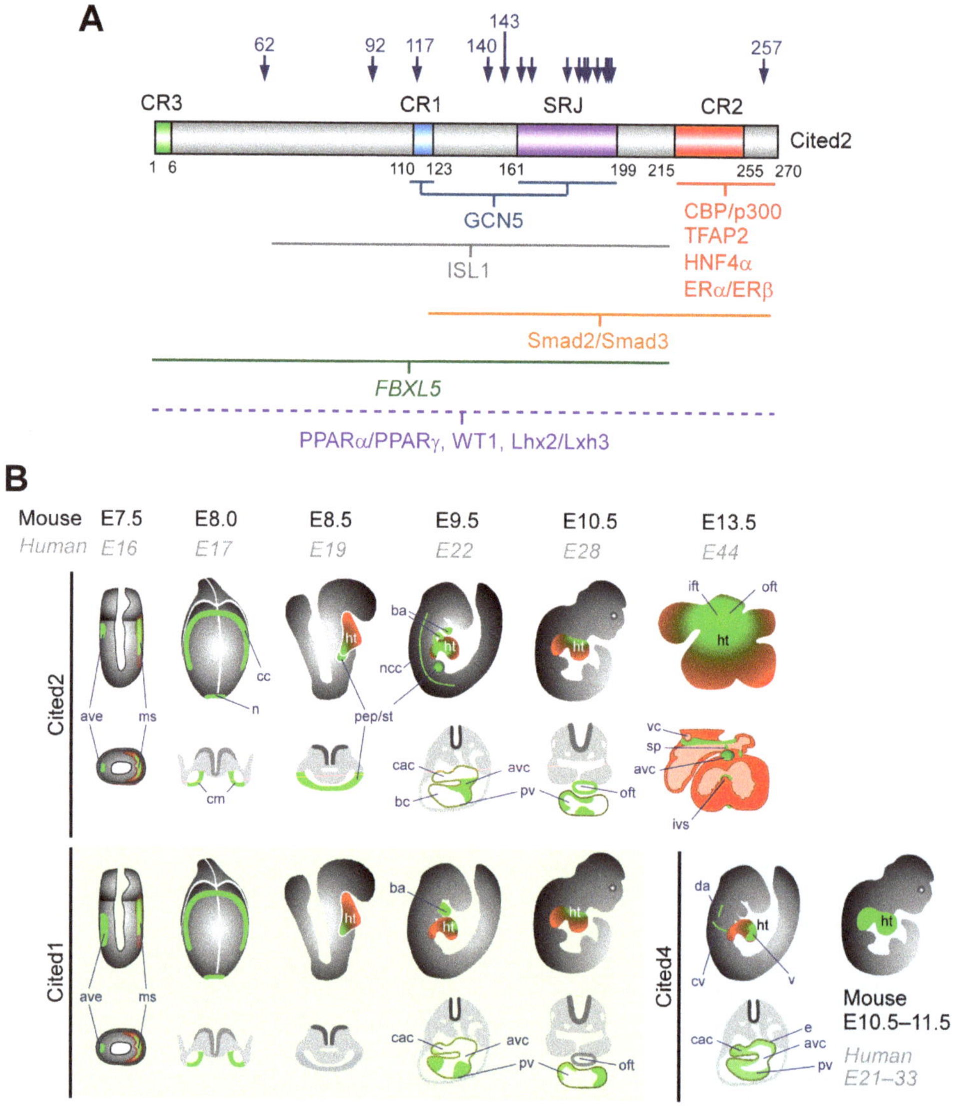

Figure 2. CITED interaction domains and expression during mouse embryonic development. (**A**) Representation of the human CITED2 protein showing the conserved regions (CR13). CR2 is shared by all CITED proteins, while CR1 is common to CITED1 and CITED2, and CR3 is found in CITED2 and CITED4. The serine-glycine-rich junction (SRJ), unique to CITED2, is also indicated. CITED2 protein interactors and their interaction domains with CITED2 are indicated below the CITED2 diagram. The CITED2 domains and its interacting proteins are indicated. Blue arrows mark the locations of CITED2 variants identified in CHD patients. (**B**) Illustrations of the temporal and spatial expression of *Cited2* transcripts represented by green areas (top panel) in cardiac-related regions with the corresponding transverse sections below. At E7.5, Cited2 is expressed in the anterior

visceral endoderm (ave) and mesoderm (ms), and at E8.0 in the cardiogenic mesoderm (cm), cardiac crescent (cc), and node (n). From E8.5 to E9.5, its expression is detected in regions containing cardiac progenitors of the proepicardium (pep) and hepatic progenitors of the septum transversum (st). At E9.5, *Cited2* expression extends to the myocardium near the proepicardium, including the outflow tract (oft), bulbus cordis (bc), primitive ventricle (pv), common atrioventricular canal (cac), cardiac neural crest cells (ncc), brachial arches (ba), and atrioventricular canal (avc). By E10.5, *Cited2* is detected in the trabeculae of the primitive outflow tract (oft) and the myocardium of the common ventricular chamber (pv). At E13.5, low transcripts levels are found throughout the myocardium of the prospective left and right atria and ventricles, with stronger expression in the septum primum, endocardial cushion tissue in the AVC, and around the vena cava (vc). Additional labelled structures include the common cardinal vein (cv), dorsal aorta (da), ventricles (v), atria (a), superior part of the atrial septum (sp), intraventricular septum (ivs), and endocardium (e). At later stages, Cited2 expression becomes more homogeneous throughout the heart [11,13]. The bottom left panel indicates *Cited1* expression from E7.5 to E10.5, and the bottom right panel indicates *Cited4* expression from E10.5 to E11.5, adapted from [13,49,50].

At early stages (E8.0), *Cited4* transcripts are only detected in the yolk sac and in the blood islands, but by E9.5 they are present in the cardinal vein and dorsal aorta, and in the developing atria and ventricles, particularly in the endocardium [18], and persist in the whole heart by E10.5 and E11.5 [50]. Between E9.5 and E10.5, Cited2 expression is broadly distributed and highly enriched within the developing cardiac structures (Figure 2B), including the aortic sac, the compact myocardium and trabeculae of the ventricles and the myocardium adjacent to the endocardial cushions of the OFT, the AVC, the presumptive atria, the inflow tract (IFT), and in the fourth branchial arch [13,49]. *Cited1* transcripts are also present in the future presumptive right ventricle and atrium by E10.5 to E12.5 [49]. By E13.5, *Cited2* expression is primarily confined to the OFT, the IFT, the septum primum, regions surrounding the vena cava, the endocardial cushions of the atrioventricular canal, and the apex of the interventricular septum [13].

Despite the considerable overlap in expression among *Cited1*, *Cited2*, and *Cited4* within cardiogenic regions during mouse embryogenesis, only embryos carrying a germline *Cited2* knockout exhibit severe developmental impairments and die during gestation with a myriad of cardiac abnormalities and defective establishment of the left–right axis, which also contributes to correct heart formation [5,9–15,17,18,51–58].

On the other hand, *Cited1*-null mice die immediately after birth due to defects in trophoblast-derived extraembryonic tissues, while *Cited4*-null mice are viable, but no apparent cardiac defects were observed in mice lacking *Cited1* or *Cited4* [18,58]. Interestingly, *Cited2* is also required for trophoblast proliferation and differentiation, as well as normal placental development and vascularization in mouse models [14,17,59]. Consequently, Cited2 dysfunction may simultaneously compromise both cardiac and placental development, further exacerbating cardiac defects and embryo outcomes.

In mammals, during foetal development and the first week after birth, cardiomyocytes are generally mononucleated with a high proliferative potential to allow the growth of heart tissue, thereby providing most of the cardiomyocytes necessary throughout the lifetime of the organism [60]. The transition from mononucleated to binucleated (or multinucleated) cardiomyocytes occurs by uncoupling of DNA synthesis/nuclear division from the cytoplasmic scission and marks the cardiomyocytes' terminal differentiation stage and loss of proliferation. Thus, subsequent increases in heart size, due to physiological or pathological stimuli, will occur by expansion of the size of the cardiomyocytes, a process termed hypertrophy [60].

The function of *Cited2* in the heart after birth and throughout adult life is still poorly understood. However, blocking *Cited2* expression in neonatal rat cardiomyocytes through miR-410 and miR-495 leads to increased DNA synthesis and proliferation via downregulation of the p57 cyclin kinase inhibitor [61]. Since Cited2 is critical for heart development in mice, its role in postnatal rat cardiomyocytes is unexpected. Further studies could clarify whether Cited2 expression functions to preserve cardiomyocytes as mononucleated rather than allowing binucleated conversion. On the other hand, Cited4 overexpression in primary cardiomyocytes drives their proliferation and heart hyperplasia, at least in part through increased expression of cyclin D1 [19]. Thus, Cited2 and Cited4 appear to have distinct and perhaps antagonistic roles in regulating postnatal cardiomyocyte proliferation. Unlike *Cited2* and *Cited4* expression, abundant in mouse and human adult hearts, *Cited1* expression is absent, and its role in adult hearts is negligeable [6,8,18,26–28]. Interestingly, the decrease in CITED2 expression has been associated with impaired cardiac function in human ischemic cardiomyopathy, emphasizing its potential importance in disease mechanisms and as a possible therapeutic target [62].

A recent study has shown that Cited2 is essential for maintaining the regenerative capacity of mouse cardiac stem cells during ageing and highlighted its potential as a therapeutic target for enhancing cardiac repair in the ageing heart [63]. However, prevailing evidence supports that heart regeneration in mammals, when it occurs, is primarily mediated by the proliferation and, in some cases, dedifferentiation of existing cardiomyocytes, not by progenitor cells [64,65]. Future research should focus on elucidating the precise molecular mechanisms by which CITED2 and CITED4 regulate cardiomyocyte function, and on exploring their potential as therapeutic targets to enhance cardiac repair and regeneration in heart disease.

4. Molecular Mechanisms of CITED-Mediated Cardiac GENE Regulation

4.1. CITED Proteins and Interacting Partners

At the molecular level, CITED2 strongly binds to transcriptional co-activators and histone acetyltransferases CBP and p300 (CBP/p300), which have also been linked to CHDs in Rubinstein–Taybi syndrome [8,66,67]. Three conserved regions (CR1–3) were described in CITED proteins (Figure 2A). A specific SMAD4-Interaction Domain (SID) has also been evidenced in CITED1 [68]. The CR2 domain is the hallmark of the CITED proteins, which encompasses the CBP/p300 binding domain and has been clearly identified as a potent transactivation domain. CITED proteins exhibit a high binding affinity to the cysteine-histidine-rich domain 1 (CH1) of CBP/p300. Binding of CITED proteins to CH1 may outcompete other transcription factors such as HIF-1α for the binding to CBP/300 and consequently repress the HIF/hypoxia signalling pathway [6–8,68–70]. In addition, *CITED2* is itself a hypoxia/HIF-target gene, and its expression may protect cells and embryos from an excessive hypoxic response [8,15]. CITED2 also acts as a negative regulator of transcription factors including RXRα, NF-κB, STAT2, p53, and ETS-1, all of which interact with the CH1 domain of CBP/p300 [8,71–76]. Conversely, CITED2 functions as a co-activator for numerous transcription factors that depend on CBP/p300 cooperation for transcriptional efficiency, including TFAP2 members, LHX2/3, SMAD2/3, PPARα/γ, HNF4α, WT1, GCN5, and ISL1 [5,9,22,77–85]. CITED2 also promotes PGC-1a activation of the hepatic gluconeogenic programme upon glucagon stimulation via prevention of its GCN5-mediated acetylation during fasting, while insulin disrupts the GCN5–CITED2 interaction, suppressing PGC-1a activity to aborting the gluconeogenic programme [83].

The CITED proteins also contain a conserved CR1 motif, which is present in CITED1, CITED2, and CITED3 and is located centrally within these proteins, as well as a shorter CR3 motif at the N-terminus of CITED2, CITED3, and CITED4 [86]. Moreover, CITED2 in placental mammals possesses a unique, serine-glycine-rich junction (SRJ) domain, which is highly conserved and represents a hotspot for mutations associated with CHDs [25]. Overall, the precise function of these conserved domains and SRJ remains largely unknown.

4.2. Regulation of CITED Expression

Little is known about the stimuli and pathways that govern the expression and function of the CITED family members during embryonic development. However, the cellular expression of Cited2 is highly sensitive to numerous extrinsic and intrinsic cellular signals, including conditions like hypoxia through a direct transactivation of HIF-1α and Forkhead box (Fox) factor FOXO3A, ischemia, interleukins, adrenocorticotropic hormones, growth factors such as PDGF, GM-CSF, TGF-β, β-FGF, and NGF, hemodynamic shear forces, oestrogens, interferon-α, insulin, elevated glucose levels, lipopolysaccharides (LPS), mechano-transduction triggered by primary cilia due to strain, indoxyl sulfate, endoplasmic reticulum stress, and DNA damage stimuli [8,73,81,82,87–95]. In addition, Foxp1 stimulates *Cited2* expression and the expression of other transcription factors required for pluripotency in mouse ESCs [23,96]. *Cited2* transcription within the mesoderm is upregulated by signalling through Wnt3/WNT3A [97]. In endothelial cells, the active insulin-receptor/PI3K/Akt pathway inhibits FoxO1 activity, leading to decreased expression of CITED2 [92], while *VEGF* modulates CITED2 expression in human coronary artery cells through the control of FoxO1 activity [98]. Additionally, FoxO3 has been shown to directly induce Cited2 expression in normoxic and hypoxic conditions in erythroid progenitors and mouse embryonic fibroblasts [95,99]. Interestingly, *Cited2* may also be upregulated by FoxO1 and FoxO3 in cardiomyocytes during heart infarction [100]. In contrast to Cited2, the regulatory signals and stimuli that control the cellular expression of Cited1 and Cited4 remain largely uncharacterized.

Cited1 co-activates Smad4 upon TGF-β/BMP pathway activation and represses the Wnt/β-catenin signalling pathway [101]. The regulation of *Cited1* expression by hypoxia in mammals has not been established, but its expression is upregulated by Wnt3a in ESCs and by the parathyroid hormone in osteoblast-lineage cells [102,103]. During mouse embryogenesis, Cited1 and Hand1 show overlapping expression domains, particularly within trophoblast and ventricular regions of the developing heart [49,58,104]. Compared to wild-type embryos at E9.5–10.5, *Cited1* expression was strongly reduced in the hearts of *Neuregulin* (*Nrg*)1-null embryos at E8.5 and in the left cardiac ventricle of *Nrg1-*, *Tbx20-*, and *Hand1*-null embryos [104–106]. These observations argue that Nrg1 (through the ERK1/2 MAP kinase pathway), Tbx20, and Hand1 act upstream of *Cited1* during cardiac development, but the exact contribution of *Cited1* downregulation to the phenotypes observed in *Nrg1-*, *Tbx20-*, and *Hand1*-null embryos remains to be clarified. *Cited4* expression is induced by training exercise in adult hearts [19,107].

Post-transcriptional and post-translational regulatory mechanisms have also been shown to modulate CITED expression. For example, TGF-β activation accelerates the degradation of *Cited2* mRNA after transcription, reducing its stability [108]. The binding of CITED1 to p300 and the co-activation of Smad4 are regulated by phosphorylation of CITED1 residues during the cell cycle [68]. In vitro studies indicated that CITED2 can be phosphorylated by MAP kinases, although the significance of this modification for its cellular and developmental functions remains unclear [25]. Recently, a non-synonymous CITED2 mutation, p.Pro101Ser, identified in a patient with CHD, was shown to increase CITED2 transcriptional activity at several downstream target genes important for cardiac development, likely due to an altered phosphorylation pattern of the mutant protein [109]. Additionally, at the protein level, CITED2 stability appears to be tightly controlled through proteasome-dependent degradation under conditions such as normoxia, hypoxia, and varying cellular iron levels [69,110]. These findings underscore the importance of post-translational regulatory mechanisms acting on CITED2 for proper heart development. However, the post-translational regulation of Cited proteins remains underexplored.

4.3. CITED Proteins and Cardiogenesis

In vitro differentiation of mouse ESCs used as a model to recapitulate cardiogenesis (Figure 1) has revealed that the loss or downregulation of *Cited2* expression in ESCs during the early stages of differentiation drastically impaired the cardiogenic process [22,111]. This observation is consistent with in vivo experiments that have indicated that *Cited2* conditional-knockout in either Brachyury/T- or Mesp1-expressing cells does not overtly affect heart development, suggesting that *Cited2* may play a major role in cardiogenesis before mesoderm specification [10]. Consistently, during mouse embryonic development, *Cited2* is highly expressed in early mesodermal cardiac Mesp1-positive progenitors in the earliest Tbx5-positive CPC of the FHF isolated from embryos prior to Nkx2.5 expression [112,113]. In addition, mesoderm progenitors that originated from human ESCs or induced pluripotent stem cells (iPSCs) reprogrammed from somatic cells also express CITED2 [114], suggesting a conservation of CITED2 function in mouse and human cells. In contrast to *Cited2*, which is present in ESCs and maintained during the entire differentiation process [22], *Cited4* expression emerges in ESC-derived cells after the transient expression of *Brachyury/T* [115]. Whether Cited4 can compensate for the absence of Cited2 activity after mesoderm specification, either in vitro or in vivo, remains to be determined.

The mechanisms by which *Cited2* exerts its functions at this stage remain unknown. However, depletion of *Cited2* at the onset of ESC differentiation leads to a marked downregulation of *Brachyury/T*, *Mesp1*, *Isl1*, and to a lesser extent *Gata4*, *Nkx2.5*, and *Tbx5* expression, as well as reduced levels of mediators of cardiogenic signalling pathways, such as Wnt5a and Wnt11 proteins (Table 1). Additionally, Cited2 is expressed in committed ventricular progenitors of the SHF co-expressing Isl1 and Nkx2.5 in developing hearts at E9.5 [22], but no major heart defects were observed in embryos with *Cited2* depletion from progenitors of the FHF and SHF and cardiac neural crest cells [11,12]. The role of Cited2 in embryonic cardiac progenitors remains elusive.

Table 1. Network of CITED protein interactions within the cardiovascular system.

CITED Protein	CITED-Interacting Protein	Cardiovascular Target Genes	References
CITED1	CBP/p300	Unknown	[7]
CITED2	CBP/p300	*Pitx2c*	[5,8]
	TFAP2	*Pitx2c*, *Vegfa*, *Lefty1* *, *Lefty2* *, *Nodal* *	[5,9,10,13,77]
	ISL1	*Mefc2**	[22]
	Unknown	*Isl1*	[22]
	Unknown	*Brachyury/T* *, *Mesp1* *, *Gata4* *, *Nkx2.5* *, *Tbx5* *, *Wnt5a* *, *Wnt11* *	[22,24]
	Unknown	*p57*	[61]
	Smad2	*Nodal* *	[12]
CITED4	CBP/p300	Unknown	[6,70]
	Unknown	*Cyclin D1* *	[19]

* A direct interaction and regulation by CITED proteins remains to be established.

During mouse embryonic development, defective regulation of *Nodal*, *Lefty1/2*, *Pitx2c*, and *Vegfa* expression due, in part, to impaired cooperation among Cited2, Tfap2a, and CBP/p300 (Table 1) has been proposed to contribute to both the cardiac malformations and disrupted establishment of left–right asymmetry observed in *Cited2*-null mouse embryos [5,9,10,13]. The Tfap2a–Cited2 complex activates the P1 promoter of Pitx2c and promotes cardiac *Vegfa* expression during mouse embryo development [9,10], while Cited2 may cooperate with Smad2/3 and Foxh1 to enhance *Nodal* transcription via its Asymmetric Sequence Element [12]. In addition, Cited2 directly regulates *Isl1* expression, physically interacts with ISL1, and the CITED2–ISL1 synergizes to promote mouse ESC differentiation toward cardiomyocytes [22]. Interestingly, the proper regulation of *Isl1* is critical for SHF-derived cardiac structures, and its dysregulation could account for the cardiac malformations observed in *Cited2*-null embryos [5]. Vascular endothelial zinc finger 1 (Vezf1), which is important for embryonic vasculature formation, may exert its role by modulating the expression of *Cited2* [116]. Collectively, these observations indicate that *Cited2* holds a critical and unique function in cardiovascular development that cannot be compensated for by other members of the *Cited* gene family.

5. *CITED2* Mutations and Congenital Heart Disease

Worldwide genetic screens of patients with CHDs have identified synonymous and non-synonymous variants in *CITED2* associated with sporadic non-syndromic CHDs [25,117–124]. Thus, CITED2 is considered a useful marker for prenatal diagnosis of CHDs [121]. The cardiac defects observed in mouse *Cited2*-null embryos are phenotypically comparable to the heart abnormalities reported in patients carrying *CITED2* mutations (Table 2). Ventricular (VSD) and atrial (ASD) septal defects, transposition of the great arteries (TGA) and tetralogy of Fallot (TOF) are the most frequent heart anomalies associated with *CITED2* dysfunction (Figure 3). Notably, most of missense mutations are concentrated within the SRJ domain, a region exclusive to CITED2 (Figure 2A). The SRJ domain is predicted to be highly unstructured, and its function remains elusive since transgenic mice expressing solely the human CITED2 and lacking the SRJ domain are viable with normal heart features [25].

Table 2. Most prevalent CHD phenotypes in CITED2 mutation carrier patients.

Cardiovascular Anomaly	Estimated Average % with CITED2 Mutations *	% of CHD Patients with CITED2 Variants (Mutated CITED2/Total CHD Patients)	References
All anomalies	~1.53%	~3.33% (4/120) ~1.69% (19/1126) ~0.71% (5/700) ~0.33% (2/605)	[125] [25] [118] [119]
Ventricular Septal Defect (VSD)	~0.94%	~1.02% (4/392)	[125]
		~0.86% (6/700)	[118]
Atrial Septal Defect (ASD)	~0.35%	~1.02% (4/392) ~0.16% (1/605) ~0.14% (1/700) ~0.09% (1/1126)	[125] [119] [118] [25]
Patent Ductus Arteriosus (PDA)	~0.35%	~0.33% (2/605	[119]
Tetralogy of Fallot (TOF)	~0.29%	~0.77% (3/392) ~0.16% (1/605) ~0.14% (1/700) ~0.09% (1/1126)	[125] [119] [118] [25]
Transposition of the Great Arteries (TGA)	~0.17%	~0.26% (1/392) ~0.16% (1/605) ~0.09% (1/1126)	[125] [119] [25]
Patent *Foramen Ovale* (PFO)	~0.16%	~0.16% (1/605)	[119]
Atrioventricular Septal Defect (AVSD)	~0.115%	~0.14% (1/700) ~0.09% (1/1126)	[118] [25]
Pulmonary Stenosis (PS)	~0.115%	~0.14% (1/700) ~0.09% (1/1126)	[118] [25]

* Percentages are the average % of CHD patients with CITED2 variants in the different cohorts referenced in the table.

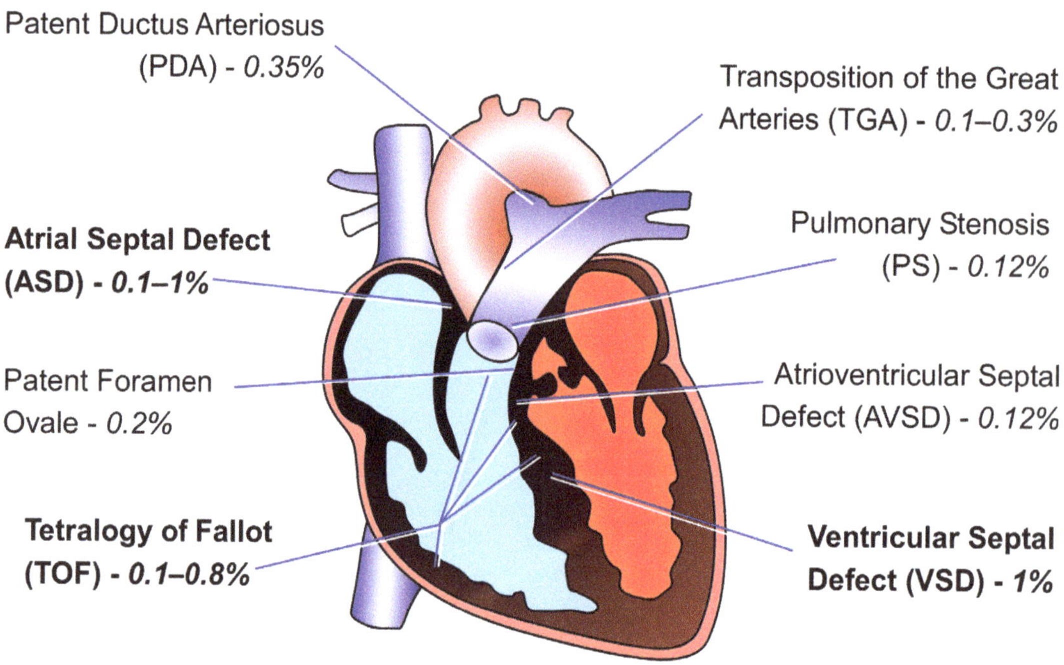

Figure 3. Illustration of the adult human heart highlighting the cardiac defects observed in CHD patients with CITED2 mutations. The percentages indicated correspond to the frequency of each defect associated with CITED2 mutations within the studied patient groups. Data was acquired from the published studies [25,118,119,125].

The majority of CITED2 mutations identified in CHD patients have minimal impact on CITED2′s ability to inhibit HIF-1α-driven transcriptional activity or to enhance TFAP2 transcriptional activity ex vivo [25,117–121,125]. Furthermore, mutations in *CITED2* identified in patients can cause significant disruption of *VEGF* expression, essential for proper vascular formation, as well as reducing the expression of the transcription factor *PITX2C*, which is critical for left–right body patterning and cardiac development [118]. Alternatively, mutations of *CITED2* may result in hyperactivity of HIF-1α and also hinder cardiogenesis in mice [15]. Considering that CITED2 interacts with key transcription factors critical for heart development, including ISL1 and SMAD2/3, it is important to assess their transcriptional defects alongside mutations in *CITED2*. Altogether, the evidence above suggests that the multifunctional roles of CITED2, when altered by mutation, may impact normal cardiac development in a non-linear manner.

The haploinsufficiency of the *Cited2* gene has been revealed in mice, since a significant part of the heterozygous embryos (harbouring both a *Cited2* functional allele and a Cited2-*null* allele, expressing half the normal levels of *Cited2* transcripts) displayed cardiac malformations [11]. This indicates that, beyond alterations in the CITED2 protein sequence or function, a reduction in CITED2 protein levels caused by genetic or epigenetic deregulations, increased protein instability, or degradation during gestation may increase the penetrance of CHDs and perhaps make embryos more sensitive to environmental stress. Thus, the three *CITED2* variants identified within the 5′-untranslated region (UTR) of the exon 1 and 3′-UTR of the exon 2, associated with ASD, VSD, and TOF [125], and another study associating decreased *CITED2* expression to abnormal hypermethylation of CpG islands on its promoter in children with CHD [117] may be a consequence of *CITED2* haploinsufficiency. Abnormal hypomethylation in the upstream regulatory regions of

CITED1 has been observed in monozygotic twins affected by double-outlet right ventricle. However, the contribution of *CITED1* to the disease aetiology remains to be clarified [126]. Overall, these observations argue in favour of the assessment of CITED2 expression levels and their impact in CHDs as a meaningful approach in both research and clinical contexts.

The embryonic and foetal environment also has a critical impact on heart development, as inadequate placental function, sporadic developmental errors, and/or maternal environmental factors, such as diabetes, some medications and drugs abuse, infections, tobacco smoke, alcohol, and harmful chemicals, are known to increase the risk of CHDs [1,127]. Interestingly, the combination of maternal high-fat diet together with embryonic *Cited2* deficiency resulted in a drastic increase in the occurrence of defects in left–right body axis patterning and heart abnormalities in comparison to *Cited2*-null embryos of gestating mice fed with a normal diet [128]. Moreover, maternal diabetes in rats results in VSD and cardiac thin ventricular walls, with embryonic hearts displaying a concomitant decrease in both *Cited2* transcript and protein expression levels [129]. Considering these observations, maternal high-fat diet and/or maternal metabolic adverse conditions such as diabetes are likely to interplay with foetal *CITED2* expression in human gestation and predispose for CHDs, particularly if the foetuses harbour mutations in the *CITED2* gene. The downregulation of *CITED2* expression by maternal diabetes/high glucose may be controlled through miR-200b, which interferes with the cardiogenic processes and targets *CITED2* [130]. On the other hand, gene expression analysis of mouse embryos exposed to maternal diabetes showed a two-fold increase in *Cited4* transcript levels in comparison to wild-type embryos [131]. The significance and the importance of diabetes-induced *Cited4* transcripts in heart development remain to be established. However, diabetes-induced *Cited4* expression is unlikely to compensate for the downregulation of *Cited2*, further indicating that *Cited* genes have distinct functions.

In vitro exposure of human cardiomyocytes to high glucose levels downregulates *CITED2* expression and increases apoptosis, while the overexpression of wild-type CITED2 confers an efficient protection to cardiomyocytes against apoptosis. Conversely, the overexpression of CITED2 harbouring the p.ser192gly mutation failed to be as effective [129], indicating that mutations of *CITED2* may affect important cellular processes, such as the support of cardiomyocyte survival under stress conditions.

Pre-eclampsia is a severe pregnancy complication characterized by placental dysfunction and reduced blood flow, which limits oxygen and nutrient delivery to the foetus and compromises foetal development of the cardiovascular system and increases the risk of CHDs. Interestingly, CITED2 expression is elevated in placental tissues from pre-eclamptic pregnancies compared to controls. Since CITED2 promotes trophoblast proliferation, migration, and invasion, while suppressing apoptosis during placental development, its increased expression in pre-eclampsia may represent a protective or compensatory mechanism to maintain placental integrity by enhancing trophoblast cell survival and invasiveness [132,133]. It would be of interest to investigate whether *CITED2* mutations are associated with a poor outcome in pre-eclamptic gestations.

Sequence variants in the *CITED2* promoter of patients with VSD or ASD displayed a significant reduction in their activity in transient transfection assays compared to control promoters [134,135]. Notably, one of these variants which disrupts an SP1 binding site is critical for CITED2 expression [134], indicating that promoter variants may create or disrupt binding sites for transcription factors, which will influence the levels of *CITED2* transcripts expressed in the cells. Surprisingly, a non-synonymous mutation, p.Pro101Ser, identified in a patient with VSD, increased CITED2 activity resulting in the upregulation of several downstream cardiac developmental genes, including *Gata4*, *Mef2c*, *Nfatc1 and*

Nfatc2, Nodal, Pitx2, and Tbx5 [109]. Furthermore, two synonymous variants were found to affect the mRNA structure and translation efficiency of *CITED2* transcripts [109].

Overall, these observations indicate that both loss and gain of *CITED2* function can disrupt cardiac development, highlighting the critical importance for precise regulation of its expression and activity. Thus, proper timing and controlled levels of *CITED2* expression are crucial to ensure the balanced activation of downstream cardiac genes during development. Any deviation, whether reduced or excessive CITED2 activity, may destabilize this regulatory network and contribute to CHDs. In addition, *CITED2* may be essential to resist environmental stresses and maintain placental function. By supporting these processes, CITED2 may also support normal embryonic development, and disturbances in its function could increase susceptibility to CHDs.

6. *CITED* Genes in ADULT Heart Physiological Adaptations and Protection Against Pathological Stress

CITED2 and *CITED4* are both expressed in adult hearts, but their specific contributions to maintaining heart homeostasis or their roles in adult cardiac pathological processes are not yet fully understood. However, patients with ischemic cardiomyopathy or a cardiomyopathy caused by infection with the protozoan *Trypanosoma cruzi* (Chagas disease) exhibit lower CITED2 transcript levels compared to control individuals. Among these patients, higher CITED2 expression is also associated with an increased left ventricular ejection fraction, a key indicator of cardiac performance and overall heart health [62,136]. In H9C2 rat cardiomyocytes subjected to hypoxia-reoxygenation, an in vitro model of ischemia–reperfusion (I/R) injury, *CITED2* expression was significantly reduced [137]. Thus, I/R injury may actively downregulate *CITED2* expression in ischemic hearts, which likely exacerbates the chronic maladaptive activation of the HIF pathway, a key mediator of I/R injury and the HIF-driven metabolic switch. Such dysregulation is likely to contribute to cardiac degeneration and heart failure progression by promoting energy deprivation [62,138]. Conversely, the overexpression of *CITED2* reduces cardiomyocyte pyroptosis (a form of inflammatory programmed cell death) by decreasing the activation of pyroptotic markers and lowering the secretion of inflammatory cytokines such as IL-1β and IL-18, primarily through the suppression of HIF-1α activity [137]. The protective role of *CITED2* in myocardial I/R injury is also closely linked to its regulation by FoxO transcription factors, particularly FoxO1 and FoxO3, which are critical mediators of oxidative stress resistance in cardiomyocytes, promoting cell survival by inducing antioxidant enzymes, anti-apoptotic proteins, and autophagy-related genes [139]. Importantly, FoxO factors directly activate CITED2 expression, which, in turn, inhibits HIF-1α transactivation, thereby reducing pyroptosis and inflammation in ischemic cardiomyocytes [100]. Thus, CITED2 is a key downstream effector of FoxO-mediated cardioprotection by modulating hypoxic responses, limiting inflammatory cell death, and enhancing survival pathways under conditions of oxidative stress. This coordinated FoxO/CITED2/HIF-1α axis highlights an important molecular mechanism by which the heart adapts to I/R stress, offering potential therapeutic targets for reducing myocardial injury. Together, these observations argue that *CITED2* expression preserves the function of adult hearts during adverse ischemic cardiomyopathy. However, in cardiac arterial endothelial cells of patients with type 2 diabetes, and in insulin-resistant or obese animal models, *CITED2* expression is increased compared to control individuals [92]. In this context, elevated CITED2 expression may inhibit HIF transactivation, thereby limiting HIF's pro-angiogenic function and impairing the adaptation of endothelial cells to hypoxia and hyperglycaemia, conditions commonly associated with diabetic complications [92]. Thus, the role of CITED2 in cardiomyocytes, where it supports cell survival and regulates metabolism, and in endothelial cells, where it inhibits angiogenesis and inflammation, illustrates the complexity of its function in heart tissue. This complexity also emphasizes the importance of considering specific cell types when evaluating CITED2 as a potential therapeutic target in heart disease.

Both iron deficiency and iron overload may impact cardiac function and are considered age-aggravated risk factors for cardiovascular disease [140]. Interestingly, FBXL5, which is an E3 ubiquitin ligase considered as an oxygen and iron sensor, targets CITED2 protein for proteasome-dependent degradation in normoxic conditions [69]. Since FBLX5 affects CITED2 expression levels, it would be of interest to investigate the impact of FBXL5 activity in heart function/protection during ageing or upon insults resulting from systemic or cellular iron content dysregulations.

On the other hand, CITED4 is a key regulator of exercise-induced physiological cardiac hypertrophy and cardiomyocyte proliferation in mice [19,107]. Indeed, exercise upregulates CITED4 expression, which promotes cardiomyocyte survival, physiological hypertrophy, and proliferative capacity. CITED4 upregulation is concomitant with the increase in GATA4 expression, a key transcription factor that promotes cardiac regeneration by stimulating cardiomyocyte proliferation, angiogenesis, and pro-regenerative gene expression. This suggests that CITED4 is part of a coordinated regulatory network supporting exercise-induced cardiac growth and regeneration [141]. Interestingly, the ectopic overexpression of CITED4 in cardiomyocytes in adult mice provokes the increase in cardiomyocyte size and heart weight, while preserving systolic function, mimicking exercise-induced effects [28]. Of interest, CITED4 also prevents excessive cardiomyocyte elongation, restraining their size to physiological limits, thereby preventing pathological hypertrophy [19,142]. Moreover, upon ischemic injury, CITED4 activates the expression of genes that facilitate myocardial repair and functional recovery. Although the overexpression of CITED4 does not reduce initial infarct size in I/R models, it attenuates adverse ventricular remodelling and fibrosis, improving long-term survival of animals [28,107]. Thus, CITED4 may be essential for protecting the heart from maladaptive remodelling due to stressors such as pressure overload. CITED4 cardioprotective effects in I/R are also attributed to a reduction in autophagosome accumulation and cardiomyocyte apoptosis after reperfusion [28]. This involves modulation of mTOR signalling, along with the upregulation of anti-fibrotic miR-30d and miR-133b, and the downregulation of pro-fibrotic miR-376c by CITED4, which collectively coordinate cardiomyocyte–fibroblast interactions to limit fibrosis and promote adaptive cardiac growth [143]. Moreover, CITED4 is positively modulated by miR-222 and negatively controlled by the transcription factor C/EBPβ, suggesting that CITED4 expression is tightly regulated during healthy heart hypertrophic remodelling [19,142]. Altogether, CITED4 functions as a critical mediator linking exercise-induced cardiomyocyte proliferation with cardioprotection, underscoring its therapeutic potential in ischemic heart disease.

7. Clinical and Translational Applications

Conventional pharmacological and surgical treatments usually aim at reducing and managing cardiovascular dysfunctions, failing to address underlying causes of cardiovascular defects and restore full cardiovascular function. However, significant progress has recently been made in the field of gene therapy and regeneration, with promising future strategies for treating both CHDs and ACDs, and to complement classical approaches.

The complexity of the gene network involved in cardiac development and timing constraints of their expression, and the environmental factors acting on developmental pathways, mean that gene therapy for CHDs is still at an investigational state and largely at preclinical or early research stages. At present, only a few key genes are targeted or compensated by gene therapy approaches for cardiovascular diseases, particularly monogenic and inherited cardiac disorders. Moreover, there are no ongoing clinical trials specifically testing gene therapy for CHDs in humans; all assays are still optimized at the preclinical stage with animal models. Genome-editing techniques based on CRISPR-Cas9 are also being developed to target specific gene mutations, along with the optimization of viral and non-viral gene delivery methods aiming to increase the expression of beneficial genes in affected heart tissues [144–146]. However, clinically successful and available therapies based on these approaches are few, although early preclinical successes and proof-of-concept clinical trials demonstrate feasibility, particularly for monogenic forms of CHD.

In ACDs, gene therapy approaches are also developed and focus on delivering genes for pro-regenerative or angiogenic factors, such as VEGF or FGF using viral vectors, nanoparticles, plasmids, or modified RNA, showing safety and some functional benefits in trials for conditions such as refractory angina [146,147]. Remarkably, an efficient gene delivery of CITED4 by AAV9-based viral vector in wild-type mice was successful and showed an increase in CITED4 levels in the heart, resulting in beneficial physiological heart hypertrophy without adverse effects [148]. This approach resulted in a decrease in cell death, fibrosis, and inflammation in mice upon I/R injury, leading to smaller scars and improved heart function in treated mice with ectopic CITED4 [148]. These encouraging results demonstrate that future gene therapy based on CITED4 expression could be translated into clinical set-ups to enhance cardiac repair and resilience following ischemic injury in humans. Since CITED2 also presents beneficial properties for heart function and protections, which may be complementary to those of CITED4, it would be interesting to develop similar approaches with CITED2 alone or in combination with CITED4. Nevertheless, durable gene expression, precise targeting, and limited immune responses of delivered genes are the main challenge that will have to be addressed in these strategies.

Stem-cell-based therapies also offer promising approaches for treating ACDs like myocardial infarction and heart failure, using sources such as mesenchymal stem cells and iPSC-derived cells, aiming to repair damaged heart tissue, improve cardiac function, and promote new blood vessel formation [149,150]. Although these therapies are not yet standard clinical practice, they hold promise as less invasive, definitive treatment options as ongoing research continues to optimize their safety and efficacy.

The discovery of multiple cardiac progenitor populations emerging during heart development and the existence of a robust network of evolutionarily conserved genes with complementary functions ensures the resilience of heart development and limits the incidence CHDs [1]. For example, mouse embryos can survive and develop normal hearts despite ablation of more than 50% of cardiac progenitors at early developmental stages, demonstrating a remarkable capacity for cellular compensation in the developing embryonic heart [151]. Moreover, emerging evidence indicates that cardiogenesis is driven primarily by intrinsic genetic programmes, which are modulated by extrinsic factors such as extracellular signals that regulate cardiac cell fate, including their spatial positioning and functional specialization, as early as during gastrulation [1]. This concept is further validated by the capacity of pluripotent stem cells to autonomously generate structured cardiac organoids, which are complex three-dimensional cardiac structures generated in vitro, when cultured in the presence of appropriate ECM components and exogenous signalling molecules [152]. Therefore, enhanced understanding of cardiovascular networks and pathways, along with their spatiotemporal dynamics, may facilitate the identification of complementary signalling pathways that could be exogenously activated, through the supplementation of proteins or molecules, to engage alternative cardiogenic mechanisms. Such strategies could serve as safeguard mechanisms to promote proper heart development and reduce the incidence of CHDs [1]. For instance, folic acid and zinc supplements have been shown to reduce the risk of CHDs, and blocking the TGF-β1 signalling pathway reduces HLHS in humans [1]. Heart malformations and mortality observed in mouse embryos lacking *Id* genes were reduced by upregulation of Igf-1 and Wnt5a upon pre-gestational ESC injection to females [1]. Loss of *ISL1* expression in non-human primate embryos and cells leads to disrupted mesoderm formation and lethality, which was partially reversed by the addition of BMP4 [153]. Remarkably, the transient supplementation before mesoderm specification of either 8R-CITED2 (human CITED2 fused to eight arginine residues allowing its diffusion through the cell membranes to the nucleus) or recombinant Wnt5a/Wnt11 proteins corrected the cardiogenic abnormalities caused by *Cited2* loss in mouse ESCs and zebrafish embryos [22,24]. These observations align with findings indicating that *Cited2* function is primarily required from the blastocyst stage to early mesoderm specification, as depletion of *Cited2* in the epiblast (blastocyst stage) of mouse embryos results in in utero lethality and cardiac malformations, and knockout of *Cited2* in mesoderm cells during gastrulation does not affect mouse embryonic development [11,22,24]. Importantly, supplementing Wnt5a/Wnt11 in wild-type zebrafish embryos decreased both natural mortality rates and heart abnormalities relative to untreated controls [24]. This observation suggests that the protective effects of Wnt5a/Wnt11 supplementation may extend beyond *Cited2*-deficient animals, suggesting also the potential for this approach to be used as a prophylactic intervention to improve cardiovascular outcomes more broadly. Given that the cardiogenic role of CITED2 is conserved across vertebrates, from fish to humans, it would be of interest to undertake further research to investigate whether a strategy of supplementation with appropriate exogenous molecules early during gestation could be adapted for mammals, particularly humans, to reduce the incidence and/or severity of CHDs.

8. Conclusions and Perspectives

CITED proteins are non-DNA-binding transcriptional modulators exhibiting distinct functional characteristics, including the modulation of specific transcription factors and regulation of distinct sets of target genes. The unifying characteristic of CITED proteins is the ability to bind with high affinity to the CH1 domain of the transcriptional co-activators and histone acetylases CBP/p300 and act either as transcriptional inhibitors or co-activators. In mice, *Cited1*, *Cited2*, and *Cited4* play distinct, stage- and tissue-specific roles in cardiac, placental, and other developmental processes. *Cited2* is essential in the early stages of embryogenesis, such as mesoderm specification, early heart morphogenesis, and placental function, with its loss causing severe cardiac malformations, placental insufficiency, and embryonic lethality. *Cited1* is crucial for trophoblast differentiation but is not essential for heart development. On the other hand, *Cited4* is dispensable during embryogenesis but promotes postnatal cardiomyocyte proliferation and heart growth.

Mutations in the *CITED2* gene, as well as its overexpression or downregulation, have been associated with CHDs in numerous reports, arguing that its function and expression must be tightly regulated for correct heart development. The SRJ domain of CITED2 has been proposed to accommodate mutations affecting heart development in a way that it is still compatible with embryonic life, while mutations occurring elsewhere in CITED2 protein might affect cardiac development and be lethal, just like *Cited2*-knockout is detrimental for mouse development. Thus, *CITED2* mutations in the SRJ domain may not always be causative of CHDs, but they might exacerbate the effect of other combined genetic mutations or environmental stressors to cause CHDs.

At present, all studies have associated CITED2 variants with CHDs in live children and may have overlooked mutations with dramatic consequences for foetal survival and heart development, before CHD detection or testing is feasible, consistent with findings from *Cited2*-null mouse models, which exhibit embryonic lethality. Moreover, CHDs may arise from, or be exacerbated by, underexplored interactions between CITED2 mutations and other genetic or environmental factors. Indeed, environmental factors to which parents are exposed before and during pregnancy, such as a high-fat diet, diabetes, obesity, alcohol consumption, viral infections, air pollution, and deficiencies in riboflavin or folic acid, are likely to influence the expression of genes critical for heart development, thereby increasing the risk of CHDs. Adverse gestational conditions are particularly relevant, as CITED2 misexpression was associated with pre-eclampsia, a severe obstetric complication that may contribute to CHDs. Thus, CITED2 dysregulation may lead to adverse pregnancy outcomes, including foetal death and CHDs due to lack of adaptive changes to unfavourable maternal environmental conditions, such as hypoxia, oxidative stress, pre-eclampsia, infections, and inflammation. In addition, foetal microenvironment, primarily governed by the placenta, plays a crucial role in CHD pathogenesis. Moreover, *CITED2* dysregulation, which disrupts trophoblast function and impairs the placenta's response to stresses, may contribute to embryonic growth and developmental defects. Many genes implicated in human CHDs are also expressed and have overlapping function in the placenta during development, suggesting that some genes, such as *CITED2*, may play critical roles simultaneously in cardiac and placental development and function, highlighting the interconnected nature of these two processes. Thus, the role of placental insufficiency in exacerbating CHDs should be further explored, particularly in patients which harbour mutations in genes, such as *CITED2*, which have an impact in both heart and placental development and are likely to influence foetal development and contribute to the severity of CHDs by creating an adverse prenatal environment.

Interestingly, the early function of *Cited2* in cardiovascular development may enable the development of prophylactic strategies to overcome its dysfunction through functional complementation and limit occurrences and/or severity of CHDs. Those strategies could involve supplementation with exogenous proteins, such as the engineered form of human CITED2, which can cross cell membranes and localize to the nucleus, or recombinant WNT5A/WNT11 proteins, which are target genes of CITED2. These proteins have been shown to mitigate the cardiogenic defects in *Cited2*-deficient mouse ESCs and zebrafish embryos when supplemented at early stages of differentiation or development. Although the cardiogenic function of CITED2 is evolutionarily conserved, further studies are required to determine whether similar outcomes would be observed in mouse embryos and human cellular models following treatment with these proteins or other agonistic molecules.

Most of the current understanding of CITED proteins in early trophoblast differentiation and cardiac development originates from studies in rodent models. Although CITED2 mutations are consistently associated with CHDs, the specific molecular mechanisms by which CITED2 contributes to the pathological aetiology of CHDs remain largely unresolved. Likewise, the roles of CITED1 and CITED2 in trophectoderm specification and trophoblast development, which are critical processes for placental formation, have been well documented in mice but remain poorly characterized in humans. Several stem-cell-based embryo models have surfaced recently and revolutionized the study of human development by enabling access to previously inaccessible early human developmental stages, particularly blastocyst implantation and trophoblast invasion [29,151–153]. Human blastoids derived from naïve pluripotent stem cells faithfully recapitulate blastocyst formation, embryonic lineage specification, and polar trophectoderm patterning, thereby mimicking key early implantation dynamics [154,155]. These blastoid models provide a mean to facilitate mechanistic studies of implantation, lineage segregation, and transcriptional regulation in human systems that are otherwise inaccessible in vivo. They are particularly adapted and valuable for elucidating the roles of CITED1 and CITED2, which are critical for early embryonic and trophoblast development, as well as for CHD pathogenesis. By combining CITED1 or CITED2 gene editing and multiomics approaches in stem-cell-derived 3D cell structures such as blastoids, trophodermic structures, or cardiac organoids, researchers can interrogate gene functions with high precision. Furthermore, blastoids which model trophoblast and epiblast lineage specification as it occurs in the mammalian preimplantation embryo would bridge important gaps left by rodent models. Indeed, these complex stem-cell-derived models recapitulate key features of early developmental stages, including spatial and temporal lineage segregation, thus providing an invaluable platform for mechanistic study. Importantly, blastoid formation presents a precise timeframe during which rescue assays can be performed to recover deficiencies, such as those triggered by *CITED2* deficiency, by supplementation of exogenous molecules, thereby enabling experimental interrogation of gene function within a defined developmental window in a human context.

In the adult heart, *Cited2* supports cardiac health and mitigates damage caused by I/R injury and other conditions, at least in part through anti-inflammatory mechanisms. On the other hand, elevated *Cited2* levels in diabetic endothelial cells may limit angiogenesis, contributing to impaired vascular repair and function in diabetes. Therefore, the beneficial effects of CITED2 depend on tightly regulated expression levels and are context- and cell-type dependent, varying with the nature and severity of cardiovascular injury and the specific heart tissue involved. In normal adult hearts, *Cited4* is a key driver of exercise-induced physiological hypertrophy and cardiac regeneration, through promotion of cardiomyocyte proliferation and survival. Under stress conditions, such as pressure overload or ischemic injury, Cited4 prevents pathological remodelling, supporting myocardial repair and long-term cardiac function and limiting fibrosis. Overall, these findings indicate that *Cited2* and *Cited4* fulfil distinct but essential roles in maintaining adult heart function, enabling adaptation to exercise-induced stress, and defending against cardiovascular damage. However, the intricate and nuanced regulation of these genes, particularly CITED2 with its diverse protein partners, makes it challenging to predict their precise impact on heart disease. Advancing our understanding of the molecular and cell-specific activities of CITED proteins and their interacting partners will be critical for elucidating their contributions to disease mechanisms and protective responses. This knowledge will facilitate novel therapeutic strategies aimed at preventing cardiac dysfunction or restoring normal heart function. The development of mature human cardiac organoids represents a significant advancement in modelling the adult human heart [156]. Recent studies demonstrates that these organoids recapitulate key features of adult cardiac tissue, including multi-lineage cellular composition, improved sarcomere organization, mitochondrial function, and electrophysiological properties, thus enhancing their physiological relevance compared to earlier, more foetal-like models. These organoids do not fully replicate all aspects of adult heart complexity, but they provide a robust platform for investigating adult-like cardiac disease mechanisms, drug responses, and regenerative processes. These mature human organoids could be instrumental to study gene functions such as CITED2 and CITED4 in healthy heart maintenance and in pathological contexts like inflammation and diabetic heart disease, offering potential for translational cardiovascular research and therapeutic discovery.

Overall, the exact functions of CITED proteins across embryonic and mature organisms, particularly within distinct tissues, cell types, and stem cell populations, are not yet fully defined. Advancing research to unravel the molecular and cellular mechanisms of CITED gene activity is essential for clarifying their contributions to cardiac development, disease processes, and protective responses in the heart. This knowledge will also be instrumental in developing novel therapeutic strategies aimed at limiting cardiac dysfunction and restoring normal cardiac function.

Author Contributions: Conceptualization, J.B.; writing—original draft preparation, J.B., R.L.C.P., I.V., S.F. and A.M.; writing—review and editing, J.B., R.L.C.P., I.V., S.F. and A.M.; project administration, J.B.; funding acquisition, J.B. All authors have read and agreed to the published version of the manuscript.

Funding: J.B., R.L.C.P., I.V., S.F. and A.M were supported by Fundação para a Ciência e Tecnologia (FCT) with the grant reference 2024.14693.PEX; R.L.C.P. received an FCT PhD fellowship with the reference 2023.00861.BD; J.B., R.P, I.V., A.M. and S.F. were supported by the Algarve Biomedical Center (ABC) award—"Bolsa de investigação translacional—José Mariano Gago by ABC", Santa Casa Misericórdia Lisboa for the "Prémio Nunes Correa Verdades de Faria" award 2025 in the category C "Progresso no Tratamento das Doenças do Coração", and the European University of the Seas Alliance for an award in the context of the SEA-EU 2.0 Erasmus+ Project 101089757 to J.B.

Institutional Review Board Statement: Not applicable.

Informed Consent Statement: Not applicable.

Data Availability Statement: Not applicable.

Acknowledgments: We thank the Fundação para a Ciência e Tecnologia (FCT) for financial support to the project 2024.14693.PEX to J.B. and the PhD fellowship 2023.00861.BD to R.L.C.P. We also thank the Algarve Biomedical Center (ABC) for the award—"Bolsa de investigação translacional—José Mariano Gago by ABC", the Santa Casa Misericórdia Lisboa for the "Prémio Nunes Correa Verdades de Faria" award 2025 in the category C "Progresso no Tratamento das Doenças do Coração", and the European University of the Seas Alliance for an award in the context of the SEA-EU 2.0 Erasmus+ Project 101089757 to J.B.

Conflicts of Interest: The authors declare no conflicts of interest.

References

1. Bragança, J.; Pinto, R.; Silva, B.; Marques, N.; Leitão, H.S.; Fernandes, M.T. Charting the Path: Navigating Embryonic Development to Potentially Safeguard against Congenital Heart Defects. *J. Pers. Med.* **2023**, *13*, 1263. [CrossRef] [PubMed]
2. Brown, M.A.; Rajamarthandan, S.; Francis, B.; O'Leary-Kelly, M.K.; Sinha, P. Update on stem cell technologies in congenital heart disease. *J. Card. Surg.* **2020**, *35*, 174–179. [CrossRef] [PubMed]
3. Chowdhury, D.; Elliott, P.A.; Asaki, S.Y.; Amdani, S.; Nguyen, Q.T.; Ronai, C.; Tierney, S.; Levy, V.Y.; Puri, K.; Altman, C.A.; et al. Addressing Disparities in Pediatric Congenital Heart Disease: A Call for Equitable Health Care. *J. Am. Heart Assoc.* **2024**, *13*, e032415. [CrossRef] [PubMed]
4. Chong, B.; Jayabaskaran, J.; Jauhari, S.M.; Chan, S.P.; Goh, R.; Kueh, M.T.W.; Li, H.; Chin, Y.H.; Kong, G.; Anand, V.V.; et al. Global burden of cardiovascular diseases: Projections from 2025 to 2050. *Eur. J. Prev. Cardiol.* **2025**, *32*, 1001–1015. [CrossRef]
5. Bamforth/Bragança, S.D.; Bragança, J.; Eloranta, J.J.; Murdoch, J.N.; Marques, F.I.R.; Kranc, K.R.; Farza, H.; Henderson, D.J.; Hurst, H.C.; Bhattacharya, S. Cardiac malformations, adrenal agenesis, neural crest defects and exencephaly in mice lacking Cited2, a new Tfap2 co-activator. *Nat. Genet.* **2001**, *29*, 469–474. [CrossRef]
6. Bragança, J.; Swingler, T.; Marques, F.I.R.; Jones, T.; Eloranta, J.J.; Hurst, H.C.; Shioda, T.; Bhattacharya, S. Human CREB-binding Protein/p300-interacting Transactivator with ED-rich Tail (CITED) 4, a New Member of the CITED Family, Functions as a Co-activator for Transcription Factor AP-2. *J. Biol. Chem.* **2002**, *277*, 8559–8565. [CrossRef]
7. Yahata, T.; Shao, W.; Endoh, H.; Hur, J.; Coser, K.R.; Sun, H.; Ueda, Y.; Kato, S.; Isselbacher, K.J.; Brown, M.; et al. Selective coactivation of estrogen-dependent transcription by CITED1 CBP/p300-binding protein. *Genes Dev.* **2001**, *15*, 2598–2612. [CrossRef]
8. Bhattacharya, S.; Michels, C.L.; Leung, M.K.; Arany, Z.P.; Kung, A.L.; Livingston, D.M. Functional role of p35srj, a novel p300/CBP binding protein, during transactivation by HIF-1. *Genes Dev.* **1999**, *13*, 64–75. [CrossRef]
9. Bamforth/Bragança, S.D.; Bragança, J.; Farthing, C.R.; Schneider, J.E.; Broadbent, C.; Michell, A.C.; Clarke, K.; Neubauer, S.; Norris, D.; Brown, N.A.; et al. Cited2 controls left-right patterning and heart development through a Nodal-Pitx2c pathway. *Nat. Genet.* **2004**, *36*, 1189–1196. [CrossRef]
10. MacDonald, S.T.; Bamforth, S.D.; Bragança, J.; Chen, C.-M.; Broadbent, C.; Schneider, J.E.; Schwartz, R.J.; Bhattacharya, S. A cell-autonomous role of Cited2 in controlling myocardial and coronary vascular development. *Eur. Heart J.* **2013**, *34*, 2557–2567. [CrossRef]

11. MacDonald, S.T.; Bamforth, S.D.; Chen, C.-M.; Farthing, C.R.; Franklyn, A.; Broadbent, C.; Schneider, J.E.; Saga, Y.; Lewandoski, M.; Bhattacharya, S. Epiblastic Cited2 deficiency results in cardiac phenotypic heterogeneity and provides a mechanism for haploinsufficiency. *Cardiovasc. Res.* **2008**, *79*, 448–457. [CrossRef]
12. Lopes Floro, K.; Artap, S.T.; Preis, J.I.; Fatkin, D.; Chapman, G.; Furtado, M.B.; Harvey, R.P.; Hamada, H.; Sparrow, D.B.; Dunwoodie, S.L. Loss of Cited2 causes congenital heart disease by perturbing left-right patterning of the body axis. *Hum. Mol. Genet.* **2011**, *20*, 1097–1110. [CrossRef] [PubMed]
13. Weninger, W.J.; Floro, K.L.; Bennett, M.B.; Withington, S.L.; Preis, J.I.; Barbera, J.P.M.; Mohun, T.J.; Dunwoodie, S.L. Cited2 is required both for heart morphogenesis and establishment of the left-right axis in mouse development. *Development* **2005**, *132*, 1337–1348. [CrossRef] [PubMed]
14. Withington, S.L.; Scott, A.N.; Saunders, D.N.; Lopes Floro, K.; Preis, J.I.; Michalicek, J.; Maclean, K.; Sparrow, D.B.; Barbera, J.P.M.; Dunwoodie, S.L. Loss of Cited2 affects trophoblast formation and vascularization of the mouse placenta. *Dev. Biol.* **2006**, *294*, 67–82. [CrossRef] [PubMed]
15. Xu, B.; Doughman, Y.; Turakhia, M.; Jiang, W.; Landsettle, C.E.; Agani, F.H.; Semenza, G.L.; Watanabe, M.; Yang, Y.-C. Partial rescue of defects in Cited2-deficient embryos by HIF-1[alpha] heterozygosity. *Dev. Biol.* **2007**, *301*, 130. [CrossRef]
16. Kuna, M.; Dhakal, P.; Iqbal, K.; Dominguez, E.M.; Kent, L.N.; Muto, M.; Moreno-Irusta, A.; Kozai, K.; Varberg, K.M.; Okae, H.; et al. CITED2 is a conserved regulator of the uterine-placental interface. *Proc. Natl. Acad. Sci. USA* **2023**, *120*, e2213622120. [CrossRef]
17. Moreau, J.L.M.; Artap, S.T.; Shi, H.; Chapman, G.; Leone, G.; Sparrow, D.B.; Dunwoodie, S.L. Cited2 is required in trophoblasts for correct placental capillary patterning. *Dev. Biol.* **2014**, *392*, 62–79. [CrossRef]
18. Yahata, T.; Takedatsu, H.; Dunwoodie, S.L.; Bragança, J.; Swingler, T.; Withington, S.L.; Hur, J.; Coser, K.R.; Isselbacher, K.J.; Bhattacharya, S.; et al. Cloning of Mouse cited4, a Member of the CITED Family p300/CBP-Binding Transcriptional Coactivators: Induced Expression in Mammary Epithelial Cells. *Genomics* **2002**, *80*, 601–613. [CrossRef]
19. Boström, P.; Mann, N.; Wu, J.; Quintero, P.A.; Plovie, E.R.; Panáková, D.; Gupta, R.K.; Xiao, C.; MacRae, C.A.; Rosenzweig, A.; et al. C/EBP[beta] Controls Exercise-Induced Cardiac Growth and Protects against Pathological Cardiac Remodeling. *Cell* **2010**, *143*, 1072–1083. [CrossRef]
20. Guo, H.-H.; Sun, Y.; Zhang, X.-l.; Jiang, X.-Y.; Zou, S.-M. Identification of duplicated Cited3 genes and their responses to hypoxic stress in blunt snout bream (*Megalobrama amblycephala*). *Fish Physiol. Biochem.* **2019**, *45*, 1141–1152. [CrossRef]
21. Devakanmalai, G.S.; Zumrut, H.E.; Ozbudak, E.M. Cited3 activates Mef2c to control muscle cell differentiation and survival. *Biol. Open* **2013**, *2*, 505–514. [CrossRef]
22. Pacheco-Leyva, I.; Matias, A.C.; Oliveira, D.V.; Santos, J.M.A.; Nascimento, R.; Guerreiro, E.; Michell, A.C.; van De Vrugt, A.M.; Machado-Oliveira, G.; Ferreira, G.; et al. CITED2 Cooperates with ISL1 and Promotes Cardiac Differentiation of Mouse Embryonic Stem Cells. *Stem Cell Rep.* **2016**, *7*, 1037–1049. [CrossRef]
23. Kranc, K.R.; Oliveira, D.V.; Armesilla-Diaz, A.; Pacheco-Leyva, I.; Matias, A.C.; Escapa, A.L.; Subramani, C.; Wheadon, H.; Trindade, M.; Nichols, J.; et al. Acute loss of Cited2 impairs Nanog expression and decreases self-renewal of mouse embryonic stem cells. *Stem Cells* **2015**, *33*, 699–712. [CrossRef]
24. Santos, J.M.; Mendes-Silva, L.; Afonso, V.; Martins, G.; Machado, R.S.R.; Lopes, J.A.; Cancela, L.; Futschik, M.E.; Sachinidis, A.; Gavaia, P.; et al. Exogenous Wnt5a and Wnt11 proteins rescue Cited2 dysfunction in mouse embryonic stem cells and zebrafish morphants. *Cell Death Dis.* **2019**, *10*, 582. [CrossRef] [PubMed]
25. Chen, C.-M.; Bentham, J.; Cosgrove, C.; Braganca, J.; Cuenda, A.; Bamforth, S.D.; Schneider, J.E.; Watkins, H.; Keavney, B.; Davies, B.; et al. Functional Significance of SRJ Domain Mutations in CITED2. *PLoS ONE* **2012**, *7*, e46256. [CrossRef] [PubMed]
26. Uhlén, M.; Fagerberg, L.; Hallström, B.M.; Lindskog, C.; Oksvold, P.; Mardinoglu, A.; Sivertsson, A.; Kampf, C.; Sjöstedt, E.; Asplund, A.; et al. Tissue-based map of the human proteome. *Science* **2015**, *347*, 1260419. [CrossRef] [PubMed]
27. Shioda, T.; Fenner, M.H.; Isselbacher, K.J. MSG1 and its related protein MRG1 share a transcription activating domain. *Gene* **1997**, *204*, 235–241. [CrossRef]
28. Bezzerides, V.J.; Platt, C.; Lerchenmuller, C.; Paruchuri, K.; Oh, N.L.; Xiao, C.; Cao, Y.; Mann, N.; Spiegelman, B.M.; Rosenzweig, A. CITED4 induces physiologic hypertrophy and promotes functional recovery after ischemic injury. *JCI Insight* **2016**, *1*, e85904. [CrossRef]
29. Dewing, J.M.; Saunders, V.; O'Kelly, I.; Wilson, D.I. Defining cardiac cell populations and relative cellular composition of the early fetal human heart. *PLoS ONE* **2022**, *17*, e0259477. [CrossRef]
30. Bello, R.O.; Frew, S.; Siddiqui, Y.; Minhas, R. Advances and Prospects in Understanding Vertebrate Cardiac Conduction System, Pacemaker Cell, and Cardiac Muscle Development: Toward Novel Biological Therapies. *Muscles* **2023**, *2*, 338–352. [CrossRef]
31. Sylva, M.; van den Hoff, M.J.B.; Moorman, A.F.M. Development of the Human Heart. *Am. J. Med. Genet. Part A* **2013**, *164*, 1347–1371. [CrossRef]
32. Krishnan, A.; Samtani, R.; Dhanantwari, P.; Lee, E.; Yamada, S.; Shiota, K.; Donofrio, M.T.; Leatherbury, L.; Lo, C.W. A Detailed Comparison of Mouse and Human Cardiac Development. *Pediatr. Res.* **2014**, *76*, 500–507. [CrossRef] [PubMed]
33. Sahara, M.; Santoro, F.; Chien, K.R. Programming and reprogramming a human heart cell. *EMBO J.* **2015**, *34*, 710–738. [CrossRef] [PubMed]

34. Bruneau, B.G. Signaling and Transcriptional Networks in Heart Development and Regeneration. *Cold Spring Harb. Perspect. Biol.* **2013**, *5*, a008292. [CrossRef] [PubMed]
35. Liau, B.; Zhang, D.; Bursac, N. Functional Cardiac Tissue Engineering. *Regen. Med.* **2012**, *7*, 187–206. [CrossRef]
36. Scuderi, G.J.; Butcher, J. Naturally Engineered Maturation of Cardiomyocytes. *Front. Cell Dev. Biol.* **2017**, *5*, 50. [CrossRef]
37. Stefanovic, S.; Laforest, B.; Desvignes, J.-P.; Lescroart, F.; Argiro, L.; Maurel-Zaffran, C.; Salgado, D.; Plaindoux, E.; De Bono, C.; Pazur, K.; et al. Hox-dependent coordination of mouse cardiac progenitor cell patterning and differentiation. *eLife* **2020**, *9*, e55124. [CrossRef]
38. Mensah, I.K.; Emerson, M.L.; Tan, H.J.; Gowher, H. Cardiomyocyte Differentiation from Mouse Embryonic Stem Cells by WNT Switch Method. *Cells* **2024**, *13*, 132. [CrossRef]
39. Bondue, A.; Tannler, S.; Chiapparo, G.; Chabab, S.; Ramialison, M.; Paulissen, C.; Beck, B.; Harvey, R.; Blanpain, C. Defining the earliest step of cardiovascular progenitor specification during embryonic stem cell differentiation. *J. Cell Biol.* **2011**, *192*, 751–765. [CrossRef]
40. Vincent, S.D.; Buckingham, M.E. How to Make a Heart: The Origin and Regulation of Cardiac Progenitor Cells. *Curr. Top. Dev. Biol.* **2010**, *90*, 1–40. [CrossRef]
41. Sizarov, A.; Ya, J.; de Boer, B.A.; Lamers, W.H.; Christoffels, V.M.; Moorman, A.F.M. Formation of the Building Plan of the Human Heart. *Circulation* **2011**, *123*, 1125–1135. [CrossRef]
42. Buijtendijk, M.F.J.; Barnett, P.; van den Hoff, M.J.B. Development of the human heart. *Am. J. Med. Genet. C Semin. Med. Genet.* **2020**, *184*, 7–22. [CrossRef] [PubMed]
43. Christoffels, V.M.; Grieskamp, T.; Norden, J.; Mommersteeg, M.T.M.; Rudat, C.; Kispert, A. Tbx18 and the fate of epicardial progenitors. *Nature* **2009**, *458*, E8. [CrossRef] [PubMed]
44. Mommersteeg, M.T.M.; DomÃnguez, J.N.; Wiese, C.; Norden, J.; de Gier-de Vries, C.; Burch, J.B.E.; Kispert, A.; Brown, N.A.; Moorman, A.F.M.; Christoffels, V.M. The sinus venosus progenitors separate and diversify from the first and second heart fields early in development. *Cardiovasc. Res.* **2010**, *87*, 92–101. [CrossRef] [PubMed]
45. Spater, D.; Hansson, E.M.; Zangi, L.; Chien, K.R. How to make a cardiomyocyte. *Development* **2014**, *141*, 4418–4431. [CrossRef]
46. Zhang, H.; Lui, K.; Zhou, B. Endocardial Cell Plasticity in Cardiac Development, Diseases and Regeneration. *Circ. Res.* **2018**, *122*, 774–789. [CrossRef]
47. Liyew, W.A.; Adane, F.; Wondemagegn, A.T.; Tsehay, B.; Deml, Y.A.; Abdu, H.M.; Animaw, Z. Roles of cardiac neural crest cells in cardiovascular development and associated congenital defects-an integrated review. *Transl. Res. Anat.* **2024**, *36*, 100304. [CrossRef]
48. Xu, Y.; Luo, X.; Fang, Z.; Zheng, X.; Zeng, Y.; Zhu, C.; Gu, J.; Tang, F.; Hu, Y.; Hu, G.; et al. Transcription coactivator Cited1 acts as an inducer of trophoblast-like state from mouse embryonic stem cells through the activation of BMP signaling. *Cell Death Dis.* **2018**, *9*, 924. [CrossRef]
49. Dunwoodie, S.L.; Rodriguez, T.A.; Beddington, R.S.P. Msg1 and Mrg1, founding members of a gene family, show distinct patterns of gene expression during mouse embryogenesis. *Mech. Dev.* **1998**, *72*, 27–40. [CrossRef]
50. Savolainen, S.M.; Foley, J.F.; Elmore, S.A. Histology Atlas of the Developing Mouse Heart with Emphasis on E11.5 to E18.5. *Toxicol. Pathol.* **2009**, *37*, 395–414. [CrossRef]
51. Howlin, J.; McBryan, J.; Napoletano, S.; Lambe, T.; McArdle, E.; Shioda, T.; Martin, F. CITED1 homozygous null mice display aberrant pubertal mammary ductal morphogenesis. *Oncogene* **2006**, *25*, 1532–1542. [CrossRef] [PubMed]
52. Novitskaya, T.; Baserga, M.; de Caestecker, M.P. Organ-Specific Defects in Insulin-Like Growth Factor and Insulin Receptor Signaling in Late Gestational Asymmetric Intrauterine Growth Restriction in Cited1 Mutant Mice. *Endocrinology* **2011**, *152*, 2503–2516. [CrossRef] [PubMed]
53. Michell, A.C.; Bragança, J.; Broadbent, C.; Joyce, B.; Franklyn, A.; Schneider, J.E.; Bhattacharya, S.; Bamforth, S.D. A novel role for transcription factor Lmo4 in thymus development through genetic interaction with Cited2. *Dev. Dyn.* **2010**, *239*, 1988–1994. [CrossRef] [PubMed]
54. Combes, A.; Spiller, C.; Harley, V.; Sinclair, A.; Dunwoodie, S.; Wilhelm, D.; Koopman, P. Gonadal defects in Cited2-mutant mice indicate a role for SF1 in both testis and ovary differentiation. *Int. J. Dev. Biol.* **2010**, *54*, 683–689. [CrossRef]
55. Xu, B.; Qu, X.; Gu, S.; Doughman, Y.-Q.; Watanabe, M.; Dunwoodie, S.L.; Yang, Y.-C. Cited2 is required for fetal lung maturation. *Dev. Biol.* **2008**, *317*, 95–105. [CrossRef]
56. Yin, Z.; Haynie, J.; Yang, X.; Han, B.; Kiatchoosakun, S.; Restivo, J.; Yuan, S.; Prabhakar, N.R.; Herrup, K.; Conlon, R.A.; et al. The essential role of Cited2, a negative regulator for HIF-1α, in heart development and neurulation. *Proc. Natl. Acad. Sci. USA* **2002**, *99*, 10488–10493. [CrossRef]
57. Barbera, J.P.M.; Rodriguez, T.A.; Greene, N.D.E.; Weninger, W.J.; Simeone, A.; Copp, A.J.; Beddington, R.S.P.; Dunwoodie, S. Folic acid prevents exencephaly in Cited2 deficient mice. *Hum. Mol. Genet.* **2002**, *11*, 283–293. [CrossRef]

58. Rodriguez, T.A.; Sparrow, D.B.; Scott, A.N.; Withington, S.L.; Preis, J.I.; Michalicek, J.; Clements, M.; Tsang, T.E.; Shioda, T.; Beddington, R.S.P.; et al. Cited1 Is Required in Trophoblasts for Placental Development and for Embryo Growth and Survival. *Mol. Cell. Biol.* **2004**, *24*, 228–244. [CrossRef]
59. Kuna, M.; Soares, M.J. Cited2 is a key regulator of placental development and plasticity. *Bioessays* **2024**, *46*, e2300118. [CrossRef]
60. Paradis, A.N.; Gay, M.S.; Zhang, L. Binucleation of cardiomyocytes: The transition from a proliferative to a terminally differentiated state. *Drug Discov. Today* **2014**, *19*, 602–609. [CrossRef]
61. Clark, A.L.; Naya, F.J. MicroRNAs in the MEF2-regulated Gtl2-Dio3 Noncoding RNA Locus Promote Cardiomyocyte Proliferation by Targeting the Transcriptional Co-activator Cited2. *J. Biol. Chem.* **2015**, *290*, 23162–23172. [CrossRef] [PubMed]
62. Herrer, I.; Roselló-Lletí, E.; Ortega, A.; Tarazón, E.; Molina-Navarro, M.M.; Triviño, J.C.; Martínez-Dolz, L.; Almenar, L.; Lago, F.; Sánchez-Lázaro, I.; et al. Gene expression network analysis reveals new transcriptional regulators as novel factors in human ischemic cardiomyopathy. *BMC Med. Genom.* **2015**, *2*, 14. [CrossRef] [PubMed]
63. Wu, Q.; Liu, Q.; Zhan, J.; Wang, Q.; Zhang, D.; He, S.; Pu, S.; Zhou, Z. Cited2 regulates proliferation and survival in young and old mouse cardiac stem cells. *BMC Mol. Cell Biol.* **2019**, *20*, 25. [CrossRef] [PubMed]
64. Derks, W.; Rode, J.; Collin, S.; Rost, F.; Heinke, P.; Hariharan, A.; Pickel, L.; Simonova, I.; Lázár, E.; Graham, E.; et al. A Latent Cardiomyocyte Regeneration Potential in Human Heart Disease. *Circulation* **2025**, *151*, 245–256. [CrossRef]
65. Chen, X.; Zhong, X.; Huang, G.N. Heart regeneration from the whole-organism perspective to single-cell resolution. *npj Regen. Med.* **2024**, *9*, 34. [CrossRef]
66. Du, C.; Li, Z.; Zou, B.; Li, X.; Chen, F.; Liang, Y.; Luo, X.; Shu, S. Novel heterozygous variants in the EP300 gene cause Rubinstein-Taybi syndrome 2: Reports from two Chinese children. *Mol. Genet. Genom. Med.* **2023**, *11*, e2192. [CrossRef]
67. Thienpont, B.; Breckpot, J.; Holvoet, M.; Vermeesch, J.R.; Devriendt, K. A microduplication of CBP in a patient with mental retardation and a congenital heart defect. *Am. J. Med. Genet. A* **2007**, *143a*, 2160–2164. [CrossRef]
68. Shi, G.; Boyle, S.C.; Sparrow, D.B.; Dunwoodie, S.L.; Shioda, T.; de Caestecker, M.P. The Transcriptional Activity of CITED1 Is Regulated by Phosphorylation in a Cell Cycle-dependent Manner. *J. Biol. Chem.* **2006**, *281*, 27426–27435. [CrossRef]
69. Machado-Oliveira, G.; Guerreiro, E.; Matias, A.C.; Facucho-Oliveira, J.; Pacheco-Leyva, I.; Bragança, J. FBXL5 modulates HIF-1α transcriptional activity by degradation of CITED2. *Arch. Biochem. Biophys.* **2015**, *576*, 61–72. [CrossRef]
70. Fox, S.B.; Bragança, J.; Turley, H.; Campo, L.; Han, C.; Gatter, K.C.; Bhattacharya, S.; Harris, A.L. CITED4 Inhibits Hypoxia-Activated Transcription in Cancer Cells, and Its Cytoplasmic Location in Breast Cancer Is Associated with Elevated Expression of Tumor Cell Hypoxia-Inducible Factor 1α. *Cancer Res.* **2004**, *64*, 6075–6081. [CrossRef]
71. Lou, X.; Sun, S.; Chen, W.; Zhou, Y.; Huang, Y.; Liu, X.; Shan, Y.; Wang, C. Negative Feedback Regulation of NF-κB Action by CITED2 in the Nucleus. *J. Immunol.* **2011**, *186*, 539–548. [CrossRef]
72. Hui, B.S. CITED2 mechanoregulation of matrix metalloproteinases. *Ann. New York Acad. Sci.* **2010**, *1192*, 429–436. [CrossRef] [PubMed]
73. Yokota, H.; Goldring, M.B.; Sun, H.B. CITED2-mediated Regulation of MMP-1 and MMP-13 in Human Chondrocytes under Flow Shear. *J. Biol. Chem.* **2003**, *278*, 47275–47280. [CrossRef] [PubMed]
74. Wojciak, J.M.; Martinez-Yamout, M.A.; Dyson, H.J.; Wright, P.E. Structural basis for recruitment of CBP/p300 coactivators by STAT1 and STAT2 transactivation domains. *EMBO J.* **2009**, *28*, 948–958. [CrossRef] [PubMed]
75. Liu, Y.-C.; Chang, P.-Y.; Chao, C.C.K. CITED2 silencing sensitizes cancer cells to cisplatin by inhibiting p53 trans-activation and chromatin relaxation on the ERCC1 DNA repair gene. *Nucleic Acids Res.* **2015**, *15*, 10760–10781. [CrossRef]
76. Mattes, K.; Berger, G.; Geugien, M.; Vellenga, E.; Schepers, H. CITED2 affects leukemic cell survival by interfering with p53 activation. *Cell Death Dis.* **2017**, *8*, e3132. [CrossRef]
77. Bragança, J.; Eloranta, J.J.; Bamforth, S.D.; Ibbitt, J.C.; Hurst, H.C.; Bhattacharya, S. Physical and Functional Interactions among AP-2 Transcription Factors, p300/CREB-binding Protein, and CITED2. *J. Biol. Chem.* **2003**, *278*, 16021–16029. [CrossRef]
78. Glenn, D.J.; Maurer, R.A. MRG1 binds to the LIM domain of Lhx2 and may function as a coactivator to stimulate glycoprotein hormone α-subunit gene expression. *J. Biol. Chem.* **1999**, *274*, 36159–36167. [CrossRef]
79. Qu, X.; Lam, E.; Doughman, Y.Q.; Chen, Y.; Chou, Y.T.; Lam, M.; Turakhia, M.; Dunwoodie, S.L.; Watanabe, M.; Xu, B.; et al. Cited2, a coactivator of HNF4alpha, is essential for liver development. *EMBO J.* **2007**, *26*, 4445–4456. [CrossRef]
80. Tien, E.S.; Davis, J.W.; Vanden Heuvel, J.P. Identification of the CREB-binding Protein/p300-interacting protein CITED2 as a peroxisome proliferator-activated receptor alpha coregulator. *J. Biol. Chem.* **2004**, *279*, 24053–24063. [CrossRef]
81. Gonzalez, Y.R.; Zhang, Y.; Behzadpoor, D.; Cregan, S.; Bamforth, S.; Slack, R.S.; Park, D.S. CITED2 Signals through Peroxisome Proliferator-Activated Receptor-{gamma} to Regulate Death of Cortical Neurons after DNA Damage. *J. Neurosci.* **2008**, *28*, 5559–5569. [CrossRef]
82. Chou, Y.T.; Wang, H.; Chen, Y.; Danielpour, D.; Yang, Y.C. Cited2 modulates TGF-beta-mediated upregulation of MMP9. *Oncogene* **2006**, *25*, 5547–5560. [CrossRef]

83. Sakai, M.; Matsumoto, M.; Tujimura, T.; Yongheng, C.; Noguchi, T.; Inagaki, K.; Inoue, H.; Hosooka, T.; Takazawa, K.; Kido, Y.; et al. CITED2 links hormonal signaling to PGC-1[alpha] acetylation in the regulation of gluconeogenesis. *Nat. Med.* **2012**, *18*, 612–617. [CrossRef]
84. Val, P.; Martinez-Barbera, J.-P.; Swain, A. Adrenal development is initiated by Cited2 and Wt1 through modulation of Sf-1 dosage. *Development* **2007**, *134*, 2349–2358. [CrossRef] [PubMed]
85. Buaas, F.W.; Val, P.; Swain, A. The transcription co-factor CITED2 functions during sex determination and early gonad development. *Hum. Mol. Genet.* **2009**, *18*, 2989–3001. [CrossRef] [PubMed]
86. Wiggins, D.A.; Maxwell, J.N.; Nelson, D.E. Exploring the role of CITED transcriptional regulators in the control of macrophage polarization. *Front. Immunol.* **2024**, *15*, 1365718. [CrossRef] [PubMed]
87. Sun, H.B.; Zhu, Y.X.; Yin, T.; Sledge, G.; Yang, Y.-C. MRG1, the product of a melanocyte-specific gene related gene, is a cytokine-inducible transcription factor with transformation activity. *Proc. Natl. Acad. Sci. USA* **1998**, *95*, 13555–13560. [CrossRef]
88. Leffers, H.; Naesby, M.; Vendelbo, B.; Skakkebæk, N.E.; Jorgensen, M. Oestrogenic potencies of Zeranol, oestradiol, diethylstilboestrol, Bisphenol-A and genistein: Implications for exposure assessment of potential endocrine disrupters. *Hum. Reprod.* **2001**, *16*, 1037–1045. [CrossRef]
89. Dijkmans, T.F.; Hooijdonk, L.W.A.V.; Schouten, T.G.; Kamphorst, J.T.; Fitzsimons, C.P.; Vreugdenhil, E. Identification of new Nerve Growth Factor-responsive immediate early genes. *Brain Res.* **2009**, *1249*, 19–33. [CrossRef]
90. Parmentier-Batteur, S.; Jin, K.; Xie, L.; Mao, X.O.; Greenberg, D.A. DNA Microarray Analysis of Cannabinoid Signaling in Mouse Brain in Vivo. *Mol. Pharmacol.* **2002**, *62*, 828–835. [CrossRef]
91. Haase, M.; Schott, M.; Bornstein, S.R.; Malendowicz, L.K.; Scherbaum, W.A.; Willenberg, H.S. CITED2 is expressed in human adrenocortical cells and regulated by basic fibroblast growth factor. *J. Endocrinol.* **2007**, *192*, 459–465. [CrossRef]
92. Wang, X.; Lockhart, S.M.; Rathjen, T.; Albadawi, H.; Sørensen, D.; Neill, B.T.; Dwivedi, N.; Preil, S.R.; Beck, H.C.; Dunwoodie, S.L.; et al. Insulin Downregulates the Transcriptional Coregulator CITED2, an Inhibitor of Proangiogenic Function in Endothelial Cells. *Diabetes* **2016**, *65*, 3680–3689. [CrossRef]
93. Tanaka, T.; Yamaguchi, J.; Higashijima, Y.; Nangaku, M. Indoxyl sulfate signals for rapid mRNA stabilization of Cbp/p300-interacting transactivator with Glu/Asp-rich carboxy-terminal domain 2 (CITED2) and suppresses the expression of hypoxia-inducible genes in experimental CKD and uremia. *FASEB J.* **2013**, *27*, 4059–4075. [CrossRef]
94. Collett, G.P.; Redman, C.W.; Sargent, I.L.; Vatish, M. Endoplasmic reticulum stress stimulates the release of extracellular vesicles carrying danger-associated molecular pattern (DAMP) molecules. *Oncotarget* **2018**, *9*, 6707–6717. [CrossRef]
95. Bakker, W.J.; Harris, I.S.; Mak, T.W. FOXO3a Is Activated in Response to Hypoxic Stress and Inhibits HIF1-Induced Apoptosis via Regulation of CITED2. *Mol. Cell* **2007**, *28*, 941–953. [CrossRef] [PubMed]
96. Gabut, M.; Samavarchi-Tehrani, P.; Wang, X.; Slobodeniuc, V.; O'Hanlon, D.; Sung, H.-K.; Alvarez, M.; Talukder, S.; Pan, Q.; Mazzoni, E.O.; et al. An Alternative Splicing Switch Regulates Embryonic Stem Cell Pluripotency and Reprogramming. *Cell* **2011**, *147*, 132–146. [CrossRef] [PubMed]
97. Aramaki, S.; Hayashi, K.; Kurimoto, K.; Ohta, H.; Yabuta, Y.; Iwanari, H.; Mochizuki, Y.; Hamakubo, T.; Kato, Y.; Shirahige, K.; et al. A Mesodermal Factor, T, Specifies Mouse Germ Cell Fate by Directly Activating Germline Determinants. *Dev. Cell* **2013**, *27*, 516–529. [CrossRef] [PubMed]
98. Abid, M.R.; Shih, S.-C.; Otu, H.H.; Spokes, K.C.; Okada, Y.; Curiel, D.T.; Minami, T.; Aird, W.C. A Novel Class of Vascular Endothelial Growth Factor-responsive Genes That Require Forkhead Activity for Expression. *J. Biol. Chem.* **2006**, *281*, 35544–35553. [CrossRef]
99. Bakker, W.J.; van Dijk, T.B.; Parren-van Amelsvoort, M.; Kolbus, A.; Yamamoto, K.; Steinlein, P.; Verhaak, R.G.W.; Mak, T.W.; Beug, H.; Lowenberg, B.; et al. Differential Regulation of Foxo3a Target Genes in Erythropoiesis. *Mol. Cell. Biol.* **2007**, *27*, 3839–3854. [CrossRef]
100. Sengupta, A.; Molkentin, J.; Paik, J.; Depinho, R.; Yutzey, K. FoxO transcription factors promote cardiomyocyte survival upon induction of oxidative stress. *J. Biol. Chem.* **2011**, *286*, 7468–7478. [CrossRef]
101. Plisov, S.; Tsang, M.; Shi, G.; Boyle, S.; Yoshino, K.; Dunwoodie, S.L.; Dawid, I.B.; Shioda, T.; Perantoni, A.O.; de Caestecker, M.P. Cited1 Is a Bifunctional Transcriptional Cofactor That Regulates Early Nephronic Patterning. *J. Am. Soc. Nephrol.* **2005**, *16*, 1632–1644. [CrossRef] [PubMed]
102. Price, F.D.; Yin, H.; Jones, A.; van Ijcken, W.; Grosveld, F.; Rudnicki, M.A. Canonical Wnt signaling induces a primitive endoderm metastable state in mouse embryonic stem cells. *Stem Cells* **2013**, *31*, 752–764. [CrossRef] [PubMed]
103. Yang, D.; Guo, J.; Divieti, P.; Shioda, T.; Bringhurst, F.R. CBP/p300-Interacting Protein CITED1 Modulates Parathyroid Hormone Regulation of Osteoblastic Differentiation. *Endocrinology* **2008**, *149*, 1728–1735. [CrossRef] [PubMed]
104. McFadden, D.G.; Barbosa, A.C.; Richardson, J.A.; Schneider, M.D.; Srivastava, D.; Olson, E.N. The Hand1 and Hand2 transcription factors regulate expansion of the embryonic cardiac ventricles in a gene dosage-dependent manner. *Development* **2005**, *132*, 189–201. [CrossRef]

105. Singh, M.K.; Christoffels, V.M.; Dias, J.M.; Trowe, M.-O.; Petry, M.; Schuster-Gossler, K.; BürGer, A.; Ericson, J.; Kispert, A. Tbx20 is essential for cardiac chamber differentiation and repression of Tbx2. *Development* **2005**, *132*, 2697–2707. [CrossRef]
106. Lai, D.; Liu, X.; Forrai, A.; Wolstein, O.; Michalicek, J.; Ahmed, I.; Garratt, A.N.; Birchmeier, C.; Zhou, M.; Hartley, L.; et al. Neuregulin 1 Sustains the Gene Regulatory Network in Both Trabecular and Nontrabecular Myocardium. *Circ. Res.* **2010**, *107*, 715–727. [CrossRef]
107. Ryall, K.A.; Bezzerides, V.J.; Rosenzweig, A.; Saucerman, J.J. Phenotypic screen quantifying differential regulation of cardiac myocyte hypertrophy identifies CITED4 regulation of myocyte elongation. *J. Mol. Cell. Cardiol.* **2014**, *72*, 74–84. [CrossRef]
108. Chou, Y.-T.; Yang, Y.-C. Post-transcriptional Control of Cited2 by Transforming Growth Factor beta: REGULATION VIA SMADS AND CITED2 CODING REGION. *J. Biol. Chem.* **2006**, *281*, 18451–18462. [CrossRef]
109. Yadav, M.L.; Jain, D.; Neelabh; Agrawal, D.; Kumar, A.; Mohapatra, B. A Gain-of-function mutation in CITED2 is associated with Congenital Heart Disease. *Mutat. Res./Fundam. Mol. Mech. Mutagen.* **2021**, *822*, 111741. [CrossRef]
110. Shin, D.H.; Li, S.H.; Chun, Y.S.; Huang, L.E.; Kim, M.S.; Park, J.W. CITED2 mediates the paradoxical responses of HIF-1alpha to proteasome inhibition. *Oncogene* **2008**, *27*, 1939–1944. [CrossRef]
111. Li, Q.; Ramirez-Bergeron, D.L.; Dunwoodie, S.L.; Yang, Y.-C. Cited2 controls pluripotency and cardiomyocyte differentiation of murine embryonic stem cells through Oct4. *J. Biol. Chem.* **2012**, *287*, 29088–29100. [CrossRef]
112. Kokkinopoulos, I.; Ishida, H.; Saba, R.; Ruchaya, P.; Cabrera, C.; Struebig, M.; Barnes, M.; Terry, A.; Kaneko, M.; Shintani, Y.; et al. Single-Cell Expression Profiling Reveals a Dynamic State of Cardiac Precursor Cells in the Early Mouse Embryo. *PLoS ONE* **2015**, *10*, e0140831. [CrossRef]
113. Liu, Y.; Chen, L.; Diaz, A.D.; Benham, A.; Xu, X.; Wijaya, C.S.; Fa'aK, F.; Luo, W.; Soibam, B.; Azares, A.; et al. Mesp1 Marked Cardiac Progenitor Cells Repair Infarcted Mouse Hearts. *Sci. Rep.* **2016**, *6*, 31457. [CrossRef]
114. Kumar, N.; Richter, J.; Cutts, J.; Bush, K.T.; Trujillo, C.; Nigam, S.K.; Gaasterland, T.; Brafman, D.; Willert, K. Generation of an expandable intermediate mesoderm restricted progenitor cell line from human pluripotent stem cells. *eLife* **2015**, *4*, e08413. [CrossRef] [PubMed]
115. Miake, J.; Notsu, T.; Higaki, K.; Hidaka, K.; Morisaki, T.; Yamamoto, K.; Hisatome, I. Cited4 is related to cardiogenic induction and maintenance of proliferation capacity of embryonic stem cell-derived cardiomyocytes during in vitro cardiogenesis. *PLoS ONE* **2017**, *12*, e0183225. [CrossRef] [PubMed]
116. Alabdi, L.; He, M.; Yang, Q.; Norvil, A.B.; Gowher, H. The transcription factor Vezf1 represses the expression of the antiangiogenic factor Cited2 in endothelial cells. *J. Biol. Chem.* **2018**, *293*, 11109–11119. [CrossRef] [PubMed]
117. Xu, M.; Wu, X.; Li, Y.; Yang, X.; Hu, J.; Zheng, M.; Tian, J. CITED2 Mutation and methylation in children with congenital heart disease. *J. Biomed. Sci.* **2014**, *21*, 7. [CrossRef]
118. Liu, Y.; Wang, F.; Wu, Y.; Tan, S.; Wen, Q.; Wang, J.; Zhu, X.; Wang, X.; Li, C.; Ma, X.; et al. Variations of CITED2 Are Associated with Congenital Heart Disease (CHD) in Chinese Population. *PLoS ONE* **2014**, *9*, e98157. [CrossRef]
119. Li, B.; Pu, T.; Liu, Y.; Xu, Y.; Xu, R. CITED2 Mutations in Conserved Regions Contribute to Conotruncal Heart Defects in Chinese Children. *DNA Cell Biol.* **2017**, *36*, 589–595. [CrossRef]
120. Liu, S.; Su, Z.; Tan, S.; Ni, B.; Pan, H.; Liu, B.; Wang, J.; Xiao, J.; Chen, Q. Functional Analyses of a Novel CITED2 Nonsynonymous Mutation in Chinese Tibetan Patients with Congenital Heart Disease. *Pediatr. Cardiol.* **2017**, *38*, 1226–1231. [CrossRef]
121. Hu, P.; Qiao, F.; Wang, Y.; Meng, L.; Ji, X.; Luo, C.; Xu, T.; Zhou, R.; Zhang, J.; Yu, B.; et al. Clinical application of targeted next-generation sequencing on fetuses with congenital heart defects. *Ultrasound Obs. Gynecol.* **2018**, *5*, 205–211. [CrossRef]
122. Yaqoob, H.; Ahmad, H.; Ali, S.I.; Patel, N.; Arif, A. Missense mutations in the CITED2 gene may contribute to congenital heart disease. *BMC Cardiovasc. Disord.* **2024**, *24*, 516. [CrossRef]
123. Imam, R.; Aizezi, M.; Yan, F.; Zhu, T.; Zhang, W. Sequence variations in GATA4 and CITED2 gene among patients with cardiac septation defects from Xinjiang, China. *Cardiol. Young* **2024**, *34*, 1506–1513. [CrossRef] [PubMed]
124. Dianatpour, S.; Khatami, M.; Heidari, M.M.; Hadadzadeh, M. Novel Point Mutations of CITED2 Gene Are Associated with Non-familial Congenital Heart Disease (CHD) in Sporadic Pediatric Patients. *Appl. Biochem. Biotechnol.* **2020**, *190*, 896–906. [CrossRef] [PubMed]
125. Sperling, S.; Grimm, C.H.; Dunkel, I.; Mebus, S.; Sperling, H.-P.; Ebner, A.; Galli, R.; Lehrach, H.; Fusch, C.; Berger, F.; et al. Identification and functional analysis of CITED2 mutations in patients with congenital heart defects. *Hum. Mutat.* **2005**, *26*, 575–582. [CrossRef] [PubMed]
126. Lyu, G.; Zhang, C.; Ling, T.; Liu, R.; Zong, L.; Guan, Y.; Huang, X.; Sun, L.; Zhang, L.; Li, C.; et al. Genome and epigenome analysis of monozygotic twins discordant for congenital heart disease. *BMC Genom.* **2018**, *19*, 428. [CrossRef]
127. Boyd, R.; McMullen, H.; Beqaj, H.; Kalfa, D. Environmental Exposures and Congenital Heart Disease. *Pediatrics* **2021**, *149*, e2021052151. [CrossRef]
128. Bentham, J.; Michell, A.C.; Lockstone, H.; Andrew, D.; Schneider, J.E.; Brown, N.A.; Bhattacharya, S. Maternal high-fat diet interacts with embryonic Cited2 genotype to reduce Pitx2c expression and enhance penetrance of left-right patterning defects. *Hum. Mol. Genet.* **2010**, *9*, 3394–3401. [CrossRef]

129. Su, D.; Song, J.-X.; Gao, Q.; Guan, L.; Li, Q.; Shi, C.; Ma, X. Cited2 participates in cardiomyocyte apoptosis and maternal diabetes-induced congenital heart abnormality. *Biochem. Biophys. Res. Commun.* **2016**, *479*, 887–892. [CrossRef]
130. Gu, H.; Yu, J.; Dong, D.; Zhou, Q.; Wang, J.-Y.; Fang, S.; Yang, P. High glucose-repressed CITED2 expression through miR-200b triggers the unfolded protein response and endoplasmic reticulum stress. *Diabetes* **2015**, *65*, 149–163. [CrossRef]
131. Pavlinkova, G.; Salbaum, J.M.; Kappen, C. Maternal diabetes alters transcriptional programs in the developing embryo. *BMC Genom.* **2009**, *10*, 274. [CrossRef]
132. Lu, X.; Lan, X.; Fu, X.; Li, J.; Wu, M.; Xiao, L.; Zeng, Y. Screening Preeclampsia Genes and the Effects of CITED2 on Trophoblastic Function. *Int. J. Gen. Med.* **2024**, *17*, 3493–3509. [CrossRef]
133. Yang, C.; Song, Z. CITED2 is highly-expressed and PRX4 is poorly-expressed in preeclampsia and have diagnostic values. *J. Hum. Hypertens.* **2025**, *39*, 293–300. [CrossRef]
134. Zheng, S.-Q.; Chen, H.-X.; Liu, X.-C.; Yang, Q.; He, G.-W. Genetic analysis of the CITED2 gene promoter in isolated and sporadic congenital ventricular septal defects. *J. Cell. Mol. Med.* **2021**, *25*, 2254–2261. [CrossRef] [PubMed]
135. Chen, Z.; Chen, H.-X.; Hou, H.-T.; Yin, X.-Y.; Yang, Q.; Han, J.; He, G.-W. Genetic Variants of CITED2 Gene Promoter in Human Atrial Septal Defects: Case-Control Study and Cellular Functional Verification. *J. Cardiovasc. Dev. Dis.* **2022**, *9*, 321. [CrossRef] [PubMed]
136. Laugier, L.; Frade, A.F.; Ferreira, F.M.; Baron, M.A.; Teixeira, P.C.; Cabantous, S.; Ferreira, L.R.P.; Louis, L.; Rigaud, V.O.C.; Gaiotto, F.A.; et al. Whole-Genome Cardiac DNA Methylation Fingerprint and Gene Expression Analysis Provide New Insights in the Pathogenesis of Chronic Chagas Disease Cardiomyopathy. *Clin. Infect. Dis.* **2017**, *65*, 1103–1111. [CrossRef] [PubMed]
137. Qian, L.; Zhao, J.; Fan, M.; Wang, J.; Ji, Z. CITED2 Attenuates Ischemia Reperfusion-Induced Pyroptosis and Injury in Cardiomyocyte. *Int. Heart J.* **2024**, *65*, 1087–1094. [CrossRef]
138. Lei, L.; Mason, S.; Liu, D.; Huang, Y.; Marks, C.; Hickey, R.; Jovin, I.S.; Pypaert, M.; Johnson, R.S.; Giordano, F.J. Hypoxia-Inducible Factor-Dependent Degeneration, Failure, and Malignant Transformation of the Heart in the Absence of the von Hippel-Lindau Protein. *Mol. Cell. Biol.* **2008**, *28*, 3790–3803. [CrossRef]
139. Orea-Soufi, A.; Paik, J.; Bragança, J.; Donlon, T.A.; Willcox, B.J.; Link, W. FOXO transcription factors as therapeutic targets in human diseases. *Trends Pharmacol. Sci.* **2022**, *43*, 1070–1084. [CrossRef]
140. Sawicki, K.T.; De Jesus, A.; Ardehali, H. Iron Metabolism in Cardiovascular Disease: Physiology, Mechanisms, and Therapeutic Targets. *Circ. Res.* **2023**, *132*, 379–396. [CrossRef]
141. Naderi, N.; Hemmatinafar, M.; Gaeini, A.A.; Bahramian, A.; Ghardashi-Afousi, A.; Kordi, M.R.; Darbandi-Azar, A.; Karimzade, F.; Mohebbi, H.; Barati, M. High-intensity interval training increase GATA4, CITED4 and c-Kit and decreases C/EBPÎ² in rats after myocardial infarction. *Life Sci.* **2019**, *221*, 319–326. [CrossRef]
142. Liu, X.; Xiao, J.; Zhu, H.; Wei, X.; Platt, C.; Damilano, F.; Xiao, C.; Bezzerides, V.; Boström, P.; Che, L.; et al. miR-222 Is Necessary for Exercise-Induced Cardiac Growth and Protects against Pathological Cardiac Remodeling. *Cell Metab.* **2015**, *21*, 584–595. [CrossRef] [PubMed]
143. Lerchenmüller, C.; Rabolli, C.; Yeri, A.; Kitchen, R.; Salvador, A.; Liu, L.; Ziegler, O.; Danielson, K.; Platt, C.; Shah, R.; et al. CITED4 Protects Against Adverse Remodeling in Response to Physiological and Pathological Stress. *Circ. Res.* **2020**, *127*, 631–646. [CrossRef] [PubMed]
144. Nappi, F.; Singh, S.S.A. Gene therapy and regenerative tissue engineering in congenital heart disease. *Transl. Pediatr.* **2019**, *8*, 356–359. [CrossRef] [PubMed]
145. Seok, H.; Deng, R.; Cowan, D.B.; Wang, D.Z. Application of CRISPR-Cas9 gene editing for congenital heart disease. *Clin. Exp. Pediatr.* **2021**, *64*, 269–279. [CrossRef]
146. Grisorio, L.; Bongianino, R.; Gianeselli, M.; Priori, S.G. Gene therapy for cardiac diseases: Methods, challenges, and future directions. *Cardiovasc. Res.* **2024**, *120*, 1664–1682. [CrossRef]
147. Romeo, F.J.; Mavropoulos, S.A.; Ishikawa, K. Progress in Clinical Gene Therapy for Cardiac Disorders. *Mol. Diagn. Ther.* **2023**, *27*, 179–191. [CrossRef]
148. Lerchenmüller, C.; Hastings, M.H.; Rabolli, C.P.; Betge, F.; Roshan, M.; Liu, L.X.; Liu, X.; Heß, C.; Roh, J.D.; Platt, C.; et al. CITED4 gene therapy protects against maladaptive cardiac remodeling after ischemia/reperfusion injury in mice. *Mol. Ther.* **2024**, *32*, 3683–3694. [CrossRef]
149. Gao, S.; Li, D.; Wang, B.; Zhang, H.; Chen, L. Two promising approaches in the treatment of myocardial infarction: Stem cells and gene therapy. *Front. Cardiovasc. Med.* **2025**, *12*, 1540066. [CrossRef]
150. Carvalho, A.B.; Kasai-Brunswick, T.H.; Campos de Carvalho, A.C. Advanced cell and gene therapies in cardiology. *eBioMedicine* **2024**, *103*, 105125. [CrossRef]
151. Sturzu, A.C.; Rajarajan, K.; Passer, D.; Plonowska, K.; Riley, A.; Tan, T.C.; Sharma, A.; Xu, A.F.; Engels, M.C.; Feistritzer, R.; et al. Fetal Mammalian Heart Generates a Robust Compensatory Response to Cell Loss. *Circulation* **2015**, *132*, 109–121. [CrossRef]
152. Hofbauer, P.; Jahnel, S.M.; Mendjan, S. In vitro models of the human heart. *Development* **2021**, *148*, dev199672. [CrossRef]

153. Yang, R.; Goedel, A.; Kang, Y.; Si, C.; Chu, C.; Zheng, Y.; Chen, Z.; Gruber, P.J.; Xiao, Y.; Zhou, C.; et al. Amnion signals are essential for mesoderm formation in primates. *Nat. Commun.* **2021**, *12*, 5126. [CrossRef]
154. Rivron, N.C.; Frias-Aldeguer, J.; Vrij, E.J.; Boisset, J.-C.; Korving, J.; Vivié, J.; Truckenmüller, R.K.; van Oudenaarden, A.; van Blitterswijk, C.A.; Geijsen, N. Blastocyst-like structures generated solely from stem cells. *Nature* **2018**, *557*, 106–111. [CrossRef]
155. Yu, L.; Wei, Y.; Duan, J.; Schmitz, D.A.; Sakurai, M.; Wang, L.; Wang, K.; Zhao, S.; Hon, G.C.; Wu, J. Blastocyst-like structures generated from human pluripotent stem cells. *Nature* **2021**, *591*, 620–626. [CrossRef]
156. Pocock, M.W.; Reid, J.D.; Robinson, H.R.; Charitakis, N.; Krycer, J.R.; Foster, S.R.; Fitzsimmons, R.L.; Lor, M.; Devilée, L.A.C.; Batho, C.A.P.; et al. Maturation of human cardiac organoids enables complex disease modeling and drug discovery. *Nat. Cardiovasc. Res.* **2025**, *4*, 821–840. [CrossRef]

Journal of
Personalized Medicine

MDPI

Review

Growth Differentiation Factor-15 as an Emerging Biomarker in Cardiology: Diagnostic and Prognostic Implications

Carla Lombardi [1,†], Martina Marandola [2,†], Valentina Loria [3], Andrea Urbani [1,2] and Silvia Baroni [1,2,*]

[1] Unit of Chemistry, Biochemistry and Molecular Biology, "A. Gemelli" Hospital Foundation IRCCS, Largo A. Gemelli, 8, 00168 Rome, Italy; carla.lombardi@guest.policlinicogemelli.it (C.L.); andrea.urbani@policlinicogemelli.it (A.U.)
[2] Department of Basic Biotechnological Sciences, Intensive Care and Perioperative Clinics, Catholic University of Sacred Heart, Largo F. Vito, 1, 00168 Rome, Italy; martina.marandola01@icatt.it
[3] Department of Emergency, Anesthesiological and Reanimation Sciences, "A. Gemelli" Hospital Foundation IRCCS, Largo A. Gemelli, 8, 00168 Rome, Italy; valentina.loria@policlinicogemelli.it
* Correspondence: silvia.baroni@unicatt.it
† These authors contributed equally to this work.

Abstract

Growth Differentiation Factor-15 (GDF-15) is a stress-responsive cytokine belonging to the Transforming Growth Factor-beta (TGF-β) superfamily. Initially identified as macrophage inhibitory cytokine-1 (MIC-1), GDF-15 is expressed in various tissues and markedly upregulated under pathological conditions involving inflammation, oxidative stress, and tissue injury. Notably, GDF-15 upregulation has been associated with several cardiovascular events, such as heart failure, atrial fibrillation, atherosclerosis, coronary artery disease, and stroke. Furthermore, it has been observed that GDF-15, either alone or in combination with other cardiac biomarkers, can provide valuable complementary information enhancing risk assessment, early detection of cardiovascular events, and prediction of adverse outcomes. GDF-15 can be measured in various body fluids, using different methods. Immunoassays are widely employed and offer good sensitivity and reproducibility; however, variability between methods and potential interference from genetic variants highlight the need for standardization. This review summarizes current insights into GDF-15, with emphasis on its quantification methods, biological functions in cardiovascular diseases, and its emerging role as a diagnostic and prognostic biomarker.

Keywords: GDF-15; cardiovascular disease; biomarker; heart failure; risk stratification

1. Introduction

Cardiovascular diseases (CVDs) comprise a heterogeneous group of disorders affecting the heart and blood vessels, including coronary artery disease, heart failure, peripheral artery disease, and hypertension. According to the World Health Organization (WHO) [1], CVDs remain the leading cause of morbidity and mortality worldwide, accounting for approximately 17.9 million deaths each year. The complex pathophysiology of cardiovascular events frequently complicates early detection and precise risk stratification, thereby highlighting the need for biomarkers with significant diagnostic and prognostic value. In recent years, novel biomarkers have been identified, which allow for differentiation among diverse cardiac conditions and optimization of therapeutic strategies. Furthermore, the development of high-sensitivity assays has significantly improved the detection of established biomarkers, enabling earlier identification of cardiovascular events [2].

Among CVDs emerging biomarkers, several research focused on Growth Differentiation Factor–15 (GDF-15), a stress-responsive cytokine belonging to the Transforming Growth Factor-beta (TGF-β) superfamily. It was first identified by Bootcov et al. [3] as an autocrine cytokine secreted by activated macrophages and was therefore initially named macrophage inhibitory cytokine-1 (MIC-1). As its pleiotropic nature and tissue-specific functions became evident, GDF-15 has been referred to by several other names over time, including nonsteroidal anti-inflammatory drug-activated gene-1 (NAG-1), placental bone morphogenetic protein (PLAB), placental transforming growth factor-β (PTGFB), and prostate-derived factor (PDF) [4,5].

GDF-15 is expressed in a broad range of physiological and pathological contexts, highlighting its multifaced role as both a cellular stress biomarker and a modulator of systemic, metabolic and inflammatory responses.

In recent years, multiple studies demonstrated that GDF-15 levels are associated with the adverse cardiovascular events across a spectrum of CVD conditions including heart failure, chest pain, acute coronary syndrome, stable ischemic heart disease, stroke and atrial fibrillation [6].

However, despite this expanding literature, the clinical interpretation and translational applicability of GDF-15 in cardiovascular medicine remain incompletely defined.

In light of these considerations, the aim of the present review is to offer a focused and critical description of the current evidence supporting the diagnostic and prognostic value of GDF-15 in cardiovascular diseases.

2. Methods

This review includes Pubmed-indexed articles, written in English and published between 2000 and 2025. Studies published before 2000 were considered only if they were of particular historical or methodological relevance, such as early pioneering work on GDF-15. The database was queried using the following keywords, either individually or in combination: GDF-15, cardiovascular disease, biomarker, heart failure, risk stratification, acute coronary syndrome, myocardial infarction, atherosclerosis, stroke, atrial fibrillation, prognosis, diagnosis, mortality. The keywords were combined using Boolean operators (AND, OR) to refine the search strategy. Data extracted from the selected studies focused on GDF-15 structure and functions, measurement methods, and its applications in cardiology settings.

3. Synthesis and Expression

Located on chromosome 19p12–13.1, the GDF-15 gene (ID9518) exhibits a two-exon structure (309 bp and 891 bp) separated by a 2.9 kb intron [7,8].

The protein is initially synthesized as an inactive propeptide, known as pre-pro-GDF-15, composed of 308 amino acids (aa) and with a molecular weight of approximately 35 kDa [9]. This precursor comprises an N-terminal signal peptide of 29 aa, with storage and trafficking functions [10]; a 167 aa pro-domain; and a C-terminal portion of 112 amino acids, which represents the mature form of the protein [11]. The signal peptide is then removed with a proteolytic cleavage, generating pro-GDF-15 (~30 kDa) which rapidly dimerizes [12] (Figure 1a). β-arrestin 1 mediates the translocation of pro-GDF-15 dimers to the Golgi apparatus, where they undergo sequential proteolytic processing by pro-protein convertase subtilisin–kexin type 3 (PCSK3), PCSK 5 and PCSK 6 [9,13], which recognize the RXXR cleavage site located between the propetide sequence and the mature domain [14] (Figure 1b). After complete processing, GDF-15 is secreted as a biologically active homodimer, in which the two molecules are linked by a disulfide bond [15,16].

 https://doi.org/10.3390/jpm16010016

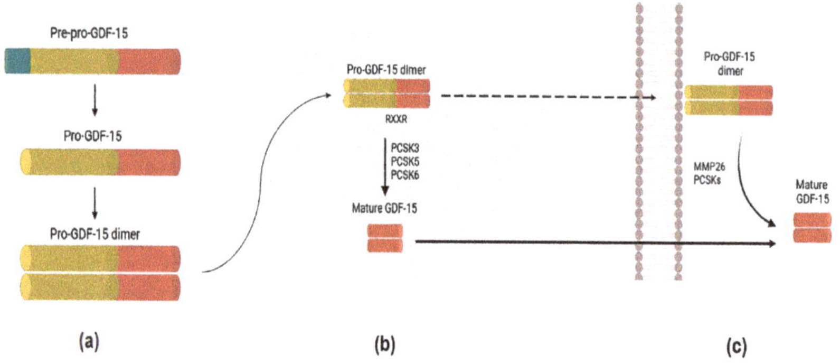

Figure 1. Schematic representation of GDF-15 biosynthesis, maturation, and secretion. (**a**) GDF-15 is synthesized as pre-pro-GDF-15, consisting of a signal peptide (blue), a pro-domain (yellow), and a mature C-terminal domain (red). Removal of the signal peptide generates pro-GDF-15, which rapidly dimerizes; (**b**) In the Golgi apparatus, pro-GDF-15 dimer is cleaved by PCSK3, PCSK5, and PCSK6 at the RXXR site, producing mature GDF-15; (**c**) Mature GDF-15 homodimers are secreted through the classical secretory pathway and released into circulation, while in specific cells pro-GDF-15 dimers may remain bound to the extracellular matrix until further cleavage by MMP26 or PCSKs. GDF-15: Growth Differentiation Factor-15; PCSK: proprotein convertase subtilisin–kexin; MMP26: matrix metalloproteinase 26.

This bond contributes to the conformational stability of the protein and occurs within a sequence of seven cysteine residues, which is conserved among members of the TGF-β family [10,17].

The secretion of GDF-15 occurs through the classical secretory pathway, in which the mature protein is packaged into vesicles within the Golgi apparatus and subsequently released into the extracellular space via exocytosis [18,19] (Figure 1c).

Given its lower affinity to the extracellular matrix (ECM), the homodimeric mature form is released into the systemic circulation [19,20]. In specific types of cells or under pathological conditions, the unprocessed form of the protein may also be secreted, although it does not enter systemic circulation [21]. For example, cancer cells and placental cytotrophoblasts secrete pro-GDF-15 dimers which remain anchored to the ECM until the pro-domain is cleaved by the matrix metalloproteinase 26 (MMP26) and PCSKs, respectively [12,22] (Figure 1c).

In healthy individuals, circulating GDF-15 levels are relatively low, with values ranging between 200 and 1200 pg/mL in adults [23,24], with expression primarily observed in kidney [25], intestine [26], liver [27], and placenta [28]. A minimal GDF-15 expression is observed in other organs as well including gallbladder, pancreas, and lung [29,30]. In physiological conditions, GDF-15 levels follow a circadian rhythm, slowly increase with aging and seem to be less influenced by sex or ethnicity [31,32]. However, in cellular stress conditions or pathological states GDF-15 expression is markedly upregulated.

Increased GDF-15 levels have been observed in association with diabetes [12], smoking [33], surgical stress [34], intense physical activity [35], cancer [36], non-alcoholic fatty liver disease (NAFLD) [37], as well as renal diseases [38].

Of note, GDF-15 upregulation has been demonstrated after various cardiovascular events triggering inflammation, endothelial activation and oxidative stress, including pressure overload, heart failure (HF), atrial fibrillation and atherosclerosis [39–41]. In these contexts, GDF-15 is abundantly expressed and secreted by a variety of cell types:

https://doi.org/10.3390/jpm16010016

macrophages, vascular smooth muscle cells (VSMCs), endothelial cells (ECs), adipocytes, and cardiomyocytes [42]. Interestingly, GDF15-specific genetic variants have been shown to cause phenotypic variation in circulating GDF-15 concentrations [8], suggesting that such polymorphisms may not only influence baseline GDF-15 expression but also modulate the individual susceptibility and response to cardiovascular stress.

4. Regulation and Signaling

As a stress-inducible cytokine, GDF-15 is regulated by several inflammatory or stress-related proteins such as interleukin (IL)-1ß, tumor necrosis factor (TNF)-α, IL-2, and macrophage colony-stimulating factor (MCSF)-1, suggesting a complex and tissue-specific regulation [43]. These molecules have been shown to promote GDF-15 expression through an intricate network of signaling pathways resulting in the activation of: activating transcription factor 4 (ATF4), C/EBP homologous protein (CHOP), p53, early growth response transcription factor 1 (EGR-1), and Nuclear Factor kappa B (NF-kB) [14,44] (Figure 2).

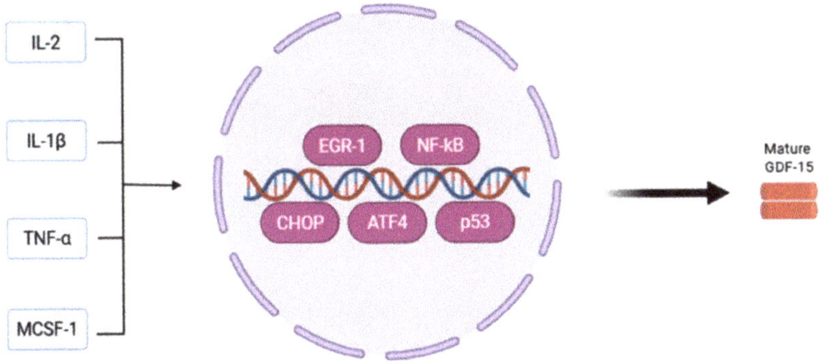

Figure 2. Molecular regulation of GDF-15. Inflammatory and stress-related mediators (IL-1β, TNF-α, IL-2, M-CSF) regulate GDF-15 expression by activating key transcription factors such as ATF4, CHOP, p53, EGR-1, and NF-κB, emphasizing the complex and tissue-dependent nature of this regulatory network. IL-1ß: interleukin-1ß; TNF-α: tumor necrosis factor-α, IL-2: interleukin-2; MCSF-1: macrophage colony-stimulating factor-1; EGR-1: early growth response transcription factor 1; NF-Kb: Nuclear Factor kappa B; CHOP: C/EBP homologous protein; ATF4: activating transcription factor 4; GDF-15: Growth Differentiation Factor-15.

Mature GDF-15 exerts its effects through the glial cell-derived neurotrophic factor (GDNF) family receptor α-like (GFRAL), which is specifically expressed in the hindbrain neurons [45]. Upon dimerization, GFRAL promotes the recruitment of rearranged during transfection (RET) tyrosine kinase, which acts as coreceptor [13]. This interaction subsequently triggers downstream signaling cascades, including the phosphorylation of extracellular signal-regulated kinase (ERK), the proto-oncogene c-Fos, phosphoinositide phospholipase C1 (PLC1), and protein kinase B (PKB) [29].

Importantly, multiple lines of evidence suggest that GDF-15 may also exert effects in peripheral tissues, including the heart [46] (Figure 3). In fact, experimental data demonstrated how GDF-15 is able to activate the Smad 2/3 and the Smad 1/5/8 signaling pathways in cultured cardiomyocytes, reducing hypertrophy and apoptosis during heart failure [47].

Moreover, there is evidence that GDF-15 may contribute to myocardial preservation by activating the signaling pathways mediated by phosphatidylinositol 3-kinase (PI3K) and PKB in rat cardiomyocytes [48].

https://doi.org/10.3390/jpm16010016

Finally, GDF-15 is thought to act as a cardioprotective factor by inhibiting c-Jun N-terminal kinase (JNK), Bcl-2-associated death promoter (Bad), and epidermal growth factor receptor (EGFR) [49].

Of note, it seems that the increase in GDF-15 levels in ischemia–reperfusion cellular models is associated with cardioprotective effects [50].

Similarly, recombinant GDF-15 administration reduces myocardial damage and inflammation [51].

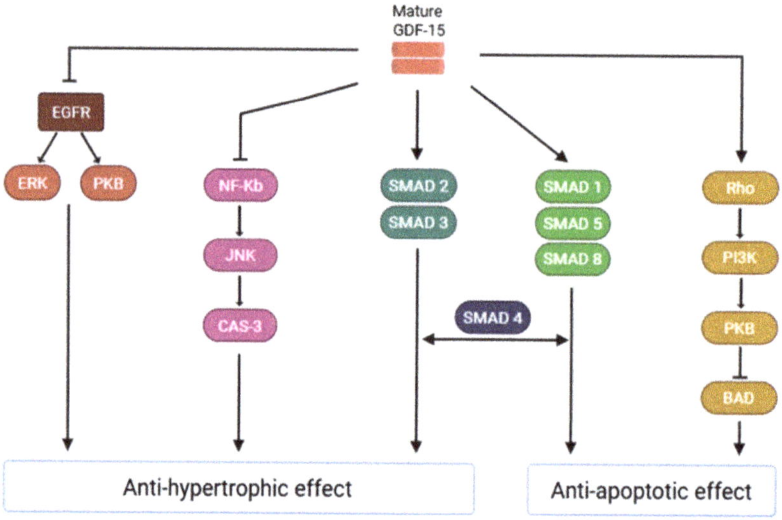

Figure 3. GDF-15–mediated mechanisms of cardiac protection. In cardiomyocytes, GDF-15 activates the Smad2/3 and Smad1/5/8 pathways to limit hypertrophy and apoptosis, enhances myocardial survival through the PI3K/PKB signaling cascade, and inhibits pro-apoptotic pathways involving JNK, Bad, and EGFR, thereby contributing to cardiac protection. GDF-15: Growth Differentiation Factor-15; EGFR: epidermal growth factor receptor; ERK: extracellular signal-regulated kinase; PKB: protein kinase B; NF-Kb: Nuclear Factor kappa B; JNK: c-Jun N-terminal kinase; CAS-3: Caspase-3; PI3K: phosphatidylinositol 3-kinase; BAD: Bcl-2-associated death promoter.

5. Measurements and Methods

GDF-15 is detectable in multiple human biological fluids, including blood, urine and seminal plasma, with varying concentration depending on the specific biological matrix and the underlying physiological or pathological conditions. Although seminal plasma and urine can provide valuable insights in specific settings [52–54], serum and plasma are the most widely used matrices for quantitative GDF-15 assessment.

All currently commercially available assays for GDF-15 quantification are based on immunometric principles employing different detection methods: enzyme-linked immunosorbent assay (ELISA), cytometric bead array, electrochemiluminescence immunoassay (ECLIA), and chemiluminescence immunoassay (CLIA) (Table 1).

Most GDF-15 assays are intended exclusively for research use, with only the Roche Elecsys ECLIA having received approval for in vitro diagnostic (IVD) applications, highlighting the limited availability of clinically validated assays for this biomarker.

https://doi.org/10.3390/jpm16010016

Table 1. Commercially available GDF-15 assays.

Assay	Manufacturer	Method	Sensitivity (pg/mL)	Measurement Range (pg/mL)
Elecsys GDF-15 [55]	Roche Diagnostics	ECLIA	400	400–20,000
Human GDF15 CLIA Kit [56]	Elabscience Biotechnology Inc.	CLIA	4.69	7.81–500
ProcartaPlex Human GDF-15 Simplex Kit [57]	Invitrogen	Bead-based	~9.65	12.21–50,000
Human GDF15/MIC-1/PTGFB [58]	AimPlex Biosciences Inc.	Bead-based	2	5–5000
Quantikine Human GDF-15 ELISA Kit [59]	R&D Systems	ELISA	4.39	23.4–1500
Human GDF-15 ELISA Kit [60]	Invitrogen	ELISA	2	1.1–800
Human GDF-15 ELISA Kit [61]	Elabscience Biotechnology Inc.	ELISA	14.06	23.44–1500
Human GDF-15 ELISA Kit [62]	FineTest	ELISA	14.063	23.44–1500
Human GDF-15 ELISA Kit [63]	Proteintech	ELISA	300	1250–40,000
Human GDF-15 ELISA Kit [64]	ACRO Biosystems	ELISA	7	11.72–1500
Human GDF-15 ELISA Kit [65]	Abcam	ELISA	2	1.1–800
Human GDF-15/MIC-1 ELISA Kit [66]	Sigma-Aldrich	ELISA	2	1.1–800

GDF-15: Growth differentiation factor-15; GDF15: Growth differentiation factor 15; ECLIA: Electrochemiluminescence Immunoassay; CLIA: Chemiluminescence Immunoassay; MIC-1: Macrophage inhibitory cytokine-1; PTGFB: Placental transforming growth factor-β; ELISA: enzyme-linked immunosorbent assay.

In 2007, Kempf et al. developed a new immunoradiometric sandwich assay (IRMA) for the detection of circulating GDF-15, showing a sensitivity of 20 pg/mL [67]. This method has been used in many studies exploring GDF-15 levels in different cardiovascular settings, showing good sensitivity and specificity [68–70].

In 2017, a multicenter study by Wollert et al. evaluated the ECLIA Elecsys GDF-15 assay (Roche Diagnostics), comparing it with the IRMA method developed by Kempf et al. and the ELISA Quantikine assay (R&D Systems). The results showed that while the Elecsys assay offers excellent precision and reproducibility, the absolute GDF-15 concentrations obtained may differ substantially from those measured using other analytical techniques [71].

These discrepancies highlight the critical need for analytical standardization to ensure consistency, accuracy, and comparability of GDF-15 measurements across populations and clinical settings. Moreover, recent evidence suggests that part of the variability in measured GDF-15 levels may not be purely methodological. Interestingly, it has been demonstrated that the genetic variant H202D alters GDF-15 antigenicity, potentially inducing antibody cross-reactivity in some ELISA measurements and thereby interfering with its quantification [72–74]. This finding implies that individual genetic differences may influence the accuracy and comparability of GDF-15 quantification.

https://doi.org/10.3390/jpm16010016

In this regard, mass spectrometry could represent a strategy to overcome antibody cross-reactivity, improving the accuracy of circulating GDF-15 quantification. For example, Lancrajan et al. [75] developed a protocol based on partial denaturation of serum proteins by organic solvents, combined with size exclusion chromatography. The absolute quantification of GDF-15 was performed by liquid chromatography electrospray ionization mass spectrometry (LC-ESI MS), using isotope labeled and concatamerized fingerprint peptides. GDF-15 quantification by this protocol has been shown to correlate well with ELISA measurements, providing higher resolution at low biomarker concentrations compared to antibody-based assays, while also enabling multiplexed analysis.

However, mass spectrometry-based approaches are generally more technically complex, time-consuming, and costly than conventional immunoassay. They also require specialized instrumentation and expertise, and pre-analytical steps such as sample enrichment and digestion can introduce variability, limiting their applicability in large-scale clinical studies. As a result, the potential of mass spectrometry for GDF-15 quantification remains poorly explored, highlighting the need for further research.

6. GDF-15 and Cardiovascular Diseases

Although its molecular mechanisms are not yet fully elucidated, preclinical studies using cellular systems and animal models suggest that increased GDF-15 expression may exert cardioprotective effects, particularly in response to cardiac stress and injury [50,51]. These experimental findings indicate a potential adaptive role for GDF-15 in limiting inflammation, cellular damage, and adverse cardiac remodeling. However, such protective effects have not been consistently confirmed in clinical studies. Elevated circulating levels of GDF-15 in CVDs patients are commonly associated with an increased risk of cardiovascular events, disease severity, and poor clinical outcomes, thus conferring a negative prognostic value. In the following sections, the role of GDF-15 will be described in detail across different cardiovascular conditions.

6.1. Heart Failure (HF)

Heart failure (HF) is a clinical syndrome in which the heart is unable to pump sufficient blood to satisfy the body's circulatory demands, resulting in symptoms such as shortness of breath and fatigue. It can develop because of various disorders affecting the myocardium or the heart valves. Heart failure occurs with roughly equal frequency in patients with reduced and preserved ventricular ejection fraction, each accounting for about 50% of all cases [76].

Elevated circulating levels of GDF-15 have been consistently linked to adverse cardiovascular outcomes, including an increased risk of heart disease, heart failure, and mortality following both ST-segment elevation and non-ST-elevation myocardial infarction [6,77]. Unlike conventional biomarkers such as B-type natriuretic peptides, which primarily reflect hemodynamic stress, GDF-15 provides complementary information about systemic and cellular stress responses. Studies directly comparing the predictive significance of GDF-15 with traditional biomarkers such as N-terminal pro-B-type natriuretic peptide (NT-proBNP) and high-sensitivity troponin T (hs-TnT), or incorporating GDF-15 into risk scores [78–80], demonstrated that it improved the prediction of adverse outcomes in patients with HF. Interestingly, Kosum et al. observed that GDF-15 levels significantly declined throughout hospitalization in patients with acute heart failure (AHF), and lower discharge GDF-15 levels were associated with a lower risk of 30-day rehospitalization, supporting its value as a dynamic marker reflecting the course of AHF with a great prognostic power [81].

Furthemore, GDF-15 emerged as the strongest predictor of HF before the first hospitalization [82]. Studies in the pre-hospitalization phase are particularly valuable, as

 https://doi.org/10.3390/jpm16010016

identifying patients at risk of adverse HF outcomes at an early stage may yield substantial clinical, societal, and economic benefits. Early detection allows intervention when underlying disease mechanisms are still modifiable, preserving the overall health status, and the high financial burden associated with HF hospitalization has not yet occurred. As the population ages and cardiometabolic comorbidities predisposing to HF become increasingly common, early risk stratification will become even more important to enable preventive strategies [83].

In this context, Bradley et al. observed that in patients at risk of HF or with HF prior to their first hospitalization, GDF-15 offers unique prognostic information and serves as a powerful predictor of HF hospitalization (HFH) and all-cause mortality [83].

6.2. *Atherosclerosis*

During the progression of atherosclerosis, GDF-15 expression is markedly increased, particularly within macrophages of atherosclerotic plaques in both humans and mice [12].

One of the first studies investigating GDF-15 in atherosclerosis was conducted in 2011. De Jager et al. identified that GDF 15 deficiency exerts protective effects in atherosclerosis by reducing C-C chemokine receptor 2 (CCR2)-mediated macrophage chemotaxis and modulating cell death. Hematopoietic GDF 15 deficiency limits early lesion formation and enhances plaque stability through increased collagen deposition and reduced necrotic core expansion [84].

Another study investigated the advanced atherogenic lipid profile using the Liposcale® test (Biosfer Teslab, Reus, Spain), highlighting that increased GDF-15 plasma concentrations are associated with a more atherogenic lipid profile. Specifically, GDF-15 increased levels were correlated to elevated Very Low-Density Lipoproteins (VLDL), Low-Density Lipoprotein (LDL) cholesterol and triglyceride content, a higher number of small and dense lipoprotein particles, and reduced High-Density Lipoproteins (HDL) cholesterol. These results indicate that elevated GDF-15 levels may reflect or contribute to lipid abnormalities that promote atherosclerosis and cardiovascular risk [85].

Park et al. reported significantly elevated circulating levels of GDF-15 in patients with atherosclerotic disease undergoing surgical revascularization, suggesting that it could facilitate earlier risk factor management to prevent disease onset and progression [86].

Furthermore, Guardiola et al. observed that GDF-15-specific genetic variants may contribute as well to the development of atherosclerosis. Specifically, carriers of the rs1054564 variant exhibited a higher prevalence of carotid atherosclerotic plaques compared with wild-type individuals [87]. In this specific case, GDF-15 serum levels were associated with diabetes and subclinical atherosclerosis in carriers of the rs1054564 variant, but no significant associations were observed with other metabolic parameters, including hypertension, obesity, metabolic syndrome, or liver steatosis [87].

6.3. *Coronary Artery Disease (CAD)*

Coronary artery disease (CAD) is one of the most prevalent cardiovascular disorders globally and continues to represent a leading cause of morbidity and mortality in both industrialized and developing countries. Its pathogenesis involves a multifactorial interplay among lifestyle, environmental, and genetic components. Among the principal determinants associated with CAD are diabetes mellitus, arterial hypertension, smoking, dyslipidemia, obesity, elevated homocysteine levels, and psychosocial stress [88].

In the context of CAD, elevated GDF-15 levels have been linked to worse clinical outcomes, including increased risks of myocardial infarction (MI), cardiovascular death, and all-cause mortality. However, high GDF-15 concentrations showed limited predictive value for myocardial infarction (MI) in patients with CAD, particularly in those with

https://doi.org/10.3390/jpm16010016

acute coronary syndrome (ACS). Only at the highest concentrations did the difference in MI risk become more apparent compared with the lowest GDF-15 levels, highlighting a concentration-dependent prognostic utility [89].

Multiple studies have shown that increased GDF-15 levels are predictive of poor prognosis in CAD patients. For instance, a meta-analysis involving over 28,000 stable CAD patients found that the highest GDF-15 levels were linked to a 42% increased risk of major adverse cardiovascular events, a 64% higher risk of cardiovascular mortality, and a 101% increased risk of all-cause mortality compared to the lowest levels [90]. The prognostic significance of GDF-15 is not limited to acute events: in stable CAD patients, higher GDF-15 levels have been found to be predictive of future cardiovascular events and mortality, independently of other established biomarkers such as N-terminal pro B-type natriuretic peptide (NT-proBNP) and high-sensitivity C-reactive protein (hs-CRP) [91]. Additionally, GDF-15 concentrations correlate with the extent of CAD, as measured by the Gensini score, and have shown high sensitivity and specificity for disease detection [92].

Nevertheless, in the context of CAD the role of GDF-15 still needs to be further elucidated.

6.4. Atrial Fibrillation (AF)

Atrial fibrillation (AF) is the most prevalent cardiac arrhythmia and represents a substantial burden on healthcare systems. AF incidence rises sharply with age, making it particularly common in elderly populations. It is also recognized as a major risk factor for thromboembolic events, including ischemic stroke, as well as for heart failure and overall mortality [93].

GDF-15 has emerged as a promising biomarker in this context. Elevated GDF-15 levels have been associated with adverse outcomes in AF patients, including increased risks of mortality, major adverse cardiac events (MACE), and thromboembolic complications. In a prospective cohort study involving 362 patients with non-valvular AF, GDF-15 levels were independently associated with all-cause mortality and MACE. Patients with higher GDF-15 concentrations had significantly lower survival probabilities over six years compared to those with lower levels, indicating its potential utility as a prognostic indicator in AF management [94].

Moreover, in patients with AF and rheumatic heart disease, elevated GDF-15 levels correlated with increased atrial fibrosis, suggesting a potential role for GDF-15 in the structural remodeling of the atria that underlies AF development and persistence [95].

6.5. Stroke

Elevated circulating GDF-15 levels have been consistently associated with acute ischemic stroke (AIS), correlating with worse functional outcomes and higher mortality. Clinical studies show that higher baseline GDF-15 predicts adverse events at 3 months post-stroke, independent of traditional risk factors, age, and stroke severity [96].

Elevated circulating levels of GDF 15 in the acute phase of ischemic stroke have been independently associated with a higher incidence of post stroke depression (PSD) at three months, suggesting that GDF-15 could be an important prognostic marker for identifying patients at higher risk of neuropsychiatric sequelae [97].

Furthermore, according to Brenière et al., admission plasma GDF-15 levels independently predict three-month mortality in ischemic stroke patients treated with acute revascularization. Deceased patients had a median GDF-15 of 2777 pg/mL, significantly higher than the 1460 pg/mL observed in survivors [98].

 https://doi.org/10.3390/jpm16010016

In hypertensive patients without prior stroke, higher plasma GDF-15 concentrations are correlated to an increased risk of first-ever ischemic stroke over follow-up periods of several years [99].

According to Alshehri et al., metformin enhances GDF-15 signaling, which mitigates inflammatory and oxidative stress responses in ischemic stroke. Targeting this pathway with selective activators may represent a promising strategy for managing both acute and chronic stroke [100].

These findings suggest that GDF-15 not only reflects ongoing cerebral injury but may also serve as a prognostic biomarker to identify high-risk patients and guide clinical management.

However, the predictive value of GDF-15 for stroke remains uncertain, and current evidence is insufficient to establish a clear association [89]. In many contexts, limited numbers of recurrent events or hemorrhagic complications reduce the power to detect meaningful associations, including the potential link between high GDF-15 levels and bleeding risk. Furthermore, incomplete mortality data and the observational nature of most investigations make it challenging to draw firm causal conclusions [98].

6.6. Cardiovascular Surgery

Cardiovascular surgery remains a pivotal element in the management of advanced cardiac and great vessel diseases, including procedures such as coronary artery bypass grafting (CABG), surgical and transcatheter valve replacement, and corrective operations for aortic pathology [101].

The field has considerably evolved, driven by an aging population, rising prevalence of cardiovascular risk factors, and rapid technological advances that allow for less invasive approaches and more complex reconstructions [102].

Despite improvements in perioperative care and risk stratification, surgical interventions still carry significant morbidity and mortality risks, making the identification of novel biomarkers and personalized strategies crucial for optimizing outcomes [34].

Ferreira et al. showed that in patients undergoing isolated surgical aortic valve replacement, GDF-15 levels peaked at 6 h post-surgery and were positively correlated with cardiopulmonary bypass and aortic cross-clamp times. Additionally, GDF-15 levels correlated with postoperative Sequential Organ Failure Assessment (SOFA) scores at 24 h after surgery, suggesting its potential utility in early risk assessment and in helping guide treatment choices for patients undergoing cardiac surgery [103].

Moreover, GDF-15 has been identified as a valuable marker for predicting long-term outcomes in cardiovascular interventions. In patients undergoing transcatheter aortic valve replacement (TAVR), increased baseline GDF-15 concentrations were linked to higher 1-year mortality rates and lack of reverse remodeling. Incorporating GDF-15 measurements into the Society of Thoracic Surgeons risk score improved the predictive accuracy for mortality, highlighting its potential role in enhancing risk assessment models for cardiovascular surgical procedures [104].

7. GDF-15 and Other Cardiovascular Biomarkers

Even though GDF-15 could represent a versatile biomarker, its clinical utility requires careful evaluation of both its strengths and limitations. This becomes particularly important when compared with biomarkers like Soluble Suppression of Tumorigenicity 2 (sST2), which reflects myocardial adverse remodeling [105], and NT-proBNP, the standard indicator of ventricular wall stretch and hemodynamic overload [106].

NT-proBNP remains the reference biomarker in heart failure, displaying a central role in screening, diagnosis, prognostic stratification, and clinical monitoring [107]. Moreover, its role in ruling out heart failure in the emergency department is well established,

https://doi.org/10.3390/jpm16010016

supported by the definition of specific age-adjusted cut-off values [108]. Furthermore, large cohort analyses show that elevated NT-proBNP levels are independently associated with higher risk of heart failure hospitalization and cardiovascular death, and that it contributes more strongly to risk prediction models than GDF-15 in diverse patient populations, including those with atrial fibrillation and heart failure risk [107].

Serial NT-proBNP measurements further improve risk assessment, reflecting changes in cardiac stress over time [109]. Despite being a highly specific marker of cardiac mechanical stress, NT-proBNP is characterized by high intra-individual biological variability [110]. In this context, other biomarkers such as sST2 and GDF-15, although less specific for cardiac stress, may help to better characterize HF patients with a more complex pathophysiological profile. Both sST2 and GDF-15 exhibit lower intra-individual biological variability compared with natriuretic peptides, but they have reduced specificity because their circulating levels are strongly influenced by systemic and local inflammatory processes [111,112]. However, this apparent limitation may represent an advantage, as these biomarkers could assist clinicians in capturing the multifactorial complexity that characterizes heart failure.

Importantly, both sST2 and GDF-15 have been shown to significantly improve prognostic assessment in heart failure patients, but they provide complementary information over different time frames. Kuster et al. observed that sST2 is primarily associated with short-term outcomes in HF, with prognostic relevance generally limited to approximately one year. In contrast, GDF-15 appears to reflect mid- to long-term risk, offering sustained prognostic information for up to five years and showing lower sensitivity to heart failure therapies. Accordingly, sST2 may be particularly useful for guiding short-term treatment decisions, whereas GDF-15 could help identify patients at risk for long-term adverse events, thereby supporting personalized long-term management strategies, including tailored rehabilitation programs [112]. Overall, a multimarker approach may provide a comprehensive assessment of HF patients, integrating hemodynamic information derived from NT-proBNP with pathophysiological insights obtained from sST2 and GDF-15. Therefore, despite its promising role, further studies are needed to better define the clinical utility of GDF-15 in cardiovascular settings. In this regard, the use of automated ECLIA platforms for GDF-15 measurement could yield more robust and reproducible results, facilitating real-time comparison with traditional biomarkers in routine clinical practice.

8. Conclusions

GDF-15 is a versatile biomarker that reflects a variety of pathophysiological processes, such as inflammation, oxidative stress, tissue damage, and metabolic imbalances. Initially recognized as a stress-responsive cytokine, GDF-15 has emerged as a comprehensive marker of cardiovascular risk and disease progression across a wide range of conditions, including heart failure, atherosclerosis, coronary artery disease, atrial fibrillation, and stroke. The main CVDs-related findings are summarized in Table 2.

The strong association between elevated levels of circulating GDF-15 and adverse cardiovascular outcomes highlights its potential as a valuable prognostic biomarker across various stages of disease (from early risk assessment to outcomes after hospitalization).

Moreover, GDF-15 has shown potential in enhancing existing risk models. Studies have demonstrated that incorporating GDF-15 improves the predictive accuracy of heart failure risk scores, provides better assessments of bleeding risk in atrial fibrillation, and offers additional prognostic insights in coronary and valvular diseases. Its dynamic variation in acute contexts, such as the observed decrease during hospitalization for acute heart failure, further underscores its value as a real-time marker of treatment response.

NT-proBNP remains the cornerstone biomarker in cardiovascular disease owing to its strong diagnostic and prognostic value, wide availability, and extensive clinical validation;

https://doi.org/10.3390/jpm16010016

however, its interpretation is limited by significant biological variability and confounding by age, renal function, and body mass index. sST2 provides complementary prognostic information, particularly in heart failure and myocardial stress, with lower intraindividual variability and reduced influence of renal function and its role in routine clinical decision-making is still evolving. In contrast, GDF-15 emerges as a robust marker of systemic cellular stress with low intraindividual biological variability and strong prognostic associations across cardiovascular conditions, although its limited disease specificity and fewer interventional data currently restrict its standalone clinical application.

Table 2. Clinical findings related to GDF-15 and cardiovascular diseases.

Condition	GDF-15	References
Heart failure (HF)	• High levels associated with adverse cardiovascular outcomes, increased mortality, and higher risk of hospitalization. • Provides additional prognostic value compared to NT-proBNP and hs-TnT. • Decreases during hospitalization in acute heart failure (AHF), improving prediction of 30-day rehospitalization. • Strong predictor of heart failure before the first hospitalization.	[6,76–83]
Atherosclerosis	• Increased expression in atherosclerotic plaques, especially in macrophages. • Deficiency reduces early lesions, improves plaque stability, and limits necrotic core expansion. • Elevated circulating levels associated with a more atherogenic lipid profile. • Higher levels observed in patients with atherosclerotic disease compared to healthy individuals. • Genetic variants (rs1054564) linked to higher prevalence of carotid plaques.	[12,84–87]
Coronary Artery Disease (CAD)	• Elevated levels predict myocardial infarction (MI), cardiovascular death, and all-cause mortality. • Elevated levels increase risk for major adverse cardiovascular events (MACE). • Correlates with CAD severity (e.g., Gensini score). • Prognostic value independent of NT-proBNP and hs-CRP.	[88–92]
Atrial Fibrillation (AF)	• High levels predict mortality, MACE, and thromboembolic complications. • Independent association with worse 6-year survival. • Correlated with the degree of atrial fibrosis.	[93–95]
Stroke	• High levels are associated with poor prognosis and higher 3-month mortality. • Predicts post-stroke depression (PSD). • Prognostic value in patients treated with acute revascularization. • Elevated levels in hypertensive patients without prior stroke predict the first ischemic event.	[96–100]
Cardiovascular surgery	• Peaks at 6 h after surgery and correlates with bypass time, cross-clamp duration, and SOFA score at 24 h. • High baseline levels in TAVR patients are associated with higher 1-year mortality and lack of reverse remodeling. • Improves the predictive accuracy for mortality if added to preoperative scores.	[34,101–104]

GDF-15: Growth Differentiation Factor-15; HF: Heart failure; NT-proBNP: N-terminal pro-B-type natriuretic peptide; hs-TnT: high-sensitivity troponin T; AHF: Acute heart failure; CAD: Coronary artery disease; MI: myocardial infarction; MACE: major adverse cardiovascular events; hs-CRP: high-sensitivity C-reactive protein; AF: atrial fibrillation; PSD: post-stroke depression; SOFA: Sequential Organ Failure Assessment; TAVR: transcatheter aortic valve replacement.

Moreover, further studies are needed to clarify the apparent discrepancy between preclinical models, in which GDF-15 seems to exert cardioprotective effects, and clinical

https://doi.org/10.3390/jpm16010016

observations, where elevated circulating GDF-15 is consistently associated with adverse outcomes and to elucidate the apparently significant role of GDF-15 in the pathophysiology of cardiovascular diseases.

In conclusion, GDF-15 represents a valuable candidate for multimarker strategies aimed at improving cardiovascular risk prediction and personalized patient care. The increasing availability of fully automated ECLIA-based assays may facilitate real-time comparison with established cardiovascular biomarkers, improve analytical harmonization, and enable the investigation of GDF-15 across diverse and well-characterized populations.

Author Contributions: Conceptualization, S.B. and V.L.; writing—original draft preparation, C.L. and M.M.; writing—review and editing, C.L., M.M., V.L., A.U. and S.B.; supervision, V.L., A.U. and S.B. All authors have read and agreed to the published version of the manuscript.

Funding: This research received no external funding.

Institutional Review Board Statement: Not applicable.

Informed Consent Statement: Not applicable.

Data Availability Statement: No new data were created or analyzed in this study. Data sharing is not applicable to this article.

Conflicts of Interest: All authors have no conflicts of interest or financial ties to disclose.

Abbreviations

The following abbreviations are used in this manuscript:

GDF-15	Growth Differentiation Factor–15
TGF-β	Transforming Growth Factor-β
MIC-1	macrophage inhibitory cytokine-1
CVDs	cardiovascular diseases
WHO	World Health Organization
NAG-1	nonsteroidal anti-inflammatory drug-activated gene-1
PLAB	placental bone morphogenetic protein
PTGFB	placental transforming growth factor-β
PDF	prostate-derived factor
aa	amino acids
PCSK	proprotein convertase subtilisin–kexin
ECM	extracellular matrix
MMP26	matrix metalloproteinase 26
NAFLD	non-alcoholic fatty liver disease
HF	heart failure
VSMCs	vascular smooth muscle cells
ECs	endothelial cells
IL-1β	interleukin-1ß
TNF-α	tumor necrosis factor-α
IL-2	interleukin-2
MCSF-1	macrophage colony-stimulating factor-1
ATF4	activating transcription factor 4
CHOP	C/EBP homologous protein
EGR-1	early growth response transcription factor-1
NF-kB	Nuclear Factor kappa B
GDNF	glial cell-derived neurotrophic factor
GFRAL	GDNF family receptor α-like

https://doi.org/10.3390/jpm16010016

RET	rearranged during transfection
ERK	extracellular signal-regulated kinase
PLC1	phosphoinositide phospholipase C 1
PKB	protein kinase B
PI3K	phosphatidylinositol 3-kinase
JNK	c-Jun N-terminal kinase
Bad	Bcl-2-associated death promoter
EGFR	epidermal growth factor receptor
CAS-3	Caspase-3
ELISA	enzyme-linked immunosorbent assay
ECLIA	electrochemiluminescence immunoassay
CLIA	chemiluminescence immunoassay
IVD	in vitro diagnostic
IRMA	immunoradiometric sandwich assay
LC-ESI MS	liquid chromatography electrospray ionization mass spectrometry
NT-proBNP	N-terminal pro-B-type natriuretic peptide
hs-TnT	high-sensitivity troponin T
AHF	acute heart failure
HFH	heart failure hospitalization
CCR2	C-C chemokine receptor 2
VLDL	Very Low-Density Lipoproteins
LDL	Low-Density Lipoproteins
HDL	High-Density Lipoproteins
CAD	coronary artery disease
MI	myocardial infarction
ACS	acute coronary syndrome
hs-CRP	high-sensitivity C-reactive protein
AF	atrial fibrillation
MACE	major adverse cardiac events
AIS	acute ischemic stroke
PSD	post-stroke depression
CABG	coronary artery bypass grafting
SOFA	Sequential Organ Failure Assessment
TAVR	transcatheter aortic valve replacement
sST2	Soluble Suppression of Tumorigenicity 2

References

1. World Health Organization (WHO). Cardiovascular Diseases. Available online: https://www.who.int/health-topics/cardiovascular-diseases (accessed on 5 November 2025).
2. Netala, V.R.; Hou, T.; Wang, Y.; Zhang, Z.; Teertam, S.K. Cardiovascular Biomarkers: Tools for Precision Diagnosis and Prognosis. *Int. J. Mol. Sci.* **2025**, *26*, 3218. [CrossRef] [PubMed]
3. Bootcov, M.R.; Bauskin, A.R.; Valenzuela, S.M.; Moore, A.G.; Bansal, M.; He, X.Y.; Zhang, H.P.; Donnellan, M.; Mahler, S.; Pryor, K.; et al. MIC-1, a novel macrophage inhibitory cytokine, is a divergent member of the TGF-beta superfamily. *Proc. Natl. Acad. Sci. USA* **1997**, *94*, 11514–11519. [CrossRef]
4. Emmerson, P.J.; Duffin, K.L.; Chintharlapalli, S.; Wu, X. GDF15 and Growth Control. *Front. Physiol.* **2018**, *9*, 1712. [CrossRef] [PubMed]
5. Spanopoulou, A.; Gkretsi, V. Growth differentiation factor 15 (GDF15) in cancer cell metastasis: From the cells to the patients. *Clin. Exp. Metastasis* **2020**, *37*, 451–464. [CrossRef]
6. Xie, S.; Lu, L.; Liu, L. Growth differentiation factor-15 and the risk of cardiovascular diseases and all-cause mortality: A meta-analysis of prospective studies. *Clin. Cardiol.* **2019**, *42*, 513–523. [CrossRef]
7. Bottner, M.; Laaff, M.; Schechinger, B.; Rappold, G.; Unsicker, K.; Suter-Crazzolara, C. Characterization of the rat, mouse, and human genes of growth/differentiation factor-15/macrophage inhibiting cytokine-1 (GDF-15/MIC-1). *Gene* **1999**, *237*, 105–111. [CrossRef]

https://doi.org/10.3390/jpm16010016

55. Roche Diagnostics. Elecsys GDF-15. Available online: https://diagnostics.roche.com/it/it/products/params/elecsys-gdf-15.html (accessed on 5 November 2025).
56. Elabscience. Human GDF15 CLIA Kit. Available online: https://www.elabscience.com/p/human-gdf15-growth-differentiation-factor-15-clia-kit--e-cl-h0080?srsltid=AfmBOorTUIsw0AmLgpqkazO2Av0Jj4tzoP4fWzYY0bzxFPZrbwF0Mr-f (accessed on 5 November 2025).
57. ProcartaPlex. Human GDF-15 Simplex Kit. Available online: https://www.thermofisher.com/order/catalog/product/EPX010-12258-901/ (accessed on 5 November 2025).
58. Aimplex. Human GDF15/MIC-1/PTGFB. Available online: https://www.aimplexbio.com/hgdf15 (accessed on 5 November 2025).
59. Quantikine. Human GDF-15 ELISA Kit. Available online: https://www.rndsystems.com/products/human-gdf-15-quantikine-elisa-kit_dgd150 (accessed on 5 November 2025).
60. Invitrogen. Human GDF-15 ELISA Kit. Available online: https://www.thermofisher.com/elisa/product/Human-GDF15-ELISA-Kit/EHGDF15 (accessed on 5 November 2025).
61. Elabscience Biotechnology Inc. Human GDF-15 ELISA Kit. Available online: https://www.elabscience.com/p/human-gdf15-growth-differentiation-factor-15-elisa-kit--e-el-0080?srsltid=AfmBOopU2_oNqgPbRMf2BWCasDmv70xUek5nrEAQfzIcYIw_3ykxKAyW (accessed on 5 November 2025).
62. FineTest. Human GDF-15 ELISA Kit. Available online: https://www.fn-test.com/product/eh0150/ (accessed on 5 November 2025).
63. Proteintech. Human GDF-15 ELISA Kit. Available online: https://www.ptglab.com/products/Human-GDF15-ELISA-Kit-KE00108.htm?srsltid=AfmBOoqn9bj_p_B6-Jf7sdg81VtOrwxgIXhpfwHu6bcbp4f8qDiZXgiF (accessed on 5 November 2025).
64. ACRO Biosystems. Human GDF-15 ELISA Kit. Available online: https://www.acrobiosystems.com/products/kits/gdf-15-human-cea-c077?srsltid=AfmBOopRwvqWrSsUDkVUUSkbybe_-ImddlhNXLQ0S-EDogYEz5TOdprb (accessed on 5 November 2025).
65. Abcam. Human GDF-15 ELISA Kit. Available online: https://www.abcam.com/en-hu/products/elisa-kits/human-gdf-15-elisa-kit-ab155432 (accessed on 5 November 2025).
66. Sigma-Aldrich. Human GDF-15/MIC-1 ELISA Kit. Available online: https://www.sigmaaldrich.com/IT/it/product/sigma/rab0204 (accessed on 5 November 2025).
67. Kempf, T.; Horn-Wichmann, R.; Brabant, G.; Peter, T.; Allhoff, T.; Klein, G.; Drexler, H.; Johnston, N.; Wallentin, L.; Wollert, K.C. Circulating concentrations of growth-differentiation factor 15 in apparently healthy elderly individuals and patients with chronic heart failure as assessed by a new immunoradiometric sandwich assay. *Clin. Chem.* **2007**, *53*, 284–291. [CrossRef]
68. Lind, L.; Wallentin, L.; Kempf, T.; Tapken, H.; Quint, A.; Lindahl, B.; Olofsson, S.; Venge, P.; Larsson, A.; Hulthe, J.; et al. Growth-differentiation factor-15 is an independent marker of cardiovascular dysfunction and disease in the elderly: Results from the Prospective Investigation of the Vasculature in Uppsala Seniors (PIVUS) Study. *Eur. Heart J.* **2009**, *30*, 2346–2353. [CrossRef]
69. Widera, C.; Pencina, M.J.; Meisner, A.; Kempf, T.; Bethmann, K.; Marquardt, I.; Katus, H.A.; Giannitsis, E.; Wollert, K.C. Adjustment of the GRACE score by growth differentiation factor 15 enables a more accurate appreciation of risk in non-ST-elevation acute coronary syndrome. *Eur. Heart J.* **2012**, *33*, 1095–1104. [CrossRef] [PubMed]
70. Anand, I.S.; Kempf, T.; Rector, T.S.; Tapken, H.; Allhoff, T.; Jantzen, F.; Kuskowski, M.; Cohn, J.N.; Drexler, H.; Wollert, K.C. Serial measurement of growth-differentiation factor-15 in heart failure: Relation to disease severity and prognosis in the Valsartan Heart Failure Trial. *Circulation* **2010**, *122*, 1387–1395. [CrossRef]
71. Wollert, K.C.; Kempf, T.; Giannitsis, E.; Bertsch, T.; Braun, S.L.; Maier, H.; Reim, M.; Christenson, R.H. An Automated Assay for Growth Differentiation Factor 15. *J. Appl. Lab. Med.* **2017**, *1*, 510–521. [CrossRef]
72. Lemmela, S.; Wigmore, E.M.; Benner, C.; Havulinna, A.S.; Ong, R.M.Y.; Kempf, T.; Wollert, K.C.; Blankenberg, S.; Zeller, T.; Peters, J.E.; et al. Integrated analyses of growth differentiation factor-15 concentration and cardiometabolic diseases in humans. *Elife* **2022**, *11*, e76272. [CrossRef]
73. Karusheva, Y.; Ratcliff, M.; Morseburg, A.; Barker, P.; Melvin, A.; Sattar, N.; Burling, K.; Backmark, A.; Roth, R.; Jermutus, L.; et al. The Common H202D Variant in GDF-15 Does Not Affect Its Bioactivity but Can Significantly Interfere with Measurement of Its Circulating Levels. *J. Appl. Lab. Med.* **2022**, *7*, 1388–1400. [CrossRef]
74. Chrysafi, P.; Valenzuela-Vallejo, L.; Stefanakis, K.; Kelesidis, T.; Connelly, M.A.; Mantzoros, C.S. Total and H-specific GDF-15 levels increase in caloric deprivation independently of leptin in humans. *Nat. Commun.* **2024**, *15*, 5190. [CrossRef]
75. Lancrajan, I.; Schneider-Stock, R.; Naschberger, E.; Schellerer, V.S.; Sturzl, M.; Enz, R. Absolute quantification of DcR3 and GDF15 from human serum by LC-ESI MS. *J. Cell Mol. Med.* **2015**, *19*, 1656–1671. [CrossRef] [PubMed]
76. Heidenreich, P.A.; Bozkurt, B.; Aguilar, D.; Allen, L.A.; Byun, J.J.; Colvin, M.M.; Deswal, A.; Drazner, M.H.; Dunlay, S.M.; Evers, L.R.; et al. 2022 AHA/ACC/HFSA Guideline for the Management of Heart Failure: A Report of the American College of Cardiology/American Heart Association Joint Committee on Clinical Practice Guidelines. *Circulation* **2022**, *145*, e895–e1032. [CrossRef]

https://doi.org/10.3390/jpm16010016

77. Rueda, F.; Lupon, J.; Garcia-Garcia, C.; Cediel, G.; Aranda Nevado, M.C.; Serra Gregori, J.; Labata, C.; Oliveras, T.; Ferrer, M.; de Diego, O.; et al. Acute-phase dynamics and prognostic value of growth differentiation factor-15 in ST-elevation myocardial infarction. *Clin. Chem. Lab. Med.* **2019**, *57*, 1093–1101. [CrossRef]
78. Lyu, L.; Xu, J.; Xv, C.; Xiao, H.; Liu, Z.; He, Y.; Gao, W.; Hao, B.; Liu, H. Prognostic value of growth differentiation factor-15 in heart failure among whole ejection fraction phenotypes. *ESC Heart Fail.* **2024**, *11*, 2295–2304. [CrossRef] [PubMed]
79. Suzuki, S.; Motoki, H.; Minamisawa, M.; Okuma, Y.; Shoin, W.; Okano, T.; Kimura, K.; Ebisawa, S.; Okada, A.; Kuwahara, K. Prognostic significance of high-sensitivity cardiac troponin in patients with heart failure with preserved ejection fraction. *Heart Vessel.* **2019**, *34*, 1650–1656. [CrossRef]
80. Woolley, R.J.; Ceelen, D.; Ouwerkerk, W.; Tromp, J.; Figarska, S.M.; Anker, S.D.; Dickstein, K.; Filippatos, G.; Zannad, F.; Metra, M.; et al. Machine learning based on biomarker profiles identifies distinct subgroups of heart failure with preserved ejection fraction. *Eur. J. Heart Fail.* **2021**, *23*, 983–991. [CrossRef]
81. Kosum, P.; Siranart, N.; Mattanapojanat, N.; Phutinart, S.; Kongruttanachok, N.; Sinphurmsukskul, S.; Siwamogsatham, S.; Puwanant, S.; Ariyachaipanich, A. GDF-15: A novel biomarker of heart failure predicts short-term and long-term heart-failure rehospitalization and short-term mortality in patients with acute heart failure syndrome. *BMC Cardiovasc. Disord.* **2024**, *24*, 151. [CrossRef]
82. Bradley, J.; Schelbert, E.B.; Bonnett, L.J.; Lewis, G.A.; Lagan, J.; Orsborne, C.; Brown, P.F.; Naish, J.H.; Williams, S.G.; McDonagh, T.; et al. Predicting hospitalisation for heart failure and death in patients with, or at risk of, heart failure before first hospitalisation: A retrospective model development and external validation study. *Lancet Digit. Health* **2022**, *4*, e445–e454. [CrossRef]
83. Bradley, J.; Schelbert, E.B.; Bonnett, L.J.; Lewis, G.A.; Lagan, J.; Orsborne, C.; Brown, P.F.; Black, N.; Naish, J.H.; Williams, S.G.; et al. Growth differentiation factor-15 in patients with or at risk of heart failure but before first hospitalisation. *Heart* **2024**, *110*, 195–201. [CrossRef]
84. De Jager, S.C.; Bermudez, B.; Bot, I.; Koenen, R.R.; Bot, M.; Kavelaars, A.; de Waard, V.; Heijnen, C.J.; Muriana, F.J.; Weber, C.; et al. Growth differentiation factor 15 deficiency protects against atherosclerosis by attenuating CCR2-mediated macrophage chemotaxis. *J. Exp. Med.* **2011**, *208*, 217–225. [CrossRef] [PubMed]
85. Girona, J.; Guardiola, M.; Barroso, E.; Garcia-Altares, M.; Ibarretxe, D.; Plana, N.; Ribalta, J.; Amigo, N.; Correig, X.; Vazquez-Carrera, M.; et al. GDF15 Circulating Levels Are Associated with Metabolic-Associated Liver Injury and Atherosclerotic Cardiovascular Disease. *Int. J. Mol. Sci.* **2025**, *26*, 2039. [CrossRef]
86. Park, J.M.; Beckman, I.; Beckman, K.; Allan, R.B.; Delaney, C.L. Investigating the Role of Growth Differentiation Factor-15 as a Biomarker of Inflammation in Patients with Atherosclerotic Vascular Disease. *J. Vasc. Res.* **2025**, 1–11. [CrossRef]
87. Guardiola, M.; Girona, J.; Barroso, E.; Garcia-Altares, M.; Ibarretxe, D.; Plana, N.; Ribalta, J.; Correig, X.; Vazquez-Carrera, M.; Masana, L.; et al. The GDF15 3′ UTR Polymorphism rs1054564 Is Associated with Diabetes and Subclinical Atherosclerosis. *Int. J. Mol. Sci.* **2024**, *25*, 11985. [CrossRef]
88. Malakar, A.K.; Choudhury, D.; Halder, B.; Paul, P.; Uddin, A.; Chakraborty, S. A review on coronary artery disease, its risk factors, and therapeutics. *J. Cell Physiol.* **2019**, *234*, 16812–16823. [CrossRef] [PubMed]
89. Zhang, S.; Hao, P.; Li, J.; Zhang, Q.; Yin, X.; Wang, J.; Chen, Y. Prognostic value of growth differentiation factor-15 in patients with coronary artery disease: A meta-analysis and systematic review. *Front. Cardiovasc. Med.* **2023**, *10*, 1054187. [CrossRef] [PubMed]
90. Li, T.; Chen, Y.; Ye, T.; Zheng, L.; Chen, L.; Fan, Y.; Lin, B. Association of growth differentiation factor-15 level with adverse outcomes in patients with stable coronary artery disease: A meta-analysis. *Atheroscler. Plus* **2022**, *47*, 1–7. [CrossRef]
91. Hagstrom, E.; James, S.K.; Bertilsson, M.; Becker, R.C.; Himmelmann, A.; Husted, S.; Katus, H.A.; Steg, P.G.; Storey, R.F.; Siegbahn, A.; et al. Growth differentiation factor-15 level predicts major bleeding and cardiovascular events in patients with acute coronary syndromes: Results from the PLATO study. *Eur. Heart J.* **2016**, *37*, 1325–1333. [CrossRef]
92. Kerkeni, M.; Weiss, I.S.; Jaisson, S.; Dandana, A.; Addad, F.; Gillery, P.; Hammami, M. Increased serum concentrations of pentosidine are related to presence and severity of coronary artery disease. *Thromb. Res.* **2014**, *134*, 633–638. [CrossRef] [PubMed]
93. Saleh, K.; Haldar, S. Atrial fibrillation: A contemporary update. *Clin. Med.* **2023**, *23*, 437–441. [CrossRef]
94. Nopp, S.; Konigsbrugge, O.; Kraemmer, D.; Pabinger, I.; Ay, C. Growth differentiation factor-15 predicts major adverse cardiac events and all-cause mortality in patients with atrial fibrillation. *Eur. J. Intern. Med.* **2021**, *88*, 35–42. [CrossRef]
95. Zhou, Y.M.; Li, M.J.; Zhou, Y.L.; Ma, L.L.; Yi, X. Growth differentiation factor-15 (GDF-15), novel biomarker for assessing atrial fibrosis in patients with atrial fibrillation and rheumatic heart disease. *Int. J. Clin. Exp. Med.* **2015**, *8*, 21201–21207.
96. Yin, J.; Zhu, Z.; Guo, D.; Wang, A.; Zeng, N.; Zheng, X.; Peng, Y.; Zhong, C.; Wang, G.; Zhou, Y.; et al. Increased Growth Differentiation Factor 15 Is Associated with Unfavorable Clinical Outcomes of Acute Ischemic Stroke. *Clin. Chem.* **2019**, *65*, 569–578. [CrossRef]
97. Lu, X.; Duan, J.; Cheng, Q.; Lu, J. The association between serum growth differentiation factor-15 and 3-month depression after acute ischemic stroke. *J. Affect. Disord.* **2020**, *260*, 695–702. [CrossRef]

 https://doi.org/10.3390/jpm16010016

98. Breniere, C.; Meloux, A.; Pedard, M.; Marie, C.; Thouant, P.; Vergely, C.; Bejot, Y. Growth Differentiation Factor-15 (GDF-15) Is Associated with Mortality in Ischemic Stroke Patients Treated with Acute Revascularization Therapy. *Front. Neurol.* **2019**, *10*, 611. [CrossRef]
99. Wang, X.; Zhu, L.; Wu, Y.; Sun, K.; Su, M.; Yu, L.; Chen, J.; Li, W.; Yang, J.; Yuan, Z.; et al. Plasma growth differentiation factor 15 predicts first-ever stroke in hypertensive patients. *Medicine* **2016**, *95*, e4342. [CrossRef]
100. Alshehri, G.H.; Al-Kuraishy, H.M.; Alsfouk, B.A.; Al-Gareeb, A.I.; Faheem, S.A.; Alexiou, A.; Papadakis, M.; Batiha, G.E. The AMPK/GDF15 Axis: A Novel Target for the Neuroprotective Effects of Metformin in Ischemic Stroke. *Mol. Neurobiol.* **2025**, *62*, 15149–15163. [CrossRef] [PubMed]
101. Abri, Q.A.; von Ballmoos, M.C.W. Cardiovascular Surgery Procedural Training and Evaluation: Current Status and Future Directions. *Methodist DeBakey Cardiovasc. J.* **2022**, *18*, 30–38. [CrossRef] [PubMed]
102. Tajdini, M.; Behnoush, A.H.; Pashang, M.; Jameie, M.; Khalaji, A.; Sadeghian, S.; Vasheghani-Farahani, A.; Poorhosseini, H.; Masoudkabir, F.; Hosseini, K.; et al. Heart surgery over two decades: What we have learned about results and changing risks. *BMC Cardiovasc. Disord.* **2024**, *24*, 195. [CrossRef]
103. Ferreira, R.; Velho, T.R.; Pereira, R.M.; Pedroso, D.; Draiblate, B.; Constantino, S.; Nobre, A.; Almeida, A.G.; Moita, L.F.; Pinto, F. Growth Differentiation Factor 15 as a Biomarker for Risk Stratification in the Cardiothoracic Surgery Intensive Care Unit. *Biomolecules* **2024**, *14*, 1593. [CrossRef] [PubMed]
104. Kim, J.B.; Kobayashi, Y.; Moneghetti, K.J.; Brenner, D.A.; O'Malley, R.; Schnittger, I.; Wu, J.C.; Murtagh, G.; Beshiri, A.; Fischbein, M.; et al. GDF-15 (Growth Differentiation Factor 15) Is Associated with Lack of Ventricular Recovery and Mortality After Transcatheter Aortic Valve Replacement. *Circ. Cardiovasc. Interv.* **2017**, *10*, e005594. [CrossRef]
105. Sciatti, E.; Merlo, A.; Scangiuzzi, C.; Limonta, R.; Gori, M.; D'Elia, E.; Aimo, A.; Vergaro, G.; Emdin, M.; Senni, M. Prognostic Value of sST2 in Heart Failure. *J. Clin. Med.* **2023**, *12*, 3970. [CrossRef]
106. Panagopoulou, V.; Deftereos, S.; Kossyvakis, C.; Raisakis, K.; Giannopoulos, G.; Bouras, G.; Pyrgakis, V.; Cleman, M.W. NT-proBNP: An Important Biomarker in Cardiac Diseases. *Curr. Top. Med. Chem.* **2013**, *13*, 82–94. [CrossRef]
107. Haller, P.M.; Jarolim, P.; Palazzolo, M.G.; Bellavia, A.; Antman, E.M.; Eikelboom, J.; Granger, C.B.; Harrington, J.; Healey, J.S.; Hijazi, Z.; et al. Heart Failure Risk Assessment Using Biomarkers in Patients with Atrial Fibrillation: Analysis From COMBINE-AF. *J. Am. Coll. Cardiol.* **2024**, *84*, 1528–1540. [CrossRef]
108. Bayes-Genis, A.; Docherty, K.F.; Petrie, M.C.; Januzzi, J.L.; Mueller, C.; Anderson, L.; Bozkurt, B.; Butler, J.; Chioncel, O.; Cleland, J.G.F.; et al. Practical algorithms for early diagnosis of heart failure and heart stress using NT-proBNP: A clinical consensus statement from the Heart Failure Association of the ESC. *Eur. J. Heart Fail.* **2023**, *25*, 1891–1898. [CrossRef]
109. Mueller, C.; Muench-Gerber, T.S.; de Boer, R.A. Growth differentiation factor 15: A biomarker searching for an indication. *Eur. Heart. J.* **2023**, *44*, 301–303. [CrossRef] [PubMed]
110. Meijers, W.C.; van der Velde, A.R.; Muller Kobold, A.C.; Dijck-Brouwer, J.; Wu, A.H.; Jaffe, A.; de Boer, R.A. Variability of biomarkers in patients with chronic heart failure and healthy controls. *Eur. J. Heart Fail.* **2017**, *19*, 357–365. [CrossRef] [PubMed]
111. Krintus, M.; Braga, F.; Kozinski, M.; Borille, S.; Kubica, J.; Sypniewska, G.; Panteghini, M. A study of biological and lifestyle factors, including within-subject variation, affecting concentrations of growth differentiation factor 15 in serum. *Clin. Chem. Lab. Med.* **2019**, *57*, 1035–1043. [CrossRef] [PubMed]
112. Kuster, N.; Huet, F.; Dupuy, A.M.; Akodad, M.; Battistella, P.; Agullo, A.; Leclercq, F.; Kalmanovich, E.; Meilhac, A.; Aguilhon, S.; et al. Multimarker approach including CRP, sST2 and GDF-15 for prognostic stratification in stable heart failure. *ESC Heart Fail.* **2020**, *7*, 2230–2239. [CrossRef]

 https://doi.org/10.3390/jpm16010016

Journal of
Personalized Medicine

MDPI

Review

Current Trends in Venous Thromboprophylaxis for Inpatient Care

Maria Velliou, Vasiliki Bistola, John Parissis and Effie Polyzogopoulou *

University Emergency Department, Attikon University Hospital, 12462 Athens, Greece;
vasobistola@med.uoa.gr (V.B.)
* Correspondence: effiepol@med.uoa.gr

Abstract

Thromboprophylaxis in hospitalized patients is a critical component of care aimed at preventing venous thromboembolism (VTE), a common and potentially fatal complication during hospitalization. The risk of VTE varies substantially across patient populations, influenced by the type of illness, including both surgical procedures and medical comorbidities, and requires individualized assessment. At the same time, the implementation of pharmacological thromboprophylaxis must carefully balance the risk of thrombosis against the potential for bleeding. Commonly used risk assessment models, such as the Padua and IMPROVE scores, can help clinicians stratify patients according to their individual risk of VTE and bleeding complications. The aim of the present review is to provide a structured synthesis of the current evidence on thromboprophylaxis strategies in hospitalized patients, critically appraise the performance and applicability of existing VTE and bleeding risk models and highlight how these tools can guide a tailored illness-specific approach to prophylactic decision-making. Where relevant, the review also outlines practical, risk-adapted algorithms to optimize thromboprophylaxis across diverse clinical settings.

Keywords: venous thromboembolism; thromboprophylaxis; unfractionated heparin; low-molecular-weight heparin; fondaparinux; hospitalization

1. Introduction

Venous thromboembolism (VTE), including deep vein thrombosis (DVT) and pulmonary embolism, is among the top five vascular diseases and the third most common cause of mortality. It is estimated to affect one million subjects per year in Europe and almost 10 million people globally, while its incidence seems to be much lower in Eastern countries [1–3]. The lifetime risk of VTE is 8% in the Western world, while about 20% of affected persons die within a year after diagnosis [1].

VTE is a multifactorial disease in which clinical conditions, pharmacologic treatments, genetic factors and demographic characteristics determine the individual's thrombotic potential. Patients with cardiovascular disease, malignancies, fractures, lower limbs immobilization following trauma, heparin-induced thrombocytopenia, infection, COVID-19 disease, antiphospholipid antibody syndrome, autoimmune diseases, a previous history of VTE, obesity and a recent surgical procedure are at a greater risk for VTE [2].

Hospitalization due to an acute medical illness is also considered a triggering factor, even in the absence of immobilization. A previous observational cohort study has shown that hospital admission was associated with a 38-fold higher risk of VTE and the risk remained 3-fold greater up to three months after discharge [4]. Given that VTE is a major cause of morbidity and mortality, identification of patients at high VTE risk in the

Emergency Department and initiation of thromboprophylaxis is an essential intervention to ensure patients' safety during hospitalization.

Despite the well-recognized burden of VTE in hospitalized patients and the availability of validated risk assessment tools, their application in routine clinical practice remains inconsistent, and uncertainty persists regarding how best to integrate thrombotic and bleeding risks across diverse clinical scenarios. Variability in patient profiles, differences between surgical and medical conditions, and continually evolving evidence further complicate decision-making at the bedside. To address these challenges, the present review examines the widely adopted thrombotic and bleeding risk models used in hospitalized patients, evaluates their effectiveness in different clinical contexts, and synthesizes current evidence on optimal thromboprophylaxis strategies. It also aims to clarify how risk-adapted approaches can be applied in everyday clinical practice and to outline practical, evidence-based decision pathways.

2. Evidence on Thromboprophylaxis in Hospitalized Patients

Hospital-acquired VTE is a common and serious complication among acutely ill medical inpatients. Landmark trials, including the MEDENOX (Prophylaxis in Medical Patients with Enoxaparin), the PREVENT (Prospective Evaluation of Dalteparin Efficacy for Prevention of VTE in Immobilized Patients Trial) and the ARTEMIS (Arixtra for Thromboembolism Prevention in a Medical Indication Study), have demonstrated that pharmacologic thromboprophylaxis with low-molecular-weight heparin (LMWH) or fondaparinux significantly reduces the VTE risk in this population (Table 1) [5–7].

Table 1. Landmark trials that evaluated the VTE risk in acutely ill medical patients during hospitalization.

	MEDENOX [5], 1999	PREVENT [6], 2004	ARTEMIS [7], 2006	ADOPT [8], 2011	MAGELLAN [9], 2013	APEX [10], 2016
Patients (*n*)	1102	3706	849	6528	8101	7513
Age (years)	>40	>40	>60	>40	>40	>40
Anticoagulant	Enoxaparin 20 mg or 40 mg for 7 days	Dalteparin 5000 IU for 14 days	Fondaparinux 2.5 mg for 6–14 days	Apixaban 2.5 mg for 30 days	Rivaroxaban 10 mg for 35 ± 4 days	Betrixaban 80 mg for 35–42 days
Comparator	Placebo	Placebo	Placebo	Enoxaparin 40 mg for 6–14 days	Enoxaparin 40 mg for 10 ± 4 days	Enoxaparin 40 mg for 10 ± 4 days
Follow-up	14 days	90 days	30 days	30 days	35 ± 4 days	47 days
Outcomes	VTE risk (5.5% vs. 14.9%) RR 0.37 (95%CI: 0.21–0.64)	VTE/sudden death risk (2.77% vs. 4.96%) RR: 0.55 (95%CI: 0.38–0.80)	VTE risk (5.6% vs. 10.5%) RR: 0.54 (95%CI: 0.31–0.92)	No superiority (2.71% vs. 3.05%) RR: 0.87 (95%CI: 0.62–1.23)	VTE risk (4.4% vs. 5.7%) RR: 0.77 (95%CI: 0.62–0.96)	VTE risk (5.3% vs. 7%) RR: 0.76 (95%CI: 0.63–0.92)

Abbreviations: RR: relative risk; VTE: venous thromboembolism.

The MEDENOX study included 1102 hospitalized patients aged > 40 years that were randomly assigned to receive enoxaparin 40 mg, enoxaparin 20 mg or placebo once daily for 6–14 days. The study showed that the incidence of VTE was significantly lower in the group of enoxaparin 40 mg compared to the placebo group (5.5% versus 14.9%). Importantly, there was no significant difference in the incidence of VTE between the groups, showing that enoxaparin 40 mg is effective in preventing VTE without increasing serious bleeding risk [5].

Similarly, the PREVENT study was a randomized, double-blind, placebo-controlled, multicenter trial of 3706 patients aged ≥ 40 years admitted to the hospital due to an acute medical condition (acute heart failure, acute respiratory failure, infection, rheumatologic disorder, inflammatory bowel disease) who were expected to be hospitalized for ≥4 days and remain in bed for ≥3 days, with at least one risk factor for VTE. The patients were randomly assigned to receive either dalteparin or placebo for 14 days and were followed

 https://doi.org/10.3390/jpm16010018

for 90 days. The primary endpoint was the combination of symptomatic DVT, symptomatic pulmonary embolism, asymptomatic proximal DVT detected by ultrasound at day 21 and sudden death by day 21. The study demonstrated that thromboprophylaxis with dalteparin the primary endpoint reduced by 45% and this effect was maintained by day 90 with the incidence of symptomatic VTE being 0.93% in the dalteparin group and 1.33% in the placebo group. By day 21, no patient in the dalteparin group and two patients in the placebo group had a fatal pulmonary embolism. Regarding safety outcomes, while minor bleeding events were slightly more frequent with dalteparin, rates of major and fatal bleeding remained very low, confirming that dalteparin effectively prevents VTE in medically ill, immobilized patients with minimal bleeding risk (fatal bleeding: 0.11% versus 0.05%, major bleeding: 0.49% versus 0.16%; minor bleeding: 1.03% versus 0.55%) [6].

The ARTEMIS trial included 849 patients aged $\geq$ 60 years that were hospitalized due to congestive heart failure, acute respiratory illness, acute infectious disease or acute inflammatory disease and had $\geq$4 days of immobilization. The patients were randomly assigned to receive either fondaparinux or placebo for 6–14 days and were followed for one month. The study showed that fondaparinux reduced the risk of VTE on venography and symptomatic VTE by 46.7%. By day 15, the incidence of VTE was 5.6% among patients who received fondaparinux compared to 10.5% among those received placebo. No difference in the frequency of major bleeding episodes was recorded between the two groups. This demonstrates that fondaparinux provides substantial protection against VTE while maintaining a favorable safety profile [7].

Overall, these trials collectively show that thromboprophylaxis with LMWH or fondaparinux is both effective and safe in acutely ill medical inpatients, particularly among older, immobilized or otherwise high-risk patients.

Beyond traditional parenteral agents, several large, randomized trials have investigated extended-duration thromboprophylaxis with direct oral anticoagulants (DOACs) in this patient population [8–10]. The ADOPT study evaluated extended thromboprophylaxis using oral apixaban 2.5 mg twice daily for 30 days versus standard enoxaparin 40 mg for 6–14 days in acutely ill patients hospitalized for at least three days with congestive heart failure, respiratory failure or other medical conditions, and who had at least one additional risk factor for VTE. The study found that the prolonged apixaban regimen did not demonstrate superior efficacy; the primary composite VTE outcome occurred in 2.71% of patients receiving apixaban compared with 3.05% of those receiving enoxaparin. Additionally, apixaban was linked to a higher rate of major bleeding events (0.47% versus 0.19%) [8].

The MAGELLAN trial enrolled 8101 patients who had been hospitalized within 72 h for an acute medical illness and had reduced mobility. Participants were randomly assigned to receive oral rivaroxaban 10 mg once daily for 35 $\pm$ 4 days or subcutaneous enoxaparin 40 mg once daily for 10 $\pm$ 4 days during hospitalization. At day 35, rivaroxaban significantly reduced the composite outcome of DVT (asymptomatic or symptomatic), symptomatic pulmonary embolism, or VTE-related death (4.4% versus 5.7% with enoxaparin), demonstrating superiority over short-term prophylaxis. However, this benefit was accompanied by a notably higher risk of clinically significant bleeding (4.1% versus 1.7%) [9].

Last but not least, the APEX trial investigated extended thromboprophylaxis with the oral factor Xa inhibitor betrixaban (80 mg once daily for 35–42 days) versus a standard shorter course of enoxaparin (40 mg for 10 $\pm$ 4 days) in patients at high risk for VTE, such as those with elevated d-dimer levels or aged 75 years and older. In the overall study population, betrixaban lowered the incidence of asymptomatic proximal DVT or symptomatic VTE compared with enoxaparin (5.3% versus 7.0%). Notably, the rates of major bleeding were comparable between the two treatment groups (0.7% versus 0.6%) [10].

https://doi.org/10.3390/jpm16010018

3. VTE and Bleeding Risk Stratification

The American Society of Hematology (ASH) has endorsed the use of risk assessment models (RAMs) as an approach to simplify VTE and bleeding risk stratification in medical inpatients and guide provision of thromboprophylaxis to those at high risk (Figure 1) [11,12]. However, despite existing guidelines [12], pharmacologic thromboprophylaxis is often either underused in high-risk patients or overused in low-risk patients. A Swiss prospective cohort study of 1352 hospitalized patients showed that 36.7% to 41.3% were categorized as high VTE risk but did not receive anticoagulants, while 37.2% to 47.6% were characterized as low VTE risk and received thromboprophylaxis, highlighting a gap between guideline recommendations and clinical practice [13]. Potential causes of underuse include limited awareness of current guidelines, uncertainty regarding individual bleeding risk, variability in clinician experience and lack of standardized institutional protocols [13,14]. Conversely, overuse may result from automated order sets that do not integrate individualized risk assessments, defensive prescribing practices or misinterpretation of VTE risk in low-risk patients [13,15,16]. Institutional protocols that mandate systematic risk assessment at admission and prior to prescribing anticoagulants can standardize care, improve adherence and reduce variability in clinical practice. These challenges highlight the importance of structured risk assessment tools and consistent clinical workflows to optimize prophylaxis.

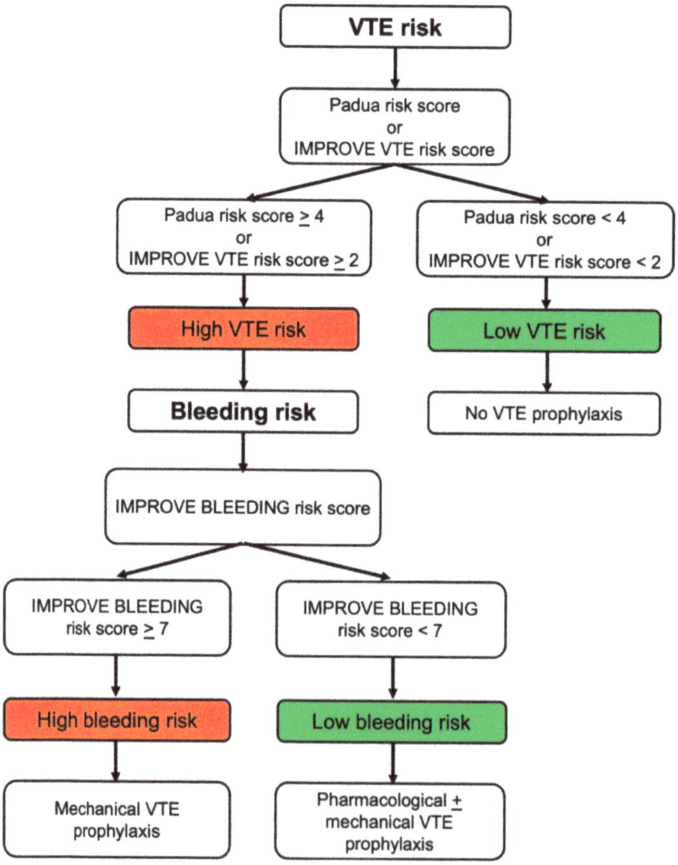

Figure 1. An individualized stepwise approach on thromboembolic prophylaxis in hospitalized patients. Abbreviation: VTE: venous thromboembolism.

https://doi.org/10.3390/jpm16010018

VTE risk scores. The Padua VTE RAM and the IMPROVE VTE RAM represent the most extensively studied validated risk scores for the identification of hospitalized patients at a greater risk for VTE. The parameters that are included in the Padua VTE RAM are: active cancer, previous VTE, reduced mobility, known thrombotic condition, recent trauma/surgery, trauma or stroke in the previous month, age > 70 years, heart or respiratory failure, acute myocardial infraction or stroke, acute infection or rheumatologic disorder, body mass index (BMI) > 30 kg/m^2 and use of hormone replacement therapy. A score of 4 or more indicates a greater VTE risk and thromboprophylaxis is recommended. The IMPROVE VTE RAM takes into account factors like previous VTE, known thrombophilia, current lower limb paralysis, active cancer, immobilization for more than seven days, age > 60 years and admission at ICU (Intensive Care Unit) or CCU (Coronary Care Unit). A score of 2 or more indicates inpatients at higher risk for VTE [12]. These tools allow clinicians to identify high-risk inpatients more accurately and target prophylaxis effectively. They can be integrated into electronic medical records (EMRs) to automatically calculate patient scores in the Emergency Department, incorporated into standardized order sets for thromboprophylaxis or included in bedside checklists for real-time risk assessment [17].

D-dimer, a fibrin degradation product, has also been recognized as a predictive factor of increased VTE risk in hospitalized patients. The MAGELLAN trial found that the incidence of VTE was 3.5-fold higher in patients with baseline d−dimer of greater than 2× the upper limit of normal (ULN). High d-dimer concentrations had similarly strong associations to already established risk factors for VTE, such as malignancy and advanced age [18]. The incorporation of d-dimer levels to the IMPROVE VTE risk score, thereby creating the modified version IMPROVEDD VTE score, was shown to improve VTE risk stratification in hospitalized patients [19]. Measuring this biomarker at admission can, thus, be combined with RAMs in EMRs or bedside checklists to further refine thromboprophylaxis decisions.

For oncology patients, the Khorana score provides validated assessment. The main parameters of the score are: stomach or pancreatic malignancy (2 points); lymphoma, lung, gynecologic, bladder or testicular cancer (1 point); pre-chemotherapy platelet count $\geq 350 \times 10^9$/L (1 point); pre-chemotherapy hemoglobin level < 10 g/dL or use of RBC (red blood cell) growth factors (1 point); pre-chemotherapy leukocyte count $> 11 \times 10^9$/L (1 point) and BMI $\geq$ 35 kg/m^2 (1 point). The Khorana score classifies cancer patients into low (0 points), intermediate (1–2 points) or high ($\geq$3 points) VTE risk [20]. Embedding this score into electronic oncology order sets allows automatic identification of high-risk patients for prophylaxis while avoiding unnecessary anticoagulation in low-risk patients.

In surgical patients, the Caprini VTE score guides thromboprophylaxis decisions by accounting 40 distinct individual VTE risk factors, such as type of surgery, and personal and family history, and distinguishes patients at low (score: 0–1), moderate (score: 2), high (score: 3–4) or very high (score $\geq$ 5) risk [21,22]. This comprehensive approach allows precise identification of surgical patients who may benefit most from prophylaxis. Integration into preoperative EMR workflows and perioperative checklists can ensure that high-risk surgical patients receive timely prophylaxis.

Table 2 summarizes the currently available VTE risk scores used in hospitalized patients.

Bleeding risk score. Even though thromboprophylaxis reduces the incidence of hospital acquired VTE, bleeding remains the most important complication in patients treated with anticoagulants. The IMPROVE (International Medical Prevention Registry on VTE) multinational, observational study demonstrated that the incidence of major and non-major bleeding within 14 days of admission was 3.2%. Active gastroduodenal ulcer, a prior bleeding event and low platelet count were the strongest independent risk factors for bleeding during hospitalization [23]. Likewise, a prospective, observational study from the Nether-

 https://doi.org/10.3390/jpm16010018

lands showed that the prevalence of in-hospital bleeding events among anticoagulant users was 7.2%, with the vast majority (78.5%) categorized as major bleeding. The median length of stay was 18 (8.5–34.5) days in patients with a bleeding event and 7 (4–13) days among those without a bleeding event. Female gender, surgical procedures (high or low bleeding risk procedures) and non-surgical interventions (endoscopic interventions, endovascular coiling) were identified as risk factors [24].

Table 2. Clinical risk scores for predicting VTE in hospitalized patients.

VTE Risk Score	Population	Risk Determinants	VTE Prophylaxis Eligibility Thresholds
Padua VTE RAM	Acutely ill medical inpatients	Active cancer, previous VTE, reduced mobility, thrombophilia, recent trauma/surgery, elderly age, heart/respiratory failure, acute MI/stroke, acute infection/rheumatologic disorder, obesity, hormone therapy	≥4: high risk
IMPROVE VTE RAM	Acutely ill medical inpatients	Previous VTE, known thrombophilia, active cancer, immobilization ≥ 7 days, ICU/CCU admission, age > 60, lower-limb paralysis	≥2: high risk
IMPROVE-DD VTE Score	Acutely ill medical inpatients	Same as IMPROVE + elevated D-dimer (≥2× ULN)	≥2: high risk
Khorana Score	Oncology patients	Cancer type, platelet count, hemoglobin or RBC growth factors use, leukocyte count, BMI ≥ 35	0: low risk 1–2: intermediate risk ≥3: high risk
Caprini VTE Score	Surgical patients	40 distinct individual VTE risk factors including age, BMI > 25, cancer, history of VTE, thrombophilia, immobilization, surgery type, pregnancy, hormonal therapy, varicose veins, edema, inflammatory conditions	0–1: low risk 2: moderate risk 3–4: high risk ≥5: very high risk

Abbreviations: BMI: body mass index; CCU: Coronary Care Unit; ICU: Intensive Care Unit; RAM: risk assessment models; RBC: red blood cells; VTE: venous thromboembolism.

The IMPROVE bleeding RAM is a validated risk score aiming to identify in-hospital patients at higher risk for bleeding. It includes 13 clinical and laboratory factors: moderate (GFR 30–59 $mL/min/m^2$) or severe (GFR < 30 $mL/min/m^2$) renal failure, male gender, age 40–84 years or ≥85 years, rheumatic disease, active malignancy, central venous catheter placement, ICU or CCU admission, liver failure (INR > 1.5), platelet count < $50 \times 10^9/L$, prior bleeding within the last three months before admission and active gastric or duodenal ulcer (Table 3). A score of 7 or more indicates patients at greater bleeding risk and should be taken into account for designing a safe and individualized thromboprophylaxis plan [12].

Integrating RAMs into routine practice has a substantial impact on healthcare resources. Accurate risk stratification reduces unnecessary use of anticoagulants, lowers the incidence of bleeding complications, optimizes pharmacy and nursing workload, and can shorten hospital stays, reducing overall costs [25–27]. Systematic implementation also enhances quality of care, ensuring evidence-based, standardized prophylaxis decisions, improving guideline adherence, reducing preventable complications, and supporting institutional performance metrics [25,28].

By combining VTE and bleeding RAMs, along with laboratory markers such as d-dimer, into electronic systems, standardized order sets and bedside checklists, clinicians can implement risk-adapted thromboprophylaxis efficiently, improving patient safety and adherence to guidelines.

https://doi.org/10.3390/jpm16010018

Table 3. IMPROVE bleeding risk score in hospitalized patients.

Predictor	Points
Active gastric or duodenal ulcer	4.5
History of bleeding within 3 months before admission	4
Platelet count < 50 × 10^9/L	4
Age 40–84 years	1.5
Age ≥ 85 years	3.5
Hepatic failure (INR > 1.5)	2.5
Moderate renal failure (GFR 30–59 mL/min)	1
Severe renal failure (GFR < 30 mL/min)	2.5
ICU or CCU admission	2.5
Central venous catheter placement	2
Rheumatic disease	2
Active cancer	2
Male sex	1

Abbreviations: CCU: Coronary Care Unit; GFR: glomerular filtration rate; ICU: Intensive Care Unit.

4. Recommendations in Specific Clinical Conditions

Heart failure. Patients with heart failure experience a greater risk for VTE, even when in sinus rhythm, mainly owing to static blood flow, hypercoagulability and endothelial dysfunction [29]. Notably, the risk is reversely correlated to left ventricular ejection fraction (LVEF). A case-control study demonstrated that a LVEF < 20% was correlated with a 38.3-fold increased risk of thromboembolic events [30]. Similarly, an analysis of the SCD-HeFT (Sudden Cardiac Death in Heart Failure Trial) showed that reduced LVEF was a significant predictor of VTE among 2114 patients without a known history of atrial fibrillation or atrial flutter. On the other hand, for every 5% rise of the LVEF, the risk of VTE decreased by 18% [31]. Hence, pharmacological prophylaxis with LMWH, fondaparinux or low-dose unfractionated heparin (UFH) is recommended in all hospitalized patients with heart failure who are not already receiving anticoagulation, unless they are at high bleeding risk [32,33].

Cancer. Malignancy is correlated with a fivefold greater hazard of VTE with the absolute risk ranging between 2% and 17% during hospitalization [34]. The risk is higher in several types of tumors, such as pancreatic, gastric, lung and primary brain cancer [35]. Therefore, thromboprophylaxis in oncological patients during hospitalization remains an important issue.

The American Society of Clinical Oncology (ASCO) [36], the European Society of Medical Oncology (ESMO) [35] and the ASH [37] have published guidelines on thromboprophylaxis among cancer inpatients. For all immobilized patients with hematologic or solid malignancies admitted to the hospital due to an acute medical illness or a planned surgical intervention, thromboprophylaxis with LMWH, fondaparinux or UFH is recommended. In non-immobilized patients, the Khorana score should be calculated and those with a score of ≤1 should not receive thromboprophylaxis, while those with a score of ≥3 are candidates for thromboprophylaxis with LMWH, fondaparinux or UFH. In patients with a Khorana score of 2 and no additional individual risk factors for VTE, including immobilization at home, thrombogenic therapy, history of VTE and hereditary thrombophilia, thromboprophylaxis is not indicated. On the other hand, in patients with a Khorana score of 2 and at least one of the aforementioned individual risk factors for VTE, thromboprophylaxis should be considered based on the presence or absence of risk factors for bleeding, such as severe thrombocytopenia, susceptibility to falls or history of bleeding. In the presence of bleeding risk factors, thromboprophylaxis is contraindicated; otherwise, thromboprophylaxis is suggested (Figure 2) [35–37].

 https://doi.org/10.3390/jpm16010018

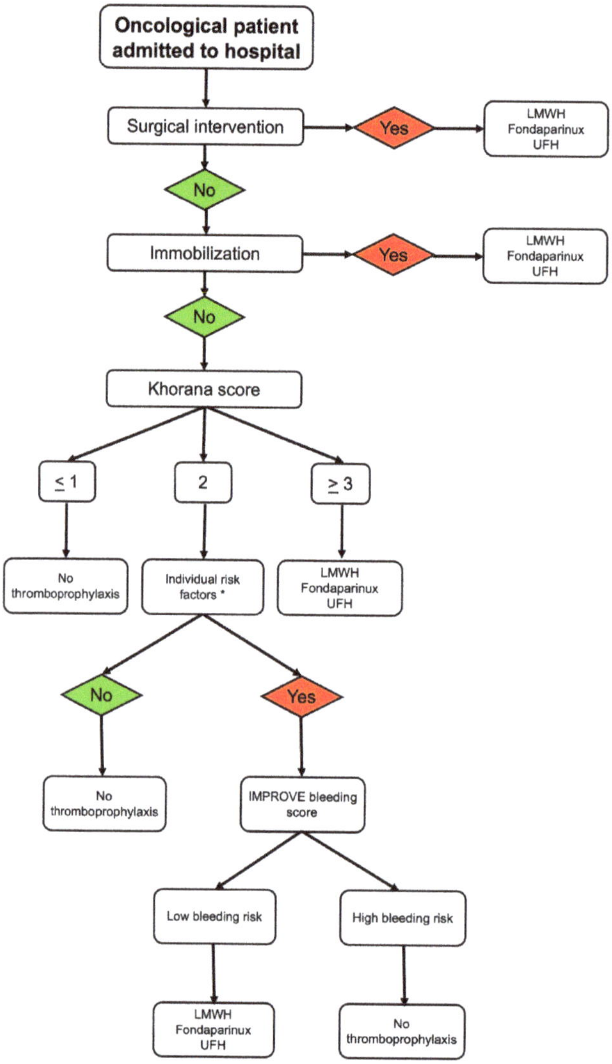

Figure 2. A proposed algorithm for thromboprophylaxis in hospitalized cancer patients. * immobilization at home, thrombogenic therapy, history of VTE, hereditary thrombophilia. Abbreviations: low-molecular-weight heparin (LMWH); unfractionated heparin (UFH); VTE: venous thromboprophylaxis.

Surgery. VTE is considered a serious complication in surgical patients receiving general anesthesia during hospitalization and it seems that the risk remains elevated up to two months following discharge [38,39]. Procedure type and duration, infectious complications and patient-specific factors, such as age, comorbidities and a personal history of VTE, play a crucial role in postoperative VTE risk [21].

The ASH recommends both mechanical and pharmacological thromboprophylaxis in patients at high VTE risk and suggests mechanical methods over pharmacological thromboprophylaxis in patients at high bleeding risk. In cases of mechanical thromboprophylaxis, intermittent compression devices are indicated over graduated compression stockings [40].

Major lower-extremity orthopedic surgeries, including total or partial knee or hip arthroplasty surgery and hip fracture repair, carry a greater risk for VTE compared to other

https://doi.org/10.3390/jpm16010018

orthopedic procedures, with the estimated incidence being approximately 4% [41]. Thus, thromboprophylaxis with aspirin or anticoagulants is suggested for patients who have undergone hip or knee arthroplasty. When anticoagulants are used, DOACs, LMWH or fondaparinux are recommended over warfarin and UFH. For patients after hip fracture repair, thromboprophylaxis with LMWH, fondaparinux or UFH is suggested [40,42].

Pharmacological thromboprophylaxis with LMWH or UFH is also preferred in patients who have undergone a major general surgery. Likewise, pharmacological prophylaxis with LMWH over UFH is recommended only in patients who have undergone major neurosurgical procedures and experiencing prolonged immobility following surgery. On the other hand, the ASH guidelines suggests against pharmacological prophylaxis in patients who have undergone laparoscopic cholecystectomy, transurethral resection of the prostate or radical prostatectomy, excluding those with known risk factors for VTE, such as a history of VTE, thrombophilia and malignancy. For those experiencing major trauma or who have undergone a major gynecological surgery, no pharmacological thromboprophylaxis is suggested [40]. Figure 3 summarizes current recommendations on thromboprophylaxis in surgical patients admitted to the hospital.

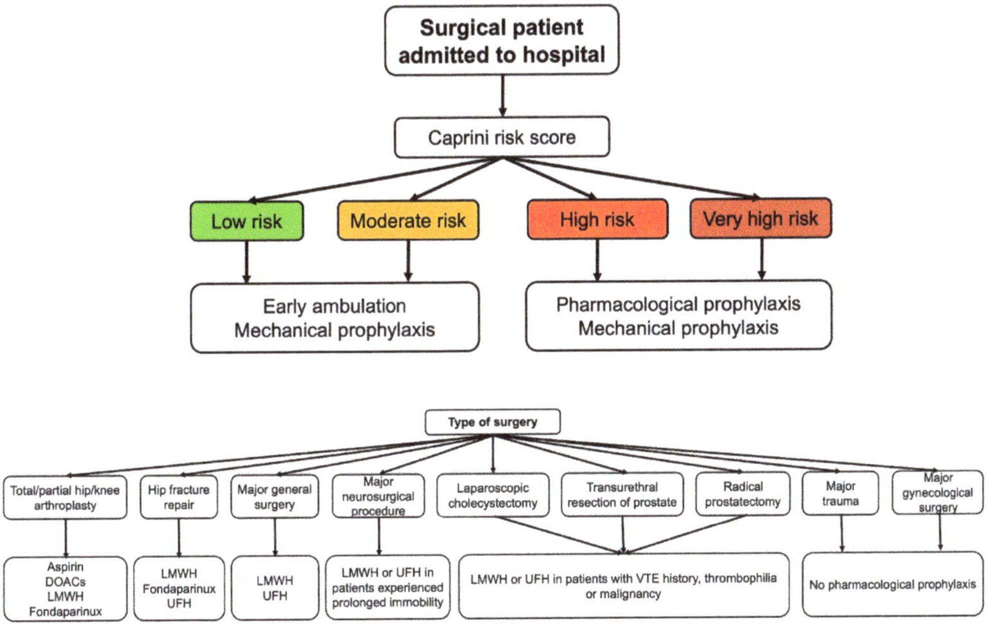

Figure 3. Thromboprophylaxis in hospitalized patients who have undergone surgical procedures. Abbreviations: DOACs: direct oral anticoagulants; LMWH: low-molecular-weight heparin; UFH: unfractionated heparin; VTE: venous thromboprophylaxis.

Stroke. VTE represents a common complication among immobile hospitalized patients with acute ischemic stroke [43]. However, these patients are at increased risk of hemorrhagic transformation [44] and managing thromboprophylaxis in this setting is a key challenge. The European Stroke Organization (ESO) advises intermittent pneumatic compression (thigh-length, sequential) combined with pharmacological prophylaxis, namely UFH, LMWH or heparinoid, for immobile patients hospitalized due to acute ischemic stroke [45]. Fondaparinux represents an alternative option since it seems to be as safe as UFH for VTE prophylaxis in this population. An analysis of 644 consecutive patients with acute ischemic stroke that were randomly assigned to receive either fondaparinux or

https://doi.org/10.3390/jpm16010018

UFH showed that major hemorrhages were less common in the fondaparinux group (1.2%) compared to the UFH group (3.7%), but this difference was not statistically significant [46].

VTE is also a serious concern in patients with acute non-traumatic intracerebral hemorrhage, affecting approximately 7% [47]. Meanwhile, the risk of DVT is four times greater than in those with acute ischemic stroke [48]. The American Heart Association (AHA) and the American Stroke Association suggest intermittent pneumatic compression from the day of diagnosis and initiating low-dose UFH or LMWH in order to reduce the risk for pulmonary embolism at 24–48 h from ICH onset in non-ambulatory patients [49].

Sepsis/septic shock. Septic patients are invariably affected by activation of coagulation and are at high risk for VTE. A study of approximately five million admissions with the diagnosis of sepsis (sepsis without shock: 4,050,824 hospitalizations, septic shock: 968,545) showed that the incidence of pulmonary embolism was 1.2% among those with sepsis and 2.3% among those with septic shock [50]. Another study of 918 hospitalized septic patients demonstrated that the incidence of DVT was 23.4% [51]. The Surviving Sepsis Campaign (SSG) guidelines recommend the use of pharmacological VTE prophylaxis with LMWH over UFH in hospitalized patients with sepsis or septic shock for VTE prevention [52].

Chronic kidney disease. Available evidence indicates that chronic kidney disease (CKD) is associated with hypercoagulability, increasing the risk of VTE in this population [53]. A large community-based study that included about 19,000 middle-aged and elderly adults demonstrated that the relative VTE risk was 1.28 among those with mild renal impairment and 2.09 among those with stage 3/4 CKD after adjustment for age, gender, race and center compared to those with normal kidney function [54]. Paradoxically, CKD is correlated with a 35% higher risk for bleeding [55]. Given that both thrombotic and bleeding risk are elevated in patients with CKD, the clinical decision on thromboprophylaxis is challenging. The National Institute for Health and Care Excellence (NICE) suggests to balance the individual VTE and bleeding risk and, if indicated, LMWH or UFH should be given in a reduced dose [56].

Table 4 summarizes the recommended thromboprophylaxis regimens for hospitalized patients across specific clinical conditions.

Table 4. Recommended thromboprophylaxis regimens for inpatients in specific clinical settings.

Clinical Condition	Recommended Thromboprophylaxis Regimens
Heart failure [32,33]	LMWH, fondaparinux, or low-dose UFH
Cancer [35–37]	LMWH, fondaparinux, or UFH
Major general surgery [40]	LMWH or UFH
Hip or knee arthroplasty [40,42]	LMWH, fondaparinux, DOACs, or aspirin
Hip fracture repair [40,42]	LMWH, fondaparinux, UFH
Major neurosurgery [40]	LMWH preferred over UFH
Acute ischemic stroke [45,46]	Intermittent pneumatic compression + LMWH, UFH, fondaparinux or heparinoid
Intracerebral hemorrhage [49]	Intermittent pneumatic compression + low-dose UFH or LMWH
Sepsis/septic shock [52]	LMWH preferred over UFH
Chronic kidney disease [56]	LMWH or UFH (dose-adjusted)

Abbreviations: DOACs: direct oral anticoagulants; UFH: unfractionated heparin; LMWH: low-molecular-weight heparin.

5. Limitations and Future Directions

Despite extensive research supporting thromboprophylaxis in hospitalized patients, several evidence gaps remain. The predictive performance and generalizability of existing RAMs, such as the Padua, IMPROVE, Caprini and Khorana scores, require further validation across diverse populations, including elderly, multi-morbid and renal-impaired patients [57]. Implementation strategies for integrating RAMs into clinical workflows,

 https://doi.org/10.3390/jpm16010018

electronic health records and standardized order sets are not fully established [58], and clinician adherence to risk-guided prophylaxis remains variable [59].

It is important to emphasize that no risk-assessment tool is perfect, and clinical judgment should remain central to decision-making. While RAMs provide structured guidance, they cannot account for all factors influencing an individual patient's thrombotic risk. These scores should be interpreted within the context of each patient's overall clinical condition, with the multidisciplinary team weighing the potential benefits and risks of anticoagulation. Engaging patients in shared decision-making is essential to ensure they understand their personalized risk–benefit profile before initiating prophylaxis. In this way, RAMs serve as a supportive tool rather than a substitute for careful, individualized clinical evaluation.

In addition, economic and patient-centered outcomes warrant further investigation. Evidence on the cost-effectiveness of RAM-guided prophylaxis, including impacts on hospital stay, drug utilization and overall healthcare resources, remains limited. Furthermore, few studies have assessed long-term patient-centered outcomes, such as quality of life, functional recovery or patient preferences. Evidence gaps also persist in special populations, including patients with obesity, sepsis or multiple comorbidities, who are often underrepresented in clinical trials. Addressing these gaps is crucial to optimizing individualized thromboprophylaxis strategies and informing future research and clinical practice.

6. Conclusions

Thromboprophylaxis plays a critical role in preventing VTE among hospitalized patients and an individualized approach is essential. The clinical decision to initiate thromboprophylaxis during hospitalization involves assessing various factors, such as the patient's thrombotic and bleeding risk and the type of medical condition or surgery. The main pharmacologic options for thromboprophylaxis include LMWH, UFH and fondaparinux. Pharmacological thromboprophylaxis is recommended in all hospitalized patients with heart failure, malignancy or sepsis/septic shock, unless they are at high bleeding risk. Patients who have undergone a major lower-extremity orthopedic surgery or a major general surgery are candidates for both mechanical and pharmacological thromboprophylaxis. Thromboprophylaxis is indicated for immobile patients hospitalized due to acute ischemic stroke. In non-ambulatory patients with ICH, intermittent pneumatic compression is recommended from the day of diagnosis while low-dose UFH or LMWH should be initiated 24–48 h from symptom onset. Anticoagulants in reduced dose are suggested in hospitalized patients with CKD.

Author Contributions: Conceptualization, J.P.; literature search and data curation, M.V.; writing—original draft preparation, M.V.; writing—review and editing, V.B., E.P. and J.P.; supervision: E.P. and J.P. All authors have read and agreed to the published version of the manuscript.

Funding: This research received no external funding.

Institutional Review Board Statement: Not applicable.

Informed Consent Statement: Not applicable.

Data Availability Statement: No new data were created or analyzed in this study. Data sharing is not applicable to this article.

Conflicts of Interest: E.P. received honoraria for lectures from Astra Zeneca, Bayer, Roche Diagnostics and GE Healthcare, unrelated to this work. J.P. received honoraria for lectures from Bayer, Pfizer, Astra and Viatris. V.B. received honoraria for lectures from Astra Zeneca, Bayer, Boehringer Ingelheim and Pfizer. M.V. declares no conflicts of interest.

https://doi.org/10.3390/jpm16010018

References

1. Lutsey, P.L.; Zakai, N.A. Epidemiology and prevention of venous thromboembolism. *Nat. Rev. Cardiol.* **2023**, *20*, 248–262. [CrossRef] [PubMed] [PubMed Central]
2. Pastori, D.; Cormaci, V.M.; Marucci, S.; Franchino, G.; Del Sole, F.; Capozza, A.; Fallarino, A.; Corso, C.; Valeriani, E.; Menichelli, D.; et al. A Comprehensive Review of Risk Factors for Venous Thromboembolism: From Epidemiology to Pathophysiology. *Int. J. Mol. Sci.* **2023**, *24*, 3169. [CrossRef]
3. Khan, F.; Tritschler, T.; Kahn, S.R.; Rodger, M.A. Venous thromboembolism. *Lancet* **2021**, *398*, 64–77. [CrossRef]
4. Jordan Bruno, X.; Koh, I.; Lutsey, P.L.; Walker, R.F.; Roetker, N.S.; Wilkinson, K.; Smith, N.L.; Plante, T.B.; Repp, A.B.; Holmes, C.E.; et al. Venous thrombosis risk during and after medical and surgical hospitalizations: The medical inpatient thrombosis and hemostasis (MITH) study. *J. Thromb. Haemost.* **2022**, *20*, 1645–1652. [CrossRef]
5. Samama, M.M.; Cohen, A.T.; Darmon, J.Y.; Desjardins, L.; Eldor, A.; Janbon, C.; Leizorovicz, A.; Nguyen, H.; Olsson, C.G.; Turpie, A.G.; et al. A comparison of enoxaparin with placebo for the prevention of venous thromboembolism in acutely ill medical patients. Prophylaxis in Medical Patients with Enoxaparin Study Group. *N. Engl. J. Med.* **1999**, *341*, 793–800. [CrossRef]
6. Leizorovicz, A.; Cohen, A.T.; Turpie, A.G.; Olsson, C.G.; Vaitkus, P.T.; Goldhaber, S.Z.; Group, P.M.T.S. Randomized, placebo-controlled trial of dalteparin for the prevention of venous thromboembolism in acutely ill medical patients. *Circulation* **2004**, *110*, 874–879. [CrossRef]
7. Cohen, A.T.; Davidson, B.L.; Gallus, A.S.; Lassen, M.R.; Prins, M.H.; Tomkowski, W.; Turpie, A.G.; Egberts, J.F.; Lensing, A.W.; Investigators, A. Efficacy and safety of fondaparinux for the prevention of venous thromboembolism in older acute medical patients: Randomised placebo controlled trial. *BMJ* **2006**, *332*, 325–329. [CrossRef]
8. Goldhaber, S.Z.; Leizorovicz, A.; Kakkar, A.K.; Haas, S.K.; Merli, G.; Knabb, R.M.; Weitz, J.I.; Investigators, A.T. Apixaban versus enoxaparin for thromboprophylaxis in medically ill patients. *N. Engl. J. Med.* **2011**, *365*, 2167–2177. [CrossRef]
9. Cohen, A.T.; Spiro, T.E.; Spyropoulos, A.C.; Committee, M.S. Rivaroxaban for thromboprophylaxis in acutely ill medical patients. *N. Engl. J. Med.* **2013**, *368*, 1945–1946. [CrossRef]
10. Cohen, A.T.; Harrington, R.A.; Goldhaber, S.Z.; Hull, R.D.; Wiens, B.L.; Gold, A.; Hernandez, A.F.; Gibson, C.M.; Investigators, A. Extended Thromboprophylaxis with Betrixaban in Acutely Ill Medical Patients. *N. Engl. J. Med.* **2016**, *375*, 534–544. [CrossRef]
11. Djulbegovic, B.; Boylan, A.; Kolo, S.; Scheurer, D.B.; Anuskiewicz, S.; Khaledi, F.; Youkhana, K.; Madgwick, S.; Maharjan, N.; Hozo, I. Converting IMPROVE bleeding and VTE risk assessment models into a fast-and-frugal decision tree for optimal hospital VTE prophylaxis. *Blood Adv.* **2024**, *8*, 3214–3224. [CrossRef]
12. Schunemann, H.J.; Cushman, M.; Burnett, A.E.; Kahn, S.R.; Beyer-Westendorf, J.; Spencer, F.A.; Rezende, S.M.; Zakai, N.A.; Bauer, K.A.; Dentali, F.; et al. American Society of Hematology 2018 guidelines for management of venous thromboembolism: Prophylaxis for hospitalized and nonhospitalized medical patients. *Blood Adv.* **2018**, *2*, 3198–3225. [CrossRef]
13. Kocher, B.; Darbellay Farhoumand, P.; Pulver, D.; Kopp, B.; Choffat, D.; Tritschler, T.; Vollenweider, P.; Reny, J.L.; Rodondi, N.; Aujesky, D.; et al. Overuse and underuse of thromboprophylaxis in medical inpatients. *Res. Pract. Thromb. Haemost.* **2023**, *7*, 102184. [CrossRef]
14. Bikdeli, B.; Sharif-Kashani, B.; Raeissi, S.; Ehteshami-Afshar, S.; Behzadnia, N.; Masjedi, M.R. Chest physicians' knowledge of appropriate thromboprophylaxis: Insights from the PROMOTE study. *Blood Coagul. Fibrinolysis* **2011**, *22*, 667–672. [CrossRef]
15. Nendaz, M.R.; Chopard, P.; Lovis, C.; Kucher, N.; Asmis, L.M.; Dorffler, J.; Spirk, D.; Bounameaux, H. Adequacy of venous thromboprophylaxis in acutely ill medical patients (IMPART): Multisite comparison of different clinical decision support systems. *J. Thromb. Haemost.* **2010**, *8*, 1230–1234. [CrossRef]
16. Khanna, R.; Vittinghoff, E.; Maselli, J.; Auerbach, A. Unintended consequences of a standard admission order set on venous thromboembolism prophylaxis and patient outcomes. *J. Gen. Intern. Med.* **2012**, *27*, 318–324. [CrossRef]
17. Loh, S.; Wijaya, K.; Rogers, M.; Asghari-Jafarabadi, M.; Wojnar, R. A clinical decision support tool for improving venous thromboembolism risk assessment and thromboprophylaxis prescribing compliance within an electronic medication management system: A retrospective observational study. *Int. J. Clin. Pharm.* **2025**, *47*, 699–707. [CrossRef]
18. Cohen, A.T.; Spiro, T.E.; Spyropoulos, A.C.; Desanctis, Y.H.; Homering, M.; Buller, H.R.; Haskell, L.; Hu, D.; Hull, R.; Mebazaa, A.; et al. D-dimer as a predictor of venous thromboembolism in acutely ill, hospitalized patients: A subanalysis of the randomized controlled MAGELLAN trial. *J. Thromb. Haemost.* **2014**, *12*, 479–487. [CrossRef]
19. Gibson, C.M.; Spyropoulos, A.C.; Cohen, A.T.; Hull, R.D.; Goldhaber, S.Z.; Yusen, R.D.; Hernandez, A.F.; Korjian, S.; Daaboul, Y.; Gold, A.; et al. The IMPROVEDD VTE Risk Score: Incorporation of D-Dimer into the IMPROVE Score to Improve Venous Thromboembolism Risk Stratification. *TH Open* **2017**, *1*, e56–e65. [CrossRef]
20. Parker, A.; Peterson, E.; Lee, A.Y.Y.; de Wit, C.; Carrier, M.; Polley, G.; Tien, J.; Wu, C. Risk stratification for the development of venous thromboembolism in hospitalized patients with cancer. *J. Thromb. Haemost.* **2018**, *16*, 1321–1326. [CrossRef]
21. Henke, P.K.; Kahn, S.R.; Pannucci, C.J.; Secemksy, E.A.; Evans, N.S.; Khorana, A.A.; Creager, M.A.; Pradhan, A.D.; American Heart Association Advocacy Coordinating Committee. Call to Action to Prevent Venous Thromboembolism in Hospitalized Patients: A Policy Statement From the American Heart Association. *Circulation* **2020**, *141*, e914–e931. [CrossRef] [PubMed]

 https://doi.org/10.3390/jpm16010018

22. Caprini, J.A.; Tapson, V.F.; Hyers, T.M.; Waldo, A.L.; Wittkowsky, A.K.; Friedman, R.; Colgan, K.J.; Shillington, A.C.; Committee, N.S. Treatment of venous thromboembolism: Adherence to guidelines and impact of physician knowledge, attitudes, and beliefs. *J. Vasc. Surg.* **2005**, *42*, 726–733. [CrossRef] [PubMed]
23. Decousus, H.; Tapson, V.F.; Bergmann, J.F.; Chong, B.H.; Froehlich, J.B.; Kakkar, A.K.; Merli, G.J.; Monreal, M.; Nakamura, M.; Pavanello, R.; et al. Factors at admission associated with bleeding risk in medical patients: Findings from the IMPROVE investigators. *Chest* **2011**, *139*, 69–79. [CrossRef]
24. Dreijer, A.R.; Diepstraten, J.; Brouwer, R.; Croles, F.N.; Kragten, E.; Leebeek, F.W.G.; Kruip, M.; van den Bemt, P. Risk of bleeding in hospitalized patients on anticoagulant therapy: Prevalence and potential risk factors. *Eur. J. Intern. Med.* **2019**, *62*, 17–23. [CrossRef]
25. Bakhsh, E. The Benefits and Imperative of Venous Thromboembolism Risk Screening for Hospitalized Patients: A Systematic Review. *J. Clin. Med.* **2023**, *12*, 7009. [CrossRef]
26. Baser, O.; Sengupta, N.; Dysinger, A.; Wang, L. Thromboembolism prophylaxis in medical inpatients: Effect on outcomes and costs. *Am. J. Manag. Care* **2012**, *18*, 294–302.
27. Davis, S.; Goodacre, S.; Horner, D.; Pandor, A.; Holland, M.; de Wit, K.; Hunt, B.J.; Griffin, X.L. Effectiveness and cost effectiveness of pharmacological thromboprophylaxis for medical inpatients: Decision analysis modelling study. *BMJ Med.* **2024**, *3*, e000408. [CrossRef]
28. Abboud, J.; Abdel Rahman, A.; Kahale, L.; Dempster, M.; Adair, P. Prevention of health care associated venous thromboembolism through implementing VTE prevention clinical practice guidelines in hospitalized medical patients: A systematic review and meta-analysis. *Implement. Sci.* **2020**, *15*, 49. [CrossRef]
29. Lin, A.Y.; Dinatolo, E.; Metra, M.; Sbolli, M.; Dasseni, N.; Butler, J.; Greenberg, B.H. Thromboembolism in Heart Failure Patients in Sinus Rhythm: Epidemiology, Pathophysiology, Clinical Trials, and Future Direction. *JACC Heart Fail.* **2021**, *9*, 243–253. [CrossRef]
30. Howell, M.D.; Geraci, J.M.; Knowlton, A.A. Congestive heart failure and outpatient risk of venous thromboembolism: A retrospective, case-control study. *J. Clin. Epidemiol.* **2001**, *54*, 810–816. [CrossRef]
31. Freudenberger, R.S.; Hellkamp, A.S.; Halperin, J.L.; Poole, J.; Anderson, J.; Johnson, G.; Mark, D.B.; Lee, K.L.; Bardy, G.H.; Investigators, S.C.-H. Risk of thromboembolism in heart failure: An analysis from the Sudden Cardiac Death in Heart Failure Trial (SCD-HeFT). *Circulation* **2007**, *115*, 2637–2641. [CrossRef]
32. McDonagh, T.A.; Metra, M.; Adamo, M.; Gardner, R.S.; Baumbach, A.; Bohm, M.; Burri, H.; Butler, J.; Celutkiene, J.; Chioncel, O.; et al. 2021 ESC Guidelines for the diagnosis and treatment of acute and chronic heart failure. *Eur. Heart J.* **2021**, *42*, 3599–3726. [CrossRef]
33. Ng, T.M.; Tsai, F.; Khatri, N.; Barakat, M.N.; Elkayam, U. Venous thromboembolism in hospitalized patients with heart failure: Incidence, prognosis, and prevention. *Circ. Heart Fail.* **2010**, *3*, 165–173. [CrossRef]
34. Patell, R.; Zwicker, J.I. Inpatient prophylaxis in cancer patients: Where is the evidence? *Thromb. Res.* **2020**, *191*, S85–S90. [CrossRef]
35. Falanga, A.; Ay, C.; Di Nisio, M.; Gerotziafas, G.; Jara-Palomares, L.; Langer, F.; Lecumberri, R.; Mandala, M.; Maraveyas, A.; Pabinger, I.; et al. Venous thromboembolism in cancer patients: ESMO Clinical Practice Guideline. *Ann. Oncol.* **2023**, *34*, 452–467. [CrossRef]
36. Key, N.S.; Khorana, A.A.; Kuderer, N.M.; Bohlke, K.; Lee, A.Y.Y.; Arcelus, J.I.; Wong, S.L.; Balaban, E.P.; Flowers, C.R.; Gates, L.E.; et al. Venous Thromboembolism Prophylaxis and Treatment in Patients With Cancer: ASCO Guideline Update. *J. Clin. Oncol.* **2023**, *41*, 3063–3071. [CrossRef]
37. Lyman, G.H.; Carrier, M.; Ay, C.; Di Nisio, M.; Hicks, L.K.; Khorana, A.A.; Leavitt, A.D.; Lee, A.Y.Y.; Macbeth, F.; Morgan, R.L.; et al. American Society of Hematology 2021 guidelines for management of venous thromboembolism: Prevention and treatment in patients with cancer. *Blood Adv.* **2021**, *5*, 927–974. [CrossRef]
38. Cohen, A.T.; Tapson, V.F.; Bergmann, J.F.; Goldhaber, S.Z.; Kakkar, A.K.; Deslandes, B.; Huang, W.; Zayaruzny, M.; Emery, L.; Anderson, F.A., Jr.; et al. Venous thromboembolism risk and prophylaxis in the acute hospital care setting (ENDORSE study): A multinational cross-sectional study. *Lancet* **2008**, *371*, 387–394. [CrossRef]
39. Exposito-Ruiz, M.; Arcelus, J.I.; Caprini, J.A.; Lopez-Espada, C.; Bura-Riviere, A.; Amado, C.; Loring, M.; Mastroiacovo, D.; Monreal, M.; Investigators, R. Timing and characteristics of venous thromboembolism after noncancer surgery. *J. Vasc. Surg. Venous Lymphat. Disord.* **2021**, *9*, 859–867 e852. [CrossRef]
40. Anderson, D.R.; Morgano, G.P.; Bennett, C.; Dentali, F.; Francis, C.W.; Garcia, D.A.; Kahn, S.R.; Rahman, M.; Rajasekhar, A.; Rogers, F.B.; et al. American Society of Hematology 2019 guidelines for management of venous thromboembolism: Prevention of venous thromboembolism in surgical hospitalized patients. *Blood Adv.* **2019**, *3*, 3898–3944. [CrossRef]
41. Jones, A.; Al-Horani, R.A. Venous Thromboembolism Prophylaxis in Major Orthopedic Surgeries and Factor XIa Inhibitors. *Med. Sci.* **2023**, *11*, 49. [CrossRef]
42. Yin, Q.; Han, L.; Wang, Y.; Kang, F.; Cai, F.; Wu, L.; Zheng, X.; Li, L.; Dong, L.E.; Dong, L.; et al. Unlocking the potential of fondaparinux: Guideline for optimal usage and clinical suggestions (2023). *Front. Pharmacol.* **2024**, *15*, 1352982. [CrossRef]

 https://doi.org/10.3390/jpm16010018

43. Rinde, L.B.; Smabrekke, B.; Mathiesen, E.B.; Lochen, M.L.; Njolstad, I.; Hald, E.M.; Wilsgaard, T.; Braekkan, S.K.; Hansen, J.B. Ischemic Stroke and Risk of Venous Thromboembolism in the General Population: The Tromso Study. *J. Am. Heart Assoc.* **2016**, *5*, 11. [CrossRef]
44. Zubair, A.S.; Sheth, K.N. Hemorrhagic Conversion of Acute Ischemic Stroke. *Neurotherapeutics* **2023**, *20*, 705–711. [CrossRef]
45. Dennis, M.; Caso, V.; Kappelle, L.J.; Pavlovic, A.; Sandercock, P.; European Stroke, O. European Stroke Organisation (ESO) guidelines for prophylaxis for venous thromboembolism in immobile patients with acute ischaemic stroke. *Eur. Stroke J.* **2016**, *1*, 6–19. [CrossRef]
46. Hackett, C.T.; Ramanathan, R.S.; Malhotra, K.; Quigley, M.R.; Kelly, K.M.; Tian, M.; Protetch, J.; Wong, C.; Wright, D.G.; Tayal, A.H. Safety of venous thromboembolism prophylaxis with fondaparinux in ischemic stroke. *Thromb. Res.* **2015**, *135*, 249–254. [CrossRef]
47. Goldstein, J.N.; Fazen, L.E.; Wendell, L.; Chang, Y.; Rost, N.S.; Snider, R.; Schwab, K.; Chanderraj, R.; Kabrhel, C.; Kinnecom, C.; et al. Risk of thromboembolism following acute intracerebral hemorrhage. *Neurocrit. Care* **2009**, *10*, 28–34. [CrossRef]
48. Raslan, A.M.; Fields, J.D.; Bhardwaj, A. Prophylaxis for venous thrombo-embolism in neurocritical care: A critical appraisal. *Neurocrit. Care* **2010**, *12*, 297–309. [CrossRef]
49. Greenberg, S.M.; Ziai, W.C.; Cordonnier, C.; Dowlatshahi, D.; Francis, B.; Goldstein, J.N.; Hemphill, J.C., 3rd; Johnson, R.; Keigher, K.M.; Mack, W.J.; et al. 2022 Guideline for the Management of Patients With Spontaneous Intracerebral Hemorrhage: A Guideline From the American Heart Association/American Stroke Association. *Stroke* **2022**, *53*, e282–e361. [CrossRef] [PubMed]
50. Hasegawa, D.; Sato, R.; Lee, Y.I.; Wang, H.Y.; Nishida, K.; Steiger, D. The prevalence, risk factors, and outcomes of acute pulmonary embolism complicating sepsis and septic shock: A national inpatient sample analysis. *Sci. Rep.* **2024**, *14*, 16049. [CrossRef]
51. Wang, L.; Ma, X.; Chen, Y.; Gao, S.; Pan, W.; Chen, J.; Su, L.; He, H.; Long, Y.; Yin, C.; et al. Factors influencing DVT formation in sepsis. *Thromb. J.* **2024**, *22*, 11. [CrossRef]
52. Evans, L.; Rhodes, A.; Alhazzani, W.; Antonelli, M.; Coopersmith, C.M.; French, C.; Machado, F.R.; McIntyre, L.; Ostermann, M.; Prescott, H.C.; et al. Surviving Sepsis Campaign: International Guidelines for Management of Sepsis and Septic Shock 2021. *Crit. Care Med.* **2021**, *49*, e1063–e1143. [CrossRef]
53. Adams, M.J.; Irish, A.B.; Watts, G.F.; Oostryck, R.; Dogra, G.K. Hypercoagulability in chronic kidney disease is associated with coagulation activation but not endothelial function. *Thromb. Res.* **2008**, *123*, 374–380. [CrossRef]
54. Wattanakit, K.; Cushman, M.; Stehman-Breen, C.; Heckbert, S.R.; Folsom, A.R. Chronic kidney disease increases risk for venous thromboembolism. *J. Am. Soc. Nephrol.* **2008**, *19*, 135–140. [CrossRef]
55. Mahady, S.E.; Polekhina, G.; Woods, R.L.; Wolfe, R.; Wetmore, J.B.; Margolis, K.L.; Wood, E.M.; Cloud, G.C.; Murray, A.M.; Polkinghorne, K.R. Association Between CKD and Major Hemorrhage in Older Persons: Data From the Aspirin in Reducing Events in the Elderly Randomized Trial. *Kidney Int. Rep.* **2023**, *8*, 737–745. [CrossRef]
56. National Guideline Centre (UK). *Venous Thromboembolism in Over 16s: Reducing the Risk of Hospital-Acquired Deep Vein Thrombosis or Pulmonary Embolism*; National Institute for Health and Care Excellence (NICE): London, UK, 2018. Available online: https://pubmed.ncbi.nlm.nih.gov/29697228/ (accessed on 1 December 2025). [PubMed]
57. Pandor, A.; Tonkins, M.; Goodacre, S.; Sworn, K.; Clowes, M.; Griffin, X.L.; Holland, M.; Hunt, B.J.; de Wit, K.; Horner, D. Risk assessment models for venous thromboembolism in hospitalised adult patients: A systematic review. *BMJ Open* **2021**, *11*, e045672. [CrossRef] [PubMed]
58. Li, R.C.; Wang, J.K.; Sharp, C.; Chen, J.H. When order sets do not align with clinician workflow: Assessing practice patterns in the electronic health record. *BMJ Qual. Saf.* **2019**, *28*, 987–996. [CrossRef]
59. Schleyer, A.M.; Schreuder, A.B.; Jarman, K.M.; Logerfo, J.P.; Goss, J.R. Adherence to guideline-directed venous thromboembolism prophylaxis among medical and surgical inpatients at 33 academic medical centers in the United States. *Am. J. Med. Qual.* **2011**, *26*, 174–180. [CrossRef] [PubMed]

https://doi.org/10.3390/jpm16010018

Journal of
Personalized Medicine

MDPI

Review

Occupational Radiation Risk Stratification and Protection in Fluoroscopy-Guided Surgeons and Interventionalists: A Multispecialty Structured Narrative Review

Nana Kwadwo Okraku-Yirenkyi †, Sri Snehita Reddy Bonthu †, Hanisha Bhakta, Oluwatoyin O. Duyile and Michael Bernas *

Anne Burnett School of Medicine, Texas Christian University, Fort Worth, TX 76104, USA; n.k.okraku@tcu.edu (N.K.O.-Y.); snehita.bonthu@tcu.edu (S.S.R.B.); hanisha.h.bhakta@tcu.edu (H.B.); o.duyile@tcu.edu (O.O.D.)

* Correspondence: m.bernas@tcu.edu

† These authors contributed equally to this work.

Abstract

Background/Objectives: Fluoroscopy-guided procedures are widely used across surgical and interventional specialties but expose operators to ionizing radiation with associated stochastic and deterministic effects. The aim is to characterize occupational radiation exposure, evaluate the effectiveness of shielding strategies, assess long-term cancer risks, and identify compliance patterns. **Methods:** This structured narrative review summarizes evidence on operator dose, shielding effectiveness, compliance with protective practices, and long-term cancer risk. A search of PubMed, Scopus, Embase, and Web of Science (limited to January 2000–March 2024) identified 62 records; 27 full texts were reviewed, and 16 studies met the inclusion criteria. **Results:** Across studies, unshielded chest exposure averaged 0.08–0.11 mSv per procedure, and eye exposure averaged 0.04–0.05 mSv. Lead aprons reduced exposure by about 90% at 0.25 mm and 99% at 0.5 mm, thyroid collars reduced neck dose by 60–70%, and lead glasses reduced ocular dose 2.5–4.5-fold. Compliance with aprons and thyroid collars was high, whereas lead glasses and lower-body shielding were inconsistently used. Limited epidemiologic data suggested a higher cancer burden in exposed surgeons, and Biologic Effects of Ionizing Radiation (BEIR) VII–based modeling projected increased lifetime risks of solid cancers in chronically exposed operators. **Conclusions:** Protective equipment substantially reduces operator dose, but exposure variability and inconsistent shielding practices persist and justify standardized monitoring, stronger enforcement of radiation safety protocols, and longitudinal studies.

Keywords: occupational radiation exposure; fluoroscopy-guided procedures; shielding effectiveness; lead aprons; thyroid collars; lead glasses; cancer risk

1. Introduction

Fluoroscopy-guided procedures are increasingly integral to modern surgical practice, particularly in specialties such as orthopedic and trauma surgery, interventional cardiology, interventional radiology, vascular surgery, and cardiothoracic surgery. These techniques offer precision and minimally invasive approaches but also expose operators to ionizing radiation, presenting a persistent occupational hazard. A recent publication by Smith-Bindman et al. has highlighted the risk to physicians from work-related exposure to radiation in some specialties utilizing medical imaging [1].

Ionizing radiation is classified as a Group I human carcinogen by the International Agency for Research on Cancer [2]. International guidelines from organizations such as the International Commission on Radiological Protection (ICRP) recommend dose limits of 20 mSv per year with limits on equivalent dose to the lens of the eye of 20 mSv and of 500 mSv to the skin, hands and feet [3,4]. Exposure to this dose is associated with an additional lifetime risk of fatal cancer of 1 in 1000 [5]. Further guidelines emphasize ALARA (As Low As Reasonably Achievable) principles involving time, distance, and shielding to reduce exposure [3,4].

Radiation exposure can lead to stochastic effects, such as genetic aberrations and cancer that can occur randomly, and deterministic effects, such as hair loss and skin changes that occur when exposure exceeds a specified limit [6]. Beyond immediate exposure, long-term health risks, including cellular damage, cataracts, and malignancies such as skin cancer, breast cancer, thyroid cancer, and leukemia, have been documented [5–7]. Modeling studies, particularly those leveraging Biological Effects of Ionizing Radiation (BEIR) VII risk estimates, project elevated lifetime attributable risks (LAR)—for example, excess incidence of solid cancers and associated mortality for long-term occupational exposure [8]. Despite this, radiation safety training and systematic compliance remain inconsistent. Surveys highlight widespread gaps in education and monitoring, and adherence to protective practices such as dosimeter or shielding use, is frequently suboptimal [9,10].

Operators across specialties experience highly variable exposure patterns because procedure type, anatomic positioning, equipment configuration, and workflow differ substantially between fields such as orthopedics, interventional cardiology, and vascular surgery. These differences create distinct exposure profiles and long-term risk trajectories for different operator groups, highlighting the importance of risk stratification in evaluating occupational hazards. Understanding these specialty-specific patterns is therefore essential for ensuring that protective strategies and monitoring practices effectively address variations in operator risk. Because exposure profiles vary substantially across specialties, procedures, and operator roles, occupational radiation risk is inherently heterogeneous. Understanding and incorporating this variability aligns with personalized medicine principles by enabling risk-stratified protective strategies tailored to operator-specific exposure patterns. Primary specialties that utilize fluoroscopy include cardiology, orthopedics, gastroenterology, urology, vascular surgery, gynecology, and pain medicine. In fluoroscopy, X-rays constitute the primary form of ionizing radiation with both bremsstrahlung radiation and characteristic X-rays [11]. The energy range for X-ray photons used in fluoroscopy is typically between 40 and 125 kilovolts peak (kVp).

Within this context, we conducted a structured narrative review encompassing a range of surgical and interventional specialties that utilize fluoroscopy, aiming to characterize occupational radiation exposure, evaluate the effectiveness of shielding strategies, assess long-term cancer risks, and identify compliance patterns.

2. Materials and Methods

This structured narrative review followed guidelines from Sukhera [12] and utilized a comprehensive literature search independently conducted between March and May 2025 using PubMed, Scopus, Embase, and Web of Science. The Boolean search strategy was used to identify relevant literature. The search string used in the electronic databases was: "radiation protection" OR "lead vest" OR "lead apron" OR "thyroid shield" OR "radiation shielding" AND "occupational exposure" OR "operator dose" OR "fluoroscopy" OR "interventional procedures" OR "surgeon" OR "interventional cardiology" OR "orthopedic surgery" OR "vascular surgery" OR "interventional radiology." This initial search strategy resulted in over 10,000 results that were a logistical challenge. Therefore, smaller, targeted Boolean variants (accomplished by reducing the number of search terms) were generated

 https://doi.org/10.3390/jpm16010050

iteratively to improve search specificity. Filters were also applied to limit results to human studies, English-language publications, and peer-reviewed articles between 2000 and 2024. Inclusion and exclusion criteria (Table 1) were also utilized (see below). Additionally, reference lists of highly relevant papers were manually screened to identify supplementary eligible studies.

Table 1. Inclusion and exclusion criteria for article selection.

	Inclusion Criteria
1. Topic Relevance	Addressed occupational radiation exposure, operator safety, or the effectiveness of protective measures (e.g., lead aprons, thyroid collars, lead glasses, leg shields, table skirts, ceiling-mounted barriers) during fluoroscopy-guided procedures.
2. Specialty Scope	Included any surgical or interventional specialty using fluoroscopy, such as orthopedics, trauma surgery, interventional cardiology, interventional radiology, vascular surgery, or cardiothoracic surgery.
3. Outcome Measures	Reported quantitative data on measured or modeled operator radiation dose, shielding-related dose reductions, procedural factors influencing exposure, or compliance with safety protocols.
4. Study Types	Peer-reviewed primary research (prospective, retrospective, or experimental), cohort studies, phantom or cadaver simulations, and high-quality narrative reviews with quantitative findings.
5. Language	English
6. Publication Time Frame	January 2000 to March 2024, ensuring relevance to modern imaging systems and protective technologies.

1. Articles that focused solely on patient radiation exposure without reporting operator outcomes
2. Articles that provided no quantitative metrics or measurable findings related to operator dose or protection effectiveness
3. Non-peer-reviewed studies (e.g., editorials, opinion pieces, conference abstracts without full texts).
4. Studies that investigated non-fluoroscopic fields (e.g., external beam radiotherapy, nuclear medicine not using fluoroscopy, dental radiography).

2.1. Article Selection

All studies identified in the search were eligible for review. The initial search yielded 62 articles after duplicate removal. Two independent authors screened titles and abstracts for relevance to occupational radiation exposure and protection strategies and retrieved 27 articles for full-text review. After applying the inclusion and exclusion criteria detailed in Table 1 at the full-text stage, 16 articles were included in the final synthesis. These studies spanned multiple specialties, procedural settings, and research methodologies, offering a broad evidence base to explore trends and best practices in occupational radiation safety during fluoroscopy-guided interventions. Although there was high methodological heterogeneity of the identified studies, inclusion and exclusion criteria is tight enough to capture relevant data.

2.2. Data Extraction

A detailed, pre-designed spreadsheet extraction template was used to collect data systematically across 25 structured fields: title, year, whether it was primary research, study design, sample size, country or region, surgical or interventional specialty, study duration or follow-up period, whether radiation exposure was measured or estimated, use of lead aprons or other shielding, consistency of lead protection use, pre- versus post-lead vest or shielding data, cancer type studied and its incidence or prevalence if applicable, whether a comparison group was included, reported risk ratios, odds ratios, or hazard ratios if applicable, confounding variables considered, lifestyle or occupational exposures assessed, statistical significance reported, whether longitudinal effects were studied, any policy or protocol recommendations, compliance with protection protocols, innovative methodologies used, inclusion of a pre-shielding or pre-vest historical baseline, and the role of that historical baseline in the paper.

https://doi.org/10.3390/jpm16010050

Manual extraction was first performed by a single reviewer with secondary reviews from additional authors with cross-checking to ensure consistency and accuracy. Emphasis was placed on numeric values (e.g., radiation dose in mSv, percentage dose reductions, fold-change effects, risk multipliers) and statistically significant results. When numeric data were not explicitly reported, dose-related information was extracted from descriptive statements when possible; otherwise, values were marked as Not Reported.

2.3. Data Analysis

Extracted data were analyzed to calculate overall and subgroup-level summary statistics–including means, medians, ranges–for operator doses, shielding-associated reductions, and compliance rates. Trends were compared across surgical and interventional specialties including orthopedics, trauma, interventional cardiology, interventional radiology, vascular surgery, and cardiothoracic surgery. Procedural factors associated with higher or lower exposure, such as fluoroscopy time, beam angle, C-arm positioning, and the use of real-time dosimetry, were identified. Common methodological strengths, weaknesses, and gaps in the existing literature were synthesized and the consistency and robustness of reported statistical significance across diverse study types were assessed.

Due to methodological heterogeneity, no formal meta-analysis or pooled effect size calculations were performed. Instead, the review presents a qualitative and quantitative synthesis of available data, highlighting both generalizable insights and areas requiring further specialty-specific investigation.

3. Results

A total of 16 studies were included in this review (Table 2). The narrative review search flow chart is depicted in Figure 1. The studies spanned a variety of surgical and interventional specialties, including orthopedic surgery [13–18], trauma surgery [14], interventional radiology [19], cardiology [20,21], and vascular surgery [22–28]. Publication dates ranged from 2000 to 2024, with the majority concentrated between 2010 and 2024. Eleven studies (69%) were primary research studies, either prospective or retrospective, while the remaining five were high-quality review or modeling articles (Table 2). Data originated from the United States, Italy, Japan, Ireland, South Korea, and multinational datasets, including large-scale analyses such as atomic bomb survivor follow-ups and BEIR VII risk models.

Table 2. Characteristics of the included studies. Reference numbers correspond to the first citation of each study, as established in this table and used consistently throughout the manuscript.

Author, Year Published	Study Type	Specialty	Summary Results	Reference
Hayda et al., 2018	Review article	Orthopaedic surgery—trauma, spine, general ortho; also referenced interventional cardiology, radiology for comparison	This article discusses the health risks associated with radiation exposure in orthopedic surgery, emphasizing the importance of protective measures to mitigate cancer risks. While focused on orthopedic surgeons, the findings are relevant to other surgical specialties that utilize fluoroscopy.	[13]
Kim et al., 2017	Prospective measurement study	Vascular surgery	Although yearly radiation hazards for vascular surgeons and scrub nurses are still within safety guidelines, protection principles can never be too stringent when aiming to minimize the cumulative harmful effects.	[22]

 https://doi.org/10.3390/jpm16010050

Table 2. *Cont.*

Author, Year Published	Study Type	Specialty	Summary Results	Reference
Hurley et al., 2022	Prospective observational study	Trauma and Orthopaedic surgery	PPE currently used by surgeons in orthopaedic trauma theatre adequately reduces radiation exposure to below recommended levels. Normative data per trauma case show specific anatomical areas of higher exposure, which may benefit from enhanced radiation protection. EPDs can be used to assess real-time radiation exposure in orthopaedic surgery.	[14]
Wan et al., 2021	Narrative review	Orthopedic surgery—trauma, spine, foot and ankle, sports medicine, general orthopedics	Fluoroscopy brings radiation hazard to the physicians and other staffs in operating theatre. Risk of leukaemia, risk to eyes, thyroid, skin, breast and fetes cannot be underestimated. Physician should properly use protective equipment including lead aprons, thyroid shields, radiation protection goggles and gloves, and dosimeter, to protect one-self from the invisible radiation hazard. The medical field should observe principles of justification and optimization, to reduce the radiation hazard to ALARA. Proper understanding of radiation risk will encourage doctors to use proper protection gear, and to clear unnecessary worries. Formal training on radiation safety and safe fluoroscopy use should also be encouraged and adopted.	[15]
Peri Ho et al., 2007	Prospective observational study	Vascular surgery—endovascular procedures	With current radiation protection practice, the radiation absorbed by vascular surgeons with a high endovascular workload did not exceed the safety limits recommended by ICRP. Variations in practice, however, can result in significant discrepancy of radiation absorption between surgeons.	[23]
Agarwal 2011	Narrative review	Orthopedic surgery—general, trauma, spine, foot and ankle	Orthopedic surgeons should use protective measures, which include lead aprons, thyroid shields, and, if at all possible, lead goggles. Techniques described to minimize direct and scatter exposure to the hands, eyes, and neck should be used. Measures to protect the patient should also be used intraoperatively, if feasible, such as shielding of the gonads. This is even more important as the awareness of patient radiation exposure increases.	[16]
Sritharan et al., 2024	Cross-sectional online survey	Vascular surgery	This survey highlights significant and concerning deficiencies in knowledge, access to personal radiation protection and failures in monitoring individual exposure to ionising radiation amongst the UK vascular surgical workforce.	[24]
Massey et al., 2022	Retrospective case-control study	Orthopedic surgery—general, trauma, C-arm fluoroscopy-assisted procedures	Institution of a PLP increased the compliance and exposure readings of radiation dosimeter badges for orthopedic surgery residents, whereas the actual monthly fluoroscopy time did not change. Teaching hospitals should consider implementing a PLP to more accurately monitor exposure.	[17]

https://doi.org/10.3390/jpm16010050

Table 2. *Cont.*

Author, Year Published	Study Type	Specialty	Summary Results	Reference
Bhinder et al., 2023	Prospective quality improvement study	Vascular surgery—endovascular, hybrid OR, angiography	Safety policies in place at vascular residency and fellowship programs were inadequate in securing the safety of their trainees. Interventions such as inventorying and ensuring availability of safety equipment, hands-on instruction to complement traditional didactics, lowering the default frame rates, and converting to real-time dosimetry to be effective measures for reducing radiation exposure.	[25]
Kirkwood et al., 2015	Prospective observational study	Vascular surgery—complex endovascular interventions	Surgeon radiation dose during FGIs depends on case type, operator position, and table skirt use but not on the level of fellow training. On the basis of these data, the primary operator could perform approximately 12 FEVARs/wk and have an annual dose <10 mSv, which would not exceed lifetime occupational dose limits during a 35-year career. With practical case loads, operator doses are relatively low and unlikely to exceed occupational limits.	[26]
Harstall et al., 2005	Prospective case-control study	Orthopaedic spine surgery	While performing percutaneous vertebroplasty, the surgeon is exposed to a significant amount of radiation. Proper surgical technique and shielding devices to decrease potentially high morbidity are mandatory. Training in radiation protection should be an integral part of the education for all surgeons using minimally invasive radiologic-guided interventional techniques.	[18]
Haqqani et al., 2012	Prospective controlled study	Vascular surgery—endovascular procedures, digital subtraction angiography	Varying imaging techniques results in different radiation exposure to members of an endovascular surgery team. Knowledge of the variable intensity of radiation exposure may allow modification of the technique to minimize radiation exposure to the team while providing suitable imaging.	[27]
Dorey et al., 2019	Controlled laboratory experiment	Interventional radiology	If the clinician's gaze is directed towards the main scattering source, a potential exists for reducing eye lens dose compared with fixed location computer monitors. Introduction of lead lined smart glasses into interventional radiology may lead to improvements in patient care, reducing the need for the clinician to look away from the patient to observe a radiographic image.	[19]
Kastrati et al., 2016	Retrospective Observational Study	Cardiology—coronary angiography and angioplasty	A new x-ray technology with image noise reduction algorithm provides a substantial reduction in radiation exposure without the need to prolong the procedure or fluoroscopy time.	[20]
Modarai 2022	Expert commentary	Vascular surgery—endovascular procedures	Vascular operators are at significant occupational risk from cumulative ionizing radiation exposure, with potential long-term health consequences. Consistent use of protective equipment, adherence to radiation-minimizing techniques, and increased awareness and education are essential to reduce exposure and improve operator safety.	[28]

 https://doi.org/10.3390/jpm16010050

Table 2. *Cont.*

Author, Year Published	Study Type	Specialty	Summary Results	Reference
Picano et al., 2024	Comprehensive review	Cardiology—diagnostic and interventional radiology, nuclear cardiology, electrophysiology	Review updates estimated societal health burden from diagnostic radiology and nuclear medicine, showing that rising population radiation exposure is associated with higher-than-previously-recognized risks of both cancer and cardiovascular disease. Emerging epidemiological evidence refutes the assumption that low-dose radiation is biologically negligible, and combined cancer and cardiovascular risks are now understood to impose a substantially greater public health impact than earlier estimates suggested.	[21]

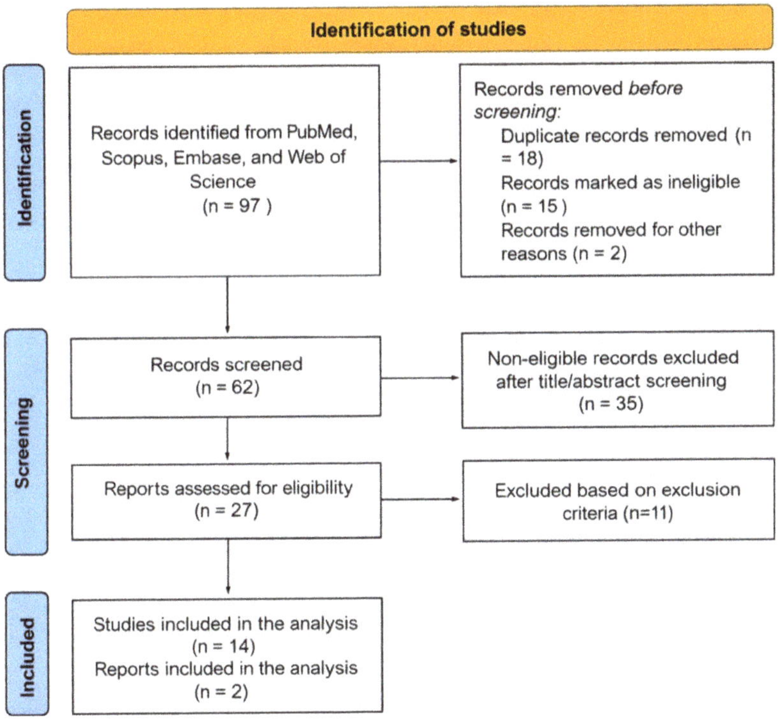

Figure 1. A PRISMA-style flow diagram of the narrative review showing the identification, screening, eligibility assessment, and inclusion of studies for final inclusion and anlaysis.

3.1. Sample Characteristics

Sample sizes ranged from large-scale epidemiological datasets ($n \approx 120{,}000$) [13] to small intraoperative measurement cohorts (n = 60 procedures) [14]. Operator-specific exposure data were reported across all studies. Vascular (7), orthopedic (6) and trauma (5) surgery represented the largest specialty groups, followed by cardiology (2), interventional radiology (1). Cardiothoracic surgery was minimally represented, largely through modeled rather than directly measured exposure data. Follow-up durations ranged from six weeks to over 50 years for studies incorporating long-term cancer risk projections, with several extrapolating annual exposure from short-term dosimetry findings.

 https://doi.org/10.3390/jpm16010050

3.2. Radiation Exposure and Shielding Effectiveness

Intraoperative exposures were consistently reported. Without protective gear, chest-level doses averaged 0.08–0.11 mSv per procedure, and eye-level doses averaged 0.04–0.05 mSv per procedure. High-volume trauma surgeons demonstrated knee-thigh doses up to 2.7 mSv annually. When shielding was employed, attenuation was substantial: 0.25 mm lead aprons reduced exposure by ~90%, while 0.5 mm aprons achieved a reduction of ~99%. Lead glasses decreased ocular doses 2.5–4.5-fold, and thyroid collars reduced neck-level exposure by approximately 60–70%. Real-time dosimetry and phantom modeling confirmed shielding efficacy, with external-to-internal dose reductions up to 91.1%.

3.3. Cancer Incidence and Modeled Risk

Direct evidence of cancer incidence was limited, largely modeled or extrapolated, but notable. One Italian orthopedic study reported a 29% cancer incidence among exposed surgeons compared with 4% in non-exposed controls [13,16]. U.S. data showed a 2.9-fold higher breast cancer rate among female orthopedic surgeons, while cardiology studies indicated a median latency of ~22 years for head and neck tumors [13]. Modeled lifetime attributable risks (LAR) per million exposed individuals, based on BEIR VII data, included colon cancer at 424 (≈1 in 236), lung cancer at 447 (≈1 in 224), all solid cancers for male surgeons at 2079 (≈1 in 48), and cancer-related mortality across all sites at 1309 (≈1 in 76) [22]. These risk estimates were based on BEIR VII reports and extrapolated occupational exposures, assuming careers spanning ages 18–65 at consistent annual doses. These extrapolated results may not imply direct causality.

3.4. Comparison Groups and Risk Ratios

Several studies incorporated internal or external comparison groups, such as non-exposed staff or population baselines [13,15,21,22]. Reported effect sizes included a relative risk (RR) of 1.6 for solid cancers per 1 Sv exposure (atomic bomb survivor data), a hazard ratio (HR) of 4.04 for high-procedure cardiologists compared to low-procedure peers, and an RR of 3.2 ($p < 0.005$) for posterior lens opacities (cataracts).

3.5. Protection Protocols and Compliance

Lead aprons and thyroid collars demonstrated high compliance rates (90–99%) [15], while lead glasses showed inconsistent use [15,22–24], often due to interference with surgical loupes [22]. Seated procedures frequently showed unshielded gaps at the apron skirt edge, raising gonadal dose exposure. Several studies highlighted routine equipment integrity checks, real-time dosimeter use, and institutional enforcement of protective protocols as key areas for improvement.

3.6. Innovative Methodologies

Methodologies included real-time electronic personal dosimeters (EPD) and thermoluminescent dosimeters (TLD) mapped across body regions, phantom models simulating scatter radiation at variable distances and angles, and procedure-specific modeling comparing exposures across endovascular aneurysm repair (EVAR), angioplasty, and trauma cases.

3.7. Summary Statistics

Summary statistics are presented in Table 3. Across studies, the mean sample size was approximately 4200 (median 1200; range 60–120,000). Mean chest-level dose was ~0.10 mSv per procedure, and mean eye-level dose without lead was ~0.05 mSv per procedure. Gonadal exposure for busy trauma surgeons averaged ~2.7 mSv annually. The estimated relative risk for solid cancer per Sv was consistently reported at 1.6 (SD 0.1).

https://doi.org/10.3390/jpm16010050

Table 3. Summary statistics for operator exposure metrics across included studies.

Metric	Mean	Median	Range	Std. Dev.
Sample Size (where reported)	~4200	~1200	60–120,000	High spread
Chest-level dose (mSv/procedure)	~0.10	0.09	0.08–0.11	0.01
Eye-level dose (mSv/procedure, no lead)	~0.05	0.045	0.04–0.07	0.01
Gonadal dose (mSv/year, busy trauma surgeons)	~2.7	2.5	2.4–3.8	0.5
Estimated risk ratios (solid cancer, per Sv)	1.6	1.6	1.5–1.7	0.1

3.8. Key Trends and Insights

Key findings included: (1) Across specialties, shielding via lead aprons, thyroid collars, and glasses provided substantial dose reductions by 60–99% depending on body region and material thickness; (2) compliance gaps persisted, particularly regarding lead glasses usage and coverage of apron skirt edges; (3) phantom and modeled data closely mirrored measured exposure patterns via dose dosimetry but highlighted variability across procedures and operator roles; (4) direct specialty-specific cancer data remain scarce, with most conclusions extrapolated from surrogate dose reductions and modeled lifetime risks; and (5) practices and safety protocols differed markedly across regions, with international comparisons often referencing U.S. and European standards.

4. Discussion

This structured narrative review across 16 studies provides valuable insights into occupational radiation exposure among surgical and interventional proceduralists. While fluoroscopy-guided techniques continue to enhance minimally invasive care, cumulative ionizing radiation exposure remains an underrecognized occupational hazard, especially due to inconsistent protective practices and insufficient long-term outcome data.

Across included studies, operator doses reported were unshielded ~0.08–0.11 mSv/procedure at the chest and ~0.04–0.05 mSv/procedure at the eye. Lead aprons reducing exposure by ~90–99% and lead glasses reducing eye dose ~2.5–4.5×) can be benchmarked against current occupational limits to judge whether fluoroscopy-guided practice is typically "acceptable." Under contemporary international guidance, the occupational effective-dose limit is 20 mSv/year averaged over 5 years (≤50 mSv in any single year), the lens limit is 20 mSv/year averaged over 5 years (≤50 mSv in any single year), and skin/extremities are limited at 500 mSv/year [2,29,30]. U.S. regulations permit a whole-body effective dose of 50 mSv/year, 150 mSv/year to the lens, and 500 mSv/year to the skin/extremities [31]. Interpreted against these thresholds, the per-procedure doses summarized here imply that routine practice with consistent shielding is generally compatible with remaining below annual effective-dose limits, while the lens and (in specific workflows) the hands are the most plausible limit-driving components. However, meeting dose limits should not be conflated with being "risk-averse"; limits are regulatory/occupational compliance thresholds, whereas stochastic effects such as cancer are probabilistic and are reduced by dose minimization rather than eliminated below any particular cutoff. Therefore, "acceptable risk" in fluoroscopy-guided practice is best interpreted as compliance plus optimization (ALARA), emphasizing consistent PPE, geometry optimization, and dosimetry strategies that specifically capture high-risk patterns of eye and extremity exposure in high-volume operators.

4.1. Shielding Efficacy and Practice Patterns

Our synthesis reaffirms that protective gear ranging from 0.25 mm to 0.5 mm lead-equivalent aprons, thyroid collars, and lead glasses provides substantial dose reduction (60–99%) across body regions. This aligns with existing recommendations that employ a combination of time, distance, and shielding (ALARA principles) to mitigate exposure risk. Additionally, newer comparative work indicates that traditional lead aprons often

https://doi.org/10.3390/jpm16010050

outperform lightweight alternatives, underscoring the importance of material integrity and equivalent thickness. These aprons should be considered for wider use.

Despite strong evidence supporting personal protective equipment (PPE), compliance gaps remain. While there is adherence to the usage of thyroid collars and aprons, lead glasses, crucial for eye protection, are underutilized, often due to interference with surgical optics (e.g., loupes). This supports broader findings that surgical trainees and attendings often express inadequate radiation safety education and concern over long-term risk, particularly regarding fertility and cancer. This area is a current actionable recommendation.

The variability observed across specialties, procedural roles, and exposed body regions highlights that occupational radiation risk is not uniform. Orthopedic trauma surgeons, interventional cardiologists, and other high-fluoroscopy practitioners demonstrate distinct exposure patterns, dose magnitudes, and long-term risk profiles. These differences underscore the need for risk-stratified approaches to occupational protection, in which monitoring practices, shielding selection, and institutional protocols are adapted to the specific exposure characteristics of different operator groups. Such stratification reflects an individualized framework consistent with modern precision-oriented occupational health. These specialty-specific exposure differences reinforce a precision-oriented approach to occupational health in which monitoring practices and protective strategies are tailored to the operator's individualized risk profile, aligning this work with core principles of personalized medicine for protection of physicians using fluoroscopy in their practices.

4.2. Risk Estimation and Long-Term Health Outcomes

Direct epidemiological data on cancer incidence among operators are limited but concerning, nonetheless. One study reported markedly higher cancer rates in exposed orthopedic surgeons than controls, and elevated breast cancer rates among female surgeons were highlighted in U.S. data. Most risk assessments, however, rely on modeling using BEIR VII data to estimate lifetime attributable risk of cancers and mortality (e.g., ~1 in 48 for solid cancers; ~1 in 76 for cancer-related mortality). These estimates reflect a need for comprehensive occupational registries and longitudinal research.

Risk estimates from atomic bomb survivors yielding an RR of 1.6 per 1 Sv may not directly apply to proceduralists, whose exposures are typically lower and chronic. Nevertheless, findings such as a hazard ratio of 4.04 for high-volume interventional cardiologists and a relative risk of approximately 3.2 for cataracts indicate that even procedural-level exposures may carry significant health risks, though study heterogeneity limits meta-analysis and strong causal inference.

4.3. Implications for Practice and Future Research

Institutional commitment to comprehensive safety measures is imperative to better protect operators. Strategies such as routine integrity checks for protective gear, standardized compliance monitoring with dosimetry, and appointing a Radiation Safety Officer (RSO) to oversee adherence to ALARA principles have proven effective in other settings. Education tailored to proceduralists, potentially through advanced tools such as virtual reality (VR)-based radiation field visualization, could further improve compliance [32]. The importance of local diagnostic reference levels (DRLs) in the context of risk stratification and optimization of radiation protection for operators is also emphasized by recent studies indicating that taking into account local procedural and equipment conditions allows for a more accurate assessment of exposure and more effective implementation of ALARA principles [33]. Additionally, procedural modifications such as maintaining modest distance from scatter sources, beam collimation, pulsed fluoroscopy, and integrating ceiling-mounted shielding in hybrid OR setups can cumulatively reduce exposure.

https://doi.org/10.3390/jpm16010050

Future research should prioritize prospective studies that track cumulative exposure and long-term outcomes such as cancer and other stochastic effects. Standardized reporting is needed to enable cross-study comparisons and meta-analysis. More studies will also reduce the heterogeneity of results and should allow subgroup analysis. Incorporating real-time dosimetry, phantom modeling, and registry-linked data can improve risk estimates, while studies testing and evaluating new shielding technologies, training strategies, and workflow changes may identify effective approaches to strengthen radiation safety practices.

4.4. Limitations

This structured narrative review has several limitations. Considerable heterogeneity was present in study designs, outcome measures, and reporting methods across the included papers. Longitudinal cancer outcome data were limited, as most studies focused on immediate or modeled radiation exposure rather than long-term health effects. Some specialties were underrepresented compared with others—for example, cardiothoracic surgery had fewer studies relative to orthopedics or interventional cardiology to generate appropriate strong data. In addition, adherence to protective equipment protocols and the rigor of monitoring practices varied substantially across institutions and operator groups. In addition, cancer risk models based on BEIR VII data may not be adequate for chronic, low-dose occupational exposure characteristic of fluoroscopy operators. Nevertheless, the aggregated findings provide valuable insights into the current state of occupational radiation safety practices in fluoroscopy-guided procedural specialties.

5. Conclusions

Operators across surgical and interventional specialties face considerable exposure to ionizing radiation during fluoroscopically guided procedures. Although protective measures achieve significant dose reductions, gaps in compliance, knowledge, and protocol implementation persist. Evidence linking exposure to long-term health outcomes remains limited, underscoring the need for standardized monitoring, rigorous safety practices, and well-designed longitudinal studies to guide future recommendations. The marked variability in exposure across specialties, procedural roles, and exposed body regions indicates that occupational risk is not uniform. Integrating risk-stratified monitoring and protective protocols may better address the distinct exposure patterns encountered by different operator groups and align with emerging precision-oriented approaches to occupational health. Anchoring these strategies within a personalized medicine framework underscores the need to tailor occupational protections to operator-specific exposure patterns, ensuring safety practices that reflect the individualized risk profiles identified in this review.

Author Contributions: Conceptualization, N.K.O.-Y.; methodology, N.K.O.-Y.; formal analysis, N.K.O.-Y.; investigation, N.K.O.-Y., S.S.R.B., H.B. and O.O.D.; data curation, N.K.O.-Y. and S.S.R.B.; writing—original draft preparation, N.K.O.-Y. and S.S.R.B.; writing—review and editing, N.K.O.-Y., S.S.R.B., H.B., O.O.D. and M.B.; supervision, M.B. All authors have read and agreed to the published version of the manuscript.

Funding: This research received no external funding.

Institutional Review Board Statement: Not applicable.

Informed Consent Statement: Not applicable.

Data Availability Statement: All data discussed in this review are drawn from previously published studies and are available within the cited literature.

Conflicts of Interest: All authors declare no conflicts of interest.

https://doi.org/10.3390/jpm16010050

Abbreviations

The following abbreviations are used in this manuscript:

BEIR	Biological Effects of Ionizing Radiation
ALARA	As Low As Reasonably Achievable
LAR	Lifetime Attributable Risks
ICRP	International Commission on Radiological Protection

References

1. Smith-Bindman, R.; Chu, P.W.; Firdaus, H.A.; Stewart, C.; Malekhedayat, M.; Alber, S.; Bolch, W.E.; Mahendra, M.; de González, A.B.; Miglioretti, D.L. Projected Lifetime Cancer Risks from Current Computed Tomography Imaging. *JAMA Intern. Med.* **2025**, *185*, 710–719, Erratum in *JAMA Intern Med.* **2025**, *185*, 747. [CrossRef] [PubMed] [PubMed Central]
2. El Ghissassi, F.; Baan, R.; Straif, K.; Grosse, Y.; Secretan, B.; Bouvard, V.; Benbrahim-Tallaa, L.; Guha, N.; Freeman, C.; Galichet, L.; et al. A review of human carcinogens--part D: Radiation. *Lancet Oncol.* **2009**, *10*, 751–752. [CrossRef]
3. López, P.O.; Dauer, L.; Loose, R.; Martin, C.; Miller, D.; Vañó, E.; Doruff, M.; Padovani, R.; Massera, G.; Yoder, C. on behalf of the ICRP. ICRP Publication 139: Occupational radiological protection in interventional procedures. *Ann. ICRP* **2018**, *47*, 1–118. [CrossRef]
4. Stewart, F.A.; Akleyev, A.V.; Hauer-Jensen, M.; Hendry, J.H.; Kleiman, N.J.; Macvittie, T.J.; Aleman, B.M.; Edgar, A.B.; Mabuchi, K.; Muirhead, C.R.; et al. ICRP publication 118: ICRP statement on tissue reactions and early and late effects of radiation in normal tissues and organs--threshold doses for tissue reactions in a radiation protection context. *Ann. ICRP* **2012**, *41*, 1–322. [CrossRef]
5. Matityahu, A.; Duffy, R.K.; Goldhahn, S.; Joeris, A.; Richter, P.H.; Gebhard, F. The Great Unknown-A systematic literature review about risk associated with intraoperative imaging during orthopaedic surgeries. *Injury* **2017**, *48*, 1727–1734. [CrossRef] [PubMed]
6. Hamid, M.A.; Younis, Z.; Raza, A.; Tauseef, A.; Khan, M.A.H.; Mir, S.; Abdulsattar, S.; Rashid, N. Radiation in the Orthopedic Operating Room: What We Know, What We Do, and What Needs Attention. *Cureus* **2025**, *17*, e90911. [CrossRef]
7. Calgary Orthopaedic Resident Research Group. Quantification of Radiation Exposure in Canadian Orthopaedic Surgery Residents. *JBJS Open Access* **2024**, *9*, e23-00170. [CrossRef] [PubMed]
8. National Research Council (US) Committee on Health Effects of Exposure to Low Levels of Ionizing Radiations (BEIR VII). *Health Effects of Exposure to Low Levels of Ionizing Radiations: Time for Reassessment?* National Academies Press: Washington, DC, USA, 1998. [PubMed]
9. Aljohmani, L.; Gaffney, A.; Kelly, L.; O'Sullivan, L.-A.; Leyva, E.; O'Connor, M.; McCavana, J.; Heffernan, E.; Quinlan, C.; Dolan, R. Knowledge gaps and radiation exposure concerns: Time for a revamp of radiation training structures for trainee surgeons. *Surgeon* **2025**, *23*, 393–398. [CrossRef]
10. Kang, S.; Cha, E.S.; Bang, Y.J.; Na, T.W.; Lee, D.; Song, S.Y.; Lee, W.J. Radiation exposure and fluoroscopically-guided interventional procedures among orthopedic surgeons in South Korea. *J. Occup. Med. Toxicol.* **2020**, *15*, 24. [CrossRef] [PubMed]
11. Rivera, K.; Ahn, S.S. Radiation Physics and Safety in Fluoroscopy: A Clinician's Guide to Principles and Practice. *Cureus* **2025**, *17*, e87245. [CrossRef]
12. Sukhera, J. Narrative Reviews: Flexible, Rigorous, and Practical. *J. Grad. Med. Educ.* **2022**, *14*, 414–417. [CrossRef] [PubMed]
13. Hayda, R.A.; Hsu, R.Y.; DePasse, J.M.; Gil, J.A. Radiation Exposure and Health Risks for Orthopaedic Surgeons. *J. Am. Acad. Orthop. Surg.* **2018**, *26*, 268–277. [CrossRef]
14. Hurley, R.J.; McCabe, F.J.; Turley, L.; Maguire, D.; Lucey, J.; Hurson, C.J. Whole-body radiation exposure in Trauma and Orthopaedic surgery. *Bone Jt. Open* **2022**, *3*, 907–912. [CrossRef] [PubMed]
15. Wan, R.C.W.; Chau, W.W.; Tso, C.Y.; Tang, N.; Chow, S.K.; Cheung, W.-H.; Wong, R.M. Occupational hazard of fluoroscopy: An invisible threat to orthopaedic surgeons. *J. Orthop. Trauma. Rehabilit.* **2021**, *28*, 22104917211035547. [CrossRef]
16. Agarwal, A. Radiation Risk in Orthopedic Surgery: Ways to Protect Yourself and the Patient. *Oper. Tech. Sports Med.* **2011**, *19*, 220–223. [CrossRef]
17. Massey, P.A.; Myers, M.E.; Guedry, R.D.; Lowery, M.T.; Perry, K.J.; Barton, R.S. Improved Radiation Exposure Monitoring of Orthopaedic Residents After Institution of a Personalized Lead Protocol. *JBJS Open Access* **2022**, *7*, e21. [CrossRef]
18. Harstall, R.; Heini, P.F.; Mini, R.L.; Orler, R. Radiation exposure to the surgeon during fluoroscopically assisted percutaneous vertebroplasty: A prospective study. *Spine* **2005**, *30*, 1893–1898. [CrossRef]
19. Dorey, S.; Gray, L.; Tootell, A.; Higgins, R.; Al-Islam, S.; Baxter, H.; Dixon, P.; Hogg, P. Radiation protection value to the operator from augmented reality smart glasses in interventional fluoroscopy procedures using phantoms. *Radiography* **2019**, *25*, 301–307. [CrossRef]
20. Kastrati, M.; Langenbrink, L.; Piatkowski, M.; Michaelsen, J.; Reimann, D.; Hoffmann, R. Reducing Radiation Dose in Coronary Angiography and Angioplasty Using Image Noise Reduction Technology. *Am. J. Cardiol.* **2016**, *118*, 353–356. [CrossRef] [PubMed]

 https://doi.org/10.3390/jpm16010050

21. Picano, E.; Vañó, E. Updated Estimates of Radiation Risk for Cancer and Cardiovascular Disease: Implications for Cardiology Practice. *J. Clin. Med.* **2024**, *13*, 2066. [CrossRef]
22. Kim, J.B.; Lee, J.; Park, K. Radiation hazards to vascular surgeon and scrub nurse in mobile fluoroscopy equipped hybrid vascular room. *Ann. Surg. Treat. Res.* **2017**, *92*, 156–163. [CrossRef]
23. Ho, P.; Cheng, S.W.K.; Wu, P.M.; Ting, A.C.; Poon, J.T.; Cheng, C.K.; Mok, J.H.; Tsang, M. Ionizing radiation absorption of vascular surgeons during endovascular procedures. *J. Vasc. Surg.* **2007**, *46*, 455–459. [CrossRef]
24. Sritharan, K.; Sheikh, Z.; Saratzis, A.; Lakshminarayan, R.; Garnham, A.; Bowbrick, G.; Morgan, R. Standards of radiation protection amongst UK vascular surgeons: A clinician's perspective. *J. Vasc. Soc. Great Br. Irel.* **2024**, *4*, 25–32. [CrossRef]
25. Bhinder, J.; O'Brien-Irr, M.; Reilly, B.; Montross, B.; Khan, S.; Rivero, M.; Cherr, G.; Harris, L. Understanding Radiation Exposure and Improving Safety for Vascular Surgery Trainees. *J. Vasc. Surg.* **2023**, *77*, 269–278. [CrossRef] [PubMed]
26. Kirkwood, M.L.; Guild, J.B.; Arbique, G.M.; Anderson, J.A.; Valentine, R.J.; Timaran, C. Surgeon radiation dose during complex endovascular procedures. *J. Vasc. Surg.* **2015**, *62*, 457–463. [CrossRef] [PubMed]
27. Haqqani, O.P.; Agarwal, P.K.; Halin, N.M.; Iafrati, M.D. Minimizing radiation exposure to the vascular surgeon. *J. Vasc. Surg.* **2012**, *55*, 799–805. [CrossRef]
28. Endovascular Today. *Radiation Exposure, Effects, and Safety Measures for Vascular Operators (with Bijan Modarai, PhD, FRCS)*; Endovascular Today: Conshohocken, PA, USA, 2022.
29. International Commission on Radiological Protection. *Statement on Tissue Reactions*; International Commission on Radiological Protection: Ottawa, ON, Canada, 2011. Available online: https://www.nrc.gov/docs/ML1326/ML13269A317.pdf (accessed on 5 January 2026).
30. International Atomic Energy Agency. *Radiation Protection and Safety of Radiation Sources: International Basic Safety Standards. IAEA Safety Standards Series No. GSR Part 3*; International Atomic Energy Agency: Vienna, Austria, 2014; STI/PUB/1578; ISBN 978-92-0-135310-8. Available online: https://www-pub.iaea.org/MTCD/Publications/PDF/Pub1578_web-57265295.pdf (accessed on 5 January 2026).
31. U.S. Nuclear Regulatory Commission. Standards for Protection Against Radiation. 10 CFR § 20.1201 Occupational Dose Limits for Adults. Electronic Code of Federal Regulations. Available online: https://unblock.federalregister.gov/ (accessed on 5 January 2026).
32. Unberath, M.; Fotouhi, J.; Hajek, J.; Maier, A.; Osgood, G.; Taylor, R.; Armand, M.; Navab, N. Augmented reality-based feedback for technician-in-the-loop C-arm repositioning. *Health Technol. Lett.* **2018**, *5*, 143–147. [CrossRef]
33. Modlińska, S.; Rojek, M.; Bielówka, M.; Kufel, J. Establishing Local Diagnostic Reference Levels for Head Computed Tomography Examinations. *Biomedicines* **2024**, *12*, 2446. [CrossRef]

 https://doi.org/10.3390/jpm16010050

Journal of
Personalized Medicine

MDPI

Review

A Multi-Axis Framework for Late-Life Alzheimer's Disease Interpretation

Yong Tae Kwak [1,*] and YoungSoon Yang [2]

[1] Department of Neurology, Hyoja Geriatric Hospital, 1-30, Jungbu-daero 874beon-gil, Giheung-gu, Yongin-si 17089, Gyeonggi-do, Republic of Korea
[2] Department of Neurology, Soonchunhyang University Cheonan Hospital, 31 Soonchunhyang 6-gil, Dongnam-gu, Cheonan-si 31151, Chungcheongnam-do, Republic of Korea; astro76@naver.com
* Correspondence: kwakdr@gmail.com; Tel.: +82-31-288-0602; Fax: +82-31-288-0539

Abstract

Late-life Alzheimer's disease (AD) is increasingly defined by biomarkers, yet in adults aged ≥65 years the relationship between amyloid positivity and near-term cognitive decline is often discordant. Amyloid PET robustly detects fibrillar plaque burden, but it incompletely captures dynamic and potentially neurotoxic amyloid processes, particularly soluble assemblies and oligomer-related "activity." This review rethinks the late-life AD spectrum by integrating four clinical lenses that frequently drive real-world interpretive uncertainty: (1) amyloid PET positivity as a measure of fibrillar plaque presence and magnitude; (2) plasma amyloid-β oligomerization tendency measured by the multimer detection system (MDS-OAβ) as an activity-oriented (i.e., a dynamic readout hypothesized to reflect ongoing processes rather than cumulative lesion burden), process-linked readout that may decouple from plaque burden; (3) postoperative delirium (POD) as a time-anchored stress-test phenotype revealing vulnerability and reduced resilience under systemic insults; and (4) drug-linked biomarker trajectories, contrasting rapid plaque removal by anti-amyloid monoclonal antibodies with observational signals raising the hypothesis that Ginkgo biloba may be associated with oligomer-related biology and, in some contexts, differences in longitudinal amyloid accumulation trajectories in the absence of observed immediate plaque reduction. We propose a pragmatic multi-axis framework—plaque burden, amyloid activity, downstream engagement, and vulnerability/resilience—to contextualize late-life discordances such as PET positivity without decline, PET negativity with elevated MDS-OAβ, delirium-associated decompensation, and clinical change without rapid PET decline. This synthesis highlights testable predictions and prioritizes longitudinal, multi-marker studies to determine whether activity-oriented biomarkers and stress phenotypes can refine late-life risk stratification beyond plaque-centered models.

Keywords: Alzheimer's disease; amyloid PET; amyloid-β oligomers; MDS-OAβ (multimer detection system); postoperative delirium

1. Introduction

Alzheimer's disease (AD) is now widely conceptualized as a biological continuum rather than a purely clinical syndrome. This shift was formalized by the NIA–AA Research Framework, which defines AD in research settings according to biomarkers of amyloid deposition (A), tau pathology (T), and neurodegeneration or neuronal injury (N), independent of clinical symptoms [1,2]. More recently, the Alzheimer's Association Workgroup updated the 2018 NIA-AA research framework by proposing revised criteria for the diagnosis and staging of Alzheimer's disease, aiming to bridge research and clinical care by incorporating advances in biomarker assessment (including fluid-based biomarkers) and providing an updated biologic diagnosis and staging scheme [3]. This biology-first approach has provided an essential foundation for therapeutic development, trial enrichment, and mechanistic clarity. However, its interpretive limits become increasingly evident in late life, where AD-related biology becomes common while dementia remains heterogeneous and far from inevitable.

In older adults, amyloid PET positivity frequently coexists with preserved cognitive function for prolonged periods, and rates of decline vary widely even among individuals with similar biomarker profiles [4,5]. Such late-life discordances are not merely statistical noise. Rather, they reflect the convergence of multiple age-dependent processes—including amyloid and tau pathology, cerebrovascular disease, systemic frailty, inflammatory states, and resilience factors—whose timing and relative dominance differ substantially across individuals. Complementing plaque-centric interpretations, late-life AD has also been framed as, at least in part, a brain expression of systemic metabolic dysfunction. In this view, cardiometabolic stressors (e.g., insulin resistance, oxidative stress, and inflammatory signaling) may shape vulnerability/reserve and contribute to symptom expression and short-term trajectory variability even when fibrillar amyloid PET burden is relatively stable [6,7]. As a result, single biomarker-defined AD in late life often fails to map cleanly onto short-term clinical trajectories.

The present review therefore adopts a late-life focus grounded in empirical observation rather than theoretical redefinition. In this context, late-life Alzheimer's disease refers to Alzheimer-spectrum biology, defined as the presence of AD-related pathological processes—most commonly amyloid positivity—across the clinical continuum, in adults aged 65 years and older. At this stage, pathological markers become increasingly prevalent, yet clinical trajectories remain highly variable and frequently discordant from biomarker status. In late life, Alzheimer-related biology intersects with aging-related vulnerability, acute physiological or cognitive stressors, and heterogeneous resilience, complicating linear interpretations that link static biomarkers directly to near-term cognitive outcomes.

This perspective emerged from a series of studies conducted by our group in older adults over 65 years, spanning perioperative cohorts as well as biomarker-confirmed Alzheimer's disease and mild cognitive impairment. Across these investigations, plasma amyloid-β oligomerization tendency (MDS-OAβ) repeatedly appeared as a convergent biological signal linking acute cognitive vulnerability—most notably postoperative delirium—to longer-term clinical trajectories, even when amyloid PET findings were stable or discordant [8,9]. Complementary studies in amyloid PET-positive AD and mild cognitive impairment (MCI) further suggested that oligomer-related biology may be modifiable, with clinical and functional changes observed in the absence of measurable plaque reduction [10,11]. In addition, our group has conducted two related analyses: (i) a large perioperative cohort study evaluating pre- and postoperative plasma MDS-OAβ for postoperative delirium risk stratification (currently under peer review); and (ii) a longitudinal amyloid-positive MCI study examining associations between Ginkgo biloba use and trajectories of amyloid PET burden and plasma Aβ oligomerization tendency (accepted for publication). These studies are referenced for context and hypothesis generation and should not be interpreted as primary evidentiary support for the framework.

Taken together, these observations motivated the present review. Rather than proposing a new disease subtype, we use the term late-life AD to emphasize an interpretive framework—one that recognizes Alzheimer-related biology as necessary but not sufficient to explain cognitive outcomes in older adults. Within this framework, late-

 https://doi.org/10.3390/jpm16030157

life discordances—such as amyloid PET positivity without near-term decline, elevated oligomer-related biomarkers in clinically normal individuals, or clinical improvement without amyloid plaque removal—are viewed not as anomalies, but as characteristic features of Alzheimer's disease as it manifests in aging brains.

Against this background, we propose a reinterpretation of late-life AD through four clinical lenses that reflect where clinical interpretation most commonly diverges in real-world practice. Rather than constituting a taxonomy derived from individual studies, each lens corresponds to a distinct and non-reducible clinical question encountered in the care of older adults with suspected or established Alzheimer-spectrum disease. (1) Amyloid PET positivity primarily addresses whether fibrillar amyloid pathology is present; (2) plasma MDS-OAβ provides a dynamic readout of amyloid oligomerization tendency and an activity-like peripheral signal (with unknown specificity for CNS oligomer burden), which may precede or decouple from plaque accumulation; (3) postoperative delirium functions as an acute stress-test phenotype, implicitly probing the brain's vulnerability to physiological or cognitive insults; and (4) drug-linked biomarker trajectories shift the focus from static diagnosis to biological response, contrasting plaque-removing anti-amyloid monoclonal antibodies with signals from biomarker-defined cohorts suggesting that Ginkgo biloba extract may be associated with oligomer-related peripheral biomarker patterns and, in some contexts, hypothesized differences in amyloid biomarker trajectories in observational settings. The proposed lenses are conceptually complementary to AT(N) while addressing dimensions that are only partly captured by it. Amyloid PET primarily reflects 'A' (fibrillar plaque burden), whereas downstream engagement may map to 'T/N'. Vulnerability/reserve —operationalized here by stress-test phenotypes such as postoperative delirium—represents an additional axis relevant to short-term trajectories in late life.

The purpose of this framework is not to replace established biomarker models, but to provide a pragmatic interpretive scaffold for late-life discordances—such as amyloid PET positivity without near-term decline, PET negativity with elevated MDS-OAβ, or clinical improvement without plaque reduction—by situating them as different positions along interacting biological and clinical trajectories that are particularly salient in late life. Although tau biomarkers (e.g., plasma or CSF phosphorylated tau) represent a critical axis in Alzheimer's disease biology, their routine clinical availability and accumulated real-world experience—particularly in blood-based assays—remain limited in current practice; therefore, detailed discussion of tau biomarkers is beyond the scope of the present review. In future work, tau biomarkers—particularly plasma p-tau species (e.g., p-tau217/p-tau231) and related markers such as NfL/GFAP—could be incorporated as an additional axis or as a modifier of downstream engagement to further refine trajectory interpretation as clinical availability matures; conceptually, PET−/high p-tau and PET+/low p-tau would represent testable discordant states expected to diverge longitudinally in symptom coupling and downstream marker trajectories. Because parts of this framework were motivated by observations from our biomarker-defined and perioperative cohorts, we present selected author-led findings as illustrative, hypothesis-generating examples rather than definitive evidence of efficacy or causality. We therefore emphasize independent and multicenter studies (including mixed or negative results) and highlight the need for replication and longitudinal validation across diverse cohorts.

1. What amyloid PET measures in late life—and what it cannot

Amyloid PET is one of the most robust in vivo tools for detecting fibrillar amyloid-β plaque deposition. Its central value is that it quantifies an accumulated burden that is otherwise accessible only at autopsy, enabling biologically anchored diagnosis, staging, and trial enrichment. Quantification has become more standardized through the Centiloid approach, which scales amyloid PET measurements across tracers and analytic pipelines

https://doi.org/10.3390/jpm16030157

onto a common 0–100 metric [12]. Centiloid thresholding has also been examined for predicting long-term progression risk in some settings [13]. Standardization strengthens longitudinal interpretation and improves cross-study comparability. It also supports a more clinically meaningful view of amyloid burden as a continuous variable rather than a binary label.

However, amyloid PET is not a direct readout of the entire amyloid system. It largely reflects fibrillar plaque, not soluble oligomeric assemblies, and it does not directly measure synaptic dysfunction, neuroinflammation, blood–brain barrier integrity, tau propagation, or vascular brain injury. These distinctions matter more in late life than they do in younger cohorts because older adults commonly have competing neurodegenerative and vascular processes, along with systemic factors that can acutely influence cognition. In an older patient, plaques may represent a long-standing biological substrate while the proximate causes of deterioration may be delirium, medication burden, sleep disruption, infection, metabolic instability, or vascular decompensation. Therefore, amyloid PET answers a crucial question—how much fibrillar plaque is present—but it does not, by itself, answer the late-life questions that families most often ask: why is decline happening now, and what will happen next?

This is precisely why binary interpretations are frequently brittle in older adults. "PET positive" can coexist with stable cognition, and "PET negative" can coexist with high vulnerability. The updated appropriate use criteria (AUC) for amyloid and tau PET emphasize that PET should be deployed in clinically appropriate scenarios and interpreted within comprehensive clinical evaluation rather than as a standalone adjudicator [14]. This guidance aligns with what the late-life clinic repeatedly teaches: interpretation should focus on axes and trajectories rather than labels.

2. How common is amyloid positivity in cognitively unimpaired older adults?

The interpretive meaning of amyloid positivity changes with age partly because the population prevalence changes with age. A large individual participant data meta-analysis demonstrated that the prevalence of amyloid pathology increases substantially with age even among individuals without dementia [4]. More recent work also provides prevalence estimates of amyloid abnormality across the Alzheimer disease clinical spectrum [15]. In practical terms, this means that a positive amyloid PET scan in an 80-year-old does not automatically have the same explanatory weight as the same scan in a 55-year-old with progressive amnestic symptoms. In late life, amyloid positivity may indicate biological AD, but it can also indicate that the individual is a plaque carrier within a mixed-pathology environment where reserve and competing conditions shape symptoms. Thresholds further complicate interpretation. PET is often dichotomized into positive/negative categories, but clinically meaningful thresholds vary by purpose: diagnostic classification, prediction of future accumulation, or trial eligibility [16]. Work focusing on lower burdens suggests that relatively low amyloid PET levels can predict future accumulation and cognitive decline in certain populations, supporting the concept of subthreshold or "early positive" states [17]. In late life, thresholds should therefore be treated as tools for probabilistic risk communication rather than deterministic labels.

3. From a single-axis cascade to interacting trajectories

The classic AD cascade model—amyloid accumulation followed by tau spread, neurodegeneration, and clinical decline—remains useful, especially in early symptomatic disease [18]. Late-life trajectories, however, often violate the simplicity of a single-axis cascade. Some older adults show high plaque burden with slow clinical change, while others experience rapid decline with modest plaque signals but strong vascular injury, inflammation, frailty, or recurrent stressors [19,20]. Rather than abandoning the cascade,

 https://doi.org/10.3390/jpm16030157

it is more faithful to treat it as one thread within a web of interacting processes. Downstream markers illustrate why the web matters. Tau pathology correlates more closely with symptoms than plaques, and blood-based phosphorylated tau markers increasingly capture amyloid-linked downstream changes and help differentiate AD from other neurodegenerative disorders [21,22]. Meanwhile, sleep and systemic physiology influence vulnerability: experimental work has demonstrated that sleep facilitates metabolite clearance in the brain [23], and human experimental/clinical studies link sleep disruption with amyloid biology [24,25]. These considerations support a practical late-life view in which processes operate at different timescales: slow plaque accumulation, intermediate tau/neurodegeneration evolution, and fast vulnerability shifts triggered by stressors. A single biomarker snapshot cannot capture all three timescales.

4. Why MDS-OAβ reframes "amyloid activity" in late life

In late-life practice, clinicians often know plaque burden but still face questions about activity: is amyloid-related biology dynamically contributing to current vulnerability, or is plaque burden a static background? Plasma MDS-OAβ is one candidate approach to address this gap. MDS-OAβ is described as a plasma-based measure of the tendency of plasma conditions to promote amyloid-β oligomer formation under assay conditions [26]. The conceptual attraction of oligomer-related markers is longstanding: soluble oligomeric assemblies are frequently considered more synaptotoxic than fibrillar plaque, and they may vary by disease stage in ways plaque burden cannot capture [27]. Blood oligomerization-based approaches have also been linked to amyloid PET positivity in some cohorts [28]. In blinded validation work, blood amyloid-β oligomerization has been reported to discriminate AD from controls in defined samples [29]. Additional plasma oligomer studies support clinical associations with severity and cerebral amyloid deposition [30]. Earlier work also proposed oligomeric forms in plasma as a potential blood-based biomarker conceptually aligned with this direction [31].

5. Why oligomers matter: bridging symptoms and vulnerability

Oligomers occupy a complicated but important place in AD biology. They are often framed as soluble assemblies that can interfere with synaptic function and potentially trigger downstream pathology [32], and emerging evidence suggests oligomer-related signals may peak early along the AD continuum and precede overt tau pathology in some biomarker-defined samples [33]. If this pattern is correct, it implies that oligomer-related markers can behave like stage-sensitive signals that do not simply mirror plaque burden. This matters in late life because older brains have reduced physiological reserve. Small perturbations in synaptic efficiency, inflammatory tone, cerebral perfusion, or sleep architecture can produce outsized clinical effects. Thus, even when plaque burden is stable, a dynamic oligomer-related signal—if validated—could help explain why symptoms worsen with intercurrent illness, hospitalization, anesthesia exposure, pain, or medication changes. This does not require assuming oligomers are the sole driver of symptoms. It requires only acknowledging that plaque burden and synaptic stress may not move in lockstep, particularly in older adults navigating multiple comorbidities.

6. What MDS-OAβ measures: a cautious functional interpretation

MDS-OAβ should be interpreted cautiously as a measure of plasma conditions influencing amyloid-β oligomer formation in the assay rather than as a direct quantitative measurement of brain oligomer concentration. Accordingly, throughout this review we treat plasma MDS-OAβ as a context-dependent dual-use marker—a peripheral 'activity-like' readout of oligomerization tendency and a systemic vulnerability phenotype—whose clinical meaning is best inferred from longitudinal trajectory and stress context (e.g., perioperative vulnerability), rather than as a direct surrogate for CNS oligomer burden (see

https://doi.org/10.3390/jpm16030157

Supplementary Box S1). In addition, genetic susceptibility (e.g., APOE ε4) may modulate oligomer dynamics and clearance across brain and peripheral compartments and has been associated with plasma/CSF oligomer patterns and MDS-OAβ–related signals. This is both a limitation and strength. It is a limitation because peripheral factors—protein binding, inflammation/acute illness, renal or hepatic function, frailty-related metabolic state—may influence signal, complicating simple inference about the brain. It is a strength because those systemic and genetic factors are precisely what shape late-life vulnerability. Late-life outcomes are shaped by brain–body coupling; therefore, peripheral dynamic signals can carry clinically meaningful information even when they are not one-to-one proxies for a single brain compartment. A pragmatic late-life use of MDS-OAβ is therefore pattern-based rather than label-based. Does the signal persist or fluctuate? Does it couple with vulnerability events? Does it align with downstream markers such as plasma p-tau? Does it predict clinical trajectories in biomarker-defined cohorts? This approach aligns with the reality that older adults often cannot be responsibly interpreted from a single timepoint result.

7. Evidence linking MDS-OAβ to Alzheimer-spectrum biology

Evidence supporting MDS-OAβ as an Alzheimer-spectrum biomarker includes methodological work demonstrating dynamic plasma oligomer signals [26], and blinded validation suggesting discriminative utility in defined samples [29]. Beyond assay feasibility, the key late-life need is to evaluate MDS-OAβ in biologically defined, ideally multicenter cohorts against clinically meaningful longitudinal outcomes, given potential variability across samples and assay conditions. As an illustrative, hypothesis-generating example in such a biologically constrained setting, we examined MDS-OAβ trajectories alongside longitudinal clinical outcomes in our cohorts. In amyloid PET-positive AD patients treated with donepezil, adjunctive Ginkgo biloba was associated with improved cognitive outcomes and greater decreases in plasma MDS-OAβ compared with donepezil alone in our cohort [10]. In amyloid PET-positive MCI patients, Ginkgo monotherapy was similarly associated with preserved cognition and reduced plasma oligomerization tendency [11]. These findings should not be overstated as definitive efficacy claims; rather, they illustrate a perspective-relevant point: in biomarker-defined late-life cohorts, dynamic oligomer-related trajectories can be studied alongside clinical outcomes, and changes in MDS-OAβ can accompany changes in symptoms. This supports the broader thesis that plaque burden and activity-like signals can diverge and that the divergence itself may be clinically informative. A concise summary distinguishing measurement scope and interpretive levels for MDS-OAβ is provided in Supplementary Box S1.

8. The key discordance—PET negative but MDS-OAβ high—and how to adjudicate it

One of the most challenging late-life patterns is discordance between amyloid PET and MDS-OAβ, particularly PET negative with high MDS-OAβ. It is tempting to force a binary resolution—either the blood-based signal is wrong or the PET missed amyloid. Late life rarely rewards such forced dichotomies. A more faithful approach treats discordance as a longitudinal question. PET negativity lowers the probability of high fibrillar plaque burden; it does not eliminate the possibility of early/subthreshold amyloid biology, nor does it exclude systemic drivers that influence the plasma signal. The responsible adjudication strategy is therefore pattern-based: repeat measurement, assess clinical trajectory, evaluate downstream markers where appropriate, and reconsider imaging if the course demands it. In late life, the primary function of an activity-like signal is often to prevent false reassurance. A negative PET scan may lower the probability that plaques are the dominant substrate, but it does not guarantee stability in an older adult with substantial vulnerability [34]. If a dynamic plasma signal remains persistently high and the individual experiences stress-test failure, the prudent conclusion is not "non-AD" but

 https://doi.org/10.3390/jpm16030157

"high vulnerability with uncertain dominant substrate," warranting careful longitudinal follow-up.

9. POD as a window into Alzheimer-spectrum vulnerability

POD represents a time-anchored clinical event that reliably exposes late-life brain vulnerability and predicts adverse long-term cognitive outcomes. Rather than being a purely transient behavioral syndrome, delirium frequently reflects failure of cerebral reserve under physiological stress and can unmask previously compensated cognitive impairment. Multiple longitudinal studies have shown that POD is associated with subsequent cognitive decline, positioning it as a meaningful inflection point along aging and Alzheimer-related trajectories [35–37]. In aging societies where surgery and hospitalization are common, POD therefore constitutes one of the most practical and reproducible stress tests of late-life brain resilience. From a biomarker perspective, POD is uniquely informative because it creates a defined before–after window in which stress-response biology can be observed. This contrasts with slowly progressive cognitive decline, where temporal coupling between biological change and clinical manifestation is often ambiguous. If Alzheimer-spectrum processes contribute to vulnerability, their influence may become most apparent when the system is acutely perturbed—as occurs during surgery and anesthesia—yet POD remains multifactorial and is also driven by perioperative factors such as anticholinergic burden, hypoxia, infection/inflammation, pain, and anesthesia depth; accordingly, this framework does not imply amyloid primacy but contextual relevance in a subset. Mechanistically, human studies increasingly implicate dynamic processes rather than fixed structural injury. Prospective cohort work has linked POD to blood–brain barrier (BBB) dysfunction [38], and other cohorts have demonstrated coupling between POD, BBB breakdown, neuroinflammatory responses, and CSF lactate shifts—pointing to a stress-responsive metabolic–inflammatory physiology rather than a plaque-driven mechanism [39]. These pathways are particularly relevant to Alzheimer-spectrum interpretation because BBB dysfunction and inflammation can amplify downstream neurodegenerative cascades and transiently worsen cognition, even in the absence of changes in plaque burden. Viewed through a multi-axis framework, POD-related mechanisms primarily map onto the vulnerability/reserve axis. They can operate independently of amyloid plaque load, contribute to symptom expression when plaque burden is stable, and accelerate decline by lowering physiological reserve. Interpreting delirium solely through a plaque-centric lens is therefore biologically incomplete; evidence from multiple perioperative cohorts instead supports stress-responsive, non-plaque pathways (e.g., BBB dysfunction, neuroinflammation, metabolic shifts) as clinically actionable dimensions of late-life brain vulnerability

10. Why amyloid plaque-centric biomarkers fail for POD, and what oligomer-related signals add

Historically, attempts to link AD biomarkers to delirium risk have focused on amyloid-centric biomarkers, such as CSF Aβ42 (often in combination with tau measures), along with tau and plasma monomeric Aβ. Results have been inconsistent across cohorts. One illustrative example is a prospective study reporting that a preoperative CSF β-amyloid/tau ratio was associated with POD risk, supporting the idea that pre-existing AD-related vulnerability can influence delirium risk, yet not reducing delirium to plaque burden alone [40]. In parallel, plasma monomeric Aβ has generally shown poor predictive performance in perioperative settings. A representative prospective study reported that perioperative changes in plasma Aβ were not strongly associated with POD, highlighting a broader limitation of monomeric plasma measures in capturing the biology underlying acute network dysfunction [41]. This pattern of negative or inconsistent findings suggests a conceptual mismatch. Delirium is best understood as failure of synaptic and network function un-

 https://doi.org/10.3390/jpm16030157

der acute physiological stress, rather than as a direct consequence of cumulative plaque burden. Biomarkers optimized to index long-term amyloid deposition may therefore be poorly suited to detect vulnerability to short-term stressors. If delirium reflects stress-induced network fragility, amyloid species more closely linked to synaptic toxicity—such as oligomer-related assemblies—may provide more relevant biological information than plaque load or monomer concentration. Emerging perioperative evidence supports this shift in focus. In an initial prospective observational study, postoperative plasma amyloid-β oligomerization tendency (MDS-OAβ) was higher in patients who developed postoperative delirium than in those who did not, and postoperative MDS-OAβ levels were correlated with delirium severity [8]. A subsequent prospective pilot study confirmed that elevated preoperative MDS-OAβ was associated with both the occurrence and severity of POD and that pre- and postoperative values were highly correlated, consistent with a predominantly trait-like vulnerability rather than a transient surgical artifact [9]. In a more recent and substantially larger prospective cohort (preliminary; under peer review), preoperative MDS-OAβ showed promising discrimination in this sample for POD, remained associated with delirium severity, and showed limited short-term perioperative change, with an exception observed among patients who developed delirium. Together, these findings support the interpretation of MDS-OAβ as indexing an underlying vulnerability that lowers the threshold for delirium when exposed to perioperative stress. Importantly, these data should be interpreted as supporting risk stratification rather than definitive causal inference. They require replication in multicenter cohorts with careful control for confounders such as frailty, vascular burden, medication exposure, and perioperative complications. Moreover, even if future work demonstrates that plasma oligomer-related signals are only indirectly related to brain oligomer burden, their association with POD would remain clinically meaningful, given the central role of brain–body coupling in late-life outcomes. Within a late-life Alzheimer-spectrum framework, these observations suggest that oligomer-related plasma signals capture a dimension of stress sensitivity that is not redundant with amyloid PET. POD may therefore serve as a biologically informative stress test that helps adjudicate discordant biomarker profiles. Elevated MDS-OAβ in PET-negative individuals who develop POD may reflect an active vulnerable state rather than a false-positive signal, whereas PET-positive individuals with low MDS-OAβ who remain delirium-free may represent a resilient or "silent amyloid" phenotype. In this way, oligomer-related measures complement plaque-centric biomarkers by providing functional insight into vulnerability, rather than duplicating information about cumulative amyloid burden.

11. Why the "activity" lens matters for therapy interpretation and why trajectories must be compared on multiple axes

In late life, the activity lens matters because it changes how we interpret therapeutic biomarker trajectories. Plaque-lowering monoclonal antibodies demonstrate that amyloid PET can show substantial target engagement while clinical effects remain modest and heterogeneous [42,43]. This should not be read as failure. It should be read as confirmation that plaque burden is one axis among several, and that late-life trajectories can be dominated by vulnerability amplification or non-AD pathology. If an older patient has high frailty burden, significant vascular disease, or recurrent stressors, plaque reduction may not translate into proportionate symptomatic benefit. Conversely, interventions that do not directly clear plaques might still influence dynamic signals and symptoms through mechanisms such as oxidative stress modulation, vascular effects, sleep stabilization, or inflammation modulation, without dramatically altering PET signals. This makes longitudinal multi-axis tracking essential: plaque burden, downstream tau markers, neurodegeneration indices, and vulnerability phenotypes should be compared rather than assumed to align. The updated appropriate use criteria reinforce that PET should be interpreted within

 https://doi.org/10.3390/jpm16030157

comprehensive clinical evaluation and evolving therapeutic contexts [14]. Importantly, late-life Alzheimer-spectrum presentations are commonly embedded in a comorbidity-rich context that can modify clinical trajectories and biomarker–symptom relationships. Co-occurring conditions—including sleep disorders, chronic pain/inflammation, neuropsychiatric syndromes, and medication effects (e.g., anticholinergic burden), as well as systemic illness—may amplify vulnerability or mimic/compound cognitive decline independent of plaque burden. Accordingly, this framework emphasizes explicit comorbidity/reserve profiling and longitudinal confirmation when adjudicating discordant profiles [44].

12. Drug-linked biomarker trajectories: anti-amyloid monoclonal antibodies versus ginkgo in a biomarker-defined framework

Drug-linked biomarker trajectories illustrate the interpretive value of a biomarker-defined, multi-axis approach. For monoclonal antibodies targeting amyloid, amyloid PET provides a direct measure of the therapy's intended biological effect and helps contextualize risk–benefit decisions [42,43]. For adjunctive or alternative strategies such as Ginkgo biloba, evaluation should not be reduced to plaque reduction alone, particularly when hypothesized mechanisms include synaptic modulation, antioxidant effects, vascular modulation, or broader resilience pathways. At the population level, systematic reviews and meta-analyses have reported variable efficacy signals of Ginkgo biloba in dementia, emphasizing heterogeneity across clinical contexts [45,46]. Large prevention trials have also reported mixed outcomes in older populations [47,48]. These broader results motivate a more biologically anchored question: in amyloid-confirmed late-life cohorts, do clinical trajectories align with changes in an activity-like biomarker axis even when plaque is unchanged? In our biomarker-defined cohorts restricted to amyloid PET-positive individuals, adjunctive Ginkgo biloba to donepezil was associated with improved cognitive outcomes and decreased plasma MDS-OAβ relative to donepezil alone [10], and Ginkgo monotherapy in amyloid PET-positive MCI was associated with preserved cognition and reduced MDS-OAβ [11] (Figure 1). In our recent 18-month extension analysis (preliminary; under peer review), baseline MDS-OAβ levels and amyloid PET burden were jointly associated with subsequent clinical trajectories, with continued Ginkgo use being linked to sustained clinical improvement. Although Ginkgo treatment was not associated with a reduction in amyloid PET burden over time, amyloid PET signal showed a progressive increase in the non-Ginkgo group, which was closely coupled with longitudinal increases in MDS-OAβ. Together, these observations suggest an apparent dissociation between amyloid plaque accumulation and plasma oligomer-related trajectories; however, causality cannot be inferred, this pattern may reflect residual confounding, and it should be interpreted as hypothesis-generating. Importantly, absence of plaque reduction does not, by itself, establish disease modification (or its absence). So, these findings should be framed as perspective-generating rather than definitive efficacy claims. Their relevance here is conceptual: selecting a biologically homogeneous cohort (PET-positive) helps clarify whether clinical trajectories align with changes in an activity-like biomarker. The broader lesson is that biomarker trajectories are not interchangeable. A drug can lower plaques without fully correcting vulnerability, and an intervention can shift dynamic biology and symptoms without large plaque changes. Definitive testing would require a randomized, biomarker-stratified trial using a standardized extract/dose, with adherence verification, safety monitoring, and clinically meaningful endpoints beyond MMSE. A multi-axis framework reduces surrogate confusion and helps define what should be measured for each mechanism.

https://doi.org/10.3390/jpm16030157

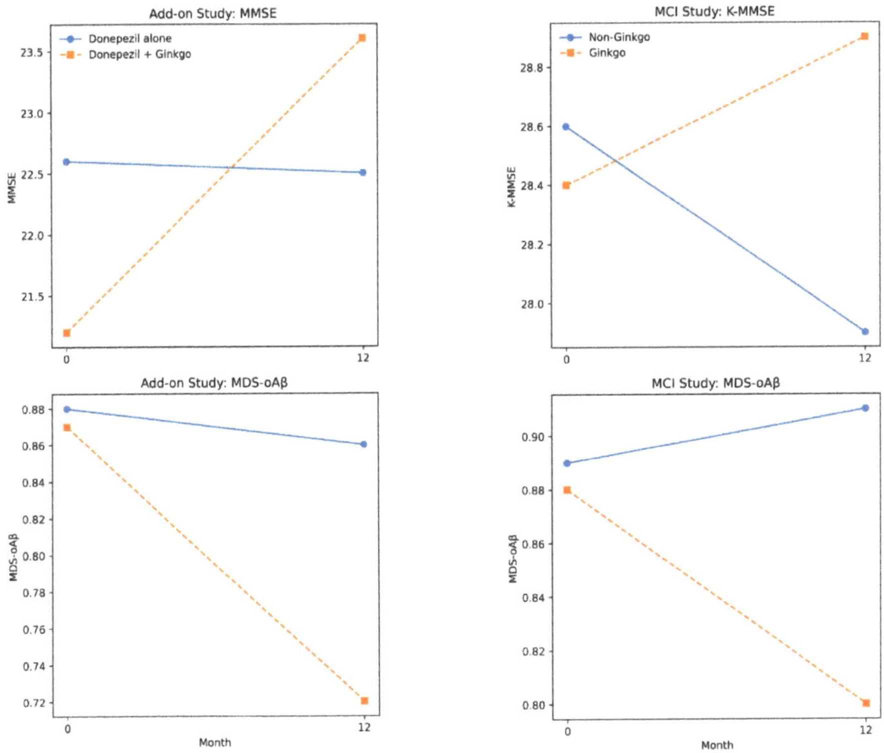

Figure 1. Effects of Ginkgo biloba on cognitive performance and plasma oligomerized amyloid-β over 12 months in different clinical contexts. The **left panels** present the add-on study evaluating the effect of Ginkgo biloba when added to donepezil treatment, while the **right panels** present the mild cognitive impairment (MCI) cohort comparing patients treated with and without Ginkgo biloba. **Upper panels** show changes in MMSE, and **lower panels** show changes in plasma oligomerized amyloid-β (MDS-oAβ). Solid lines indicate non-Ginkgo control groups (donepezil alone or non-Ginkgo), and dashed lines indicate Ginkgo-treated groups. The figure was newly generated based on previously published data.

13. Integrative late-life model—silent amyloid, active amyloid, vulnerability amplification—and what it predicts

Putting these elements together, we propose a practical late-life model with three interpretable states that can coexist and transition: silent amyloid burden, active/dynamic amyloid-related biomarker state, and vulnerability amplification (Table 1, Figure 2). "Silent amyloid" refers to individuals with amyloid PET positivity whose near-term clinical trajectory is dominated by reserve and competing pathologies; plaques function as background risk. "Active/dynamic amyloid-related biomarker state" refers to states where dynamic signals (candidate markers such as MDS-OAβ and downstream p-tau measures) suggest ongoing Alzheimer-spectrum pathophysiology that is more tightly coupled to symptoms. "Vulnerability amplification" refers to states where stress-test phenotypes such as POD reveal low reserve and heightened sensitivity to systemic perturbation, often mediated through BBB dysfunction and inflammation [38,39]. This model generates clinically useful predictions. First, late-life variance should be reduced when biomarkers are interpreted longitudinally rather than as a one-time label. Second, stress-test failures such as POD should identify a subgroup at risk for accelerated decline regardless of baseline plaque

https://doi.org/10.3390/jpm16030157

status, because vulnerability mechanisms can dominate. Third, therapy response heterogeneity should map partly onto axis alignment: individuals whose symptoms are tightly coupled to Alzheimer-spectrum dynamic biology may show more symptomatic benefit from amyloid-directed interventions than individuals whose trajectories are dominated by vulnerability or non-AD pathology. Importantly, these predictions are testable in longitudinal, biomarker-enriched cohorts; key designs and falsification criteria are summarized in Box 1. Until then, the model functions as an interpretive guardrail: it discourages over-labeling based on plaques alone, discourages false reassurance from a single negative biomarker, and discourages treating any biomarker change as a universal surrogate for clinical benefit.

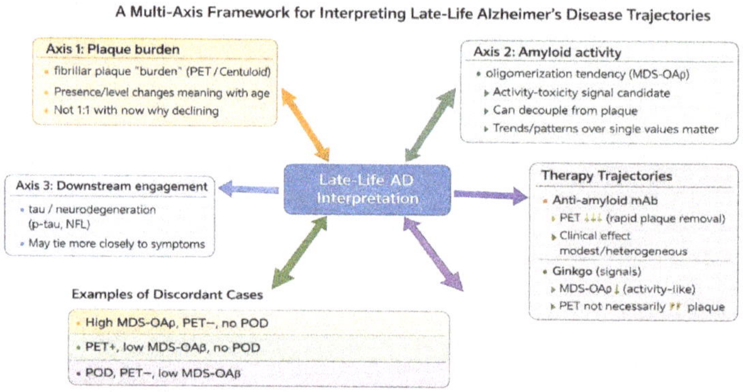

Figure 2. A Multi-Axis Framework for Interpreting Late-Life Alzheimer's Disease Trajectories. The schematic highlights three simplified discordant patterns (from Table 1): high MDS-OAβ with PET−/POD−, PET+ with MDS-OAβ−/POD− ("silent amyloid"), and POD+ with PET−/MDS-OAβ− (event-dominant vulnerability). The framework emphasizes longitudinal, multi-marker interpretation and cautions that biomarker changes may reflect different axes depending on the intervention.

Box 1. Testable Predictions and Study Designs for the Multi-Axis Framework.

Falsifiable predictions (examples)

- Discordance subgroup prediction: PET−/high MDS-OAβ individuals will show higher risk of subsequent cognitive decline than PET−/low MDS-OAβ after adjustment for age, education/reserve, and comorbidities.
- Stress-test interaction prediction: In perioperative cohorts, POD will magnify short-term cognitive worsening and accelerate longer-term decline most strongly in those with elevated vulnerability/reserve burden, regardless of baseline PET status.
- Axis-specific trajectory prediction: In PET+ biomarker-defined cohorts, within-person changes in MDS-OAβ will track symptom trajectories more closely than changes in fibrillar plaque measures, consistent with dissociable 'burden' vs. 'activity-like' signals.

Suggested study designs

- Prospective perioperative cohorts with pre- and post-event sampling (MDS-OAβ $\pm$ plasma p-tau/NfL), standardized delirium ascertainment, and multi-year cognitive follow-up.
- Biomarker-enriched PET-defined MCI/early AD samples with repeated plasma measures and longitudinal outcomes to test whether trajectory alignment predicts response heterogeneity.
- Multicenter replication using harmonized pre-analytical handling and assay protocols to evaluate robustness and generalizability.

Short-term vs. long-term expectations (hypotheses to be tested)

- Short-term outcomes: vulnerability/reserve and stress-response biology are expected to dominate (e.g., POD, intercurrent illness, frailty-related decompensation).
- Long-term outcomes: cumulative burden and downstream engagement are expected to contribute more strongly, with interactions across axes shaping heterogeneity.

https://doi.org/10.3390/jpm16030157

Table 1. Interpretation framework for late-life Alzheimer-spectrum vulnerability using MDS-OAβ, amyloid PET, and postoperative delirium (Refined Version A).

MDS-OAβ	Amyloid PET	POD	Most Plausible Interpretation (Late-Life Framework; With Modifiers)	Recommended Actions/Clinical Use
High (+)	PET+	No	Plaque-positive with elevated oligomerization tendency suggesting an activity-like amyloid milieu without observed stress-test failure in the indexed exposure. In late life, absence of POD may reflect adequate reserve, lower-intensity exposure, or effective prevention, rather than absence of vulnerability.	Longitudinal monitoring of cognition/function; emphasize trajectory (repeat MDS-OAβ when clinically indicated); consider downstream engagement (p-tau/NfL) and comorbidity/reserve profiling; avoid deterministic counseling based on PET alone.
High (+)	PET+	Yes	Convergent high-risk state: plaque burden + activity-like signal + stress-test failure phenotype, consistent with reduced resilience and potentially higher near-term risk after systemic insults.	High-priority risk pathway: delirium-prevention bundle; perioperative optimization; close post-discharge follow-up; multi-axis tracking (MDS-OAβ + downstream markers + neurodegeneration/vascular/frailty measures).
High (+)	PET−	No	Discordant "activity-high/plaque-low" pattern. In very old adults—especially those clinically stable to date—this may reflect heterogeneous biology: (i) early amyloid processes below PET detectability or (ii) non-AD/systemic drivers shaping plasma oligomerization tendency. Interpretable as a risk signal with uncertain substrate, not a diagnosis.	Reassess by trend (repeat MDS-OAβ); triangulate with clinical course and downstream markers; document as uncertain dominant substrate; reconsider imaging only if trajectory warrants.
High (+)	PET−	Yes	Stress-test failure with activity-high signal but no fibrillar plaque detected. POD remains multifactorial; elevated MDS-OAβ may mark a vulnerable milieu, but causal attribution to AD biology is uncertain when PET is negative.	Delirium evaluation/treatment; address triggers aggressively; close cognitive follow-up; broaden vulnerability assessment (frailty/vascular load, inflammatory/metabolic contributors) and consider multi-marker follow-up.
Low (−)	PET+	No	"Silent amyloid" phenotype: fibrillar plaque present with low activity-like signal and no observed stress-test failure. In late life, near-term course may be stable; symptoms (if present) may be dominated by mixed pathology or non-amyloid factors.	Risk-stratify via downstream engagement (p-tau/tau PET if available), neurodegeneration markers, vascular burden and frailty/reserve; counsel probabilistically (substrate ≠ timing).
Low (−)	PET+	Yes	Plaque-positive with stress-test failure but low activity-like signal. Suggests POD driven predominantly by non-amyloid vulnerability axes on a plaque-positive background.	Standard POD work-up/prevention; optimize precipitants; follow cognition after POD; interpret along axes rather than using PET as a single explanatory factor.
Low (−)	PET−	No	Low current AD-spectrum signal with no observed stress-test failure in the assessed window.	Usual care; investigate alternative etiologies if symptoms emerge; repeat biomarkers only if clinically indicated.
Low (−)	PET−	Yes	Event-dominant (non-amyloid) POD phenotype. Particularly in very old and/or low-education individuals, POD may reflect low cognitive reserve/resilience and non-AD mechanisms rather than amyloid-linked activity.	Standard delirium care; optimize triggers; post-event cognitive screening and follow-up (especially if prolonged/recurrent); assess frailty/vascular burden and medication risk profile.

(1) POD(−) means "no delirium observed under the indexed exposure and prevention context," not "no vulnerability." (2) Education and age are effect modifiers in late life: lower education may reflect lower cognitive reserve and influence delirium expression and cognitive testing interpretation; advanced age increases the contribution of non-amyloid vulnerability mechanisms. (3) MDS-OAβ is interpreted as an activity-oriented plasma signal (oligomerization tendency) and may be influenced by systemic factors (e.g., inflammatory/metabolic milieu). Therefore, trajectory/pattern is prioritized over a single measurement. (4) This table is a risk-interpretation scaffold rather than a diagnostic classifier; it should not be used for counseling or clinical decision-making without longitudinal confirmation, and clinical judgment remains primary. (5) Late-life discordance commonly reflects mixed pathology; key confounders and differentials to consider across patterns include vascular cognitive impairment, Lewy body disease, depression/sleep disorders, medication effects (e.g., anticholinergics/sedatives), and systemic illness/inflammation.

https://doi.org/10.3390/jpm16030157

11. Yang, Y.; Koo, M.S.; Kwak, Y.T. Efficacy of Ginkgo biloba extract in amyloid PET-positive patients with mild cognitive impairment. *Front. Neurol.* **2025**, *16*, 1639924. [CrossRef]
12. Klunk, W.E.; Koeppe, R.A.; Price, J.C.; Benzinger, T.L.S.; Devous, M.D., Sr.; Jagust, W.J.; Johnson, K.A.; Mathis, C.A.; Minhas, D.; Pontecorvo, M.J.; et al. The Centiloid Project: Standardizing quantitative amyloid plaque estimation by PET. *Alzheimers Dement.* **2015**, *11*, 1–15.e4. [CrossRef]
13. Hanseeuw, B.J.; Malotaux, V.; Dricot, L.; Quenon, L.; Sznajer, Y.; Cerman, J.; Woodard, J.L.; Buckley, C.; Farrar, G.; Ivanoiu, A.; et al. Defining a Centiloid scale threshold predicting long-term progression to dementia in patients attending the memory clinic: An [^{18}F] flutemetamol amyloid PET study. *Eur. J. Nucl. Med. Mol. Imaging* **2021**, *48*, 302–311. [CrossRef] [PubMed]
14. Rabinovici, G.D.; Knopman, D.S.; Arbizu, J.; Benzinger, T.L.S.; Donohoe, K.J.; Hansson, O.; Herscovitch, P.; Kuo, P.H.; Lingler, J.H.; Minoshima, S.; et al. Updated appropriate use criteria for amyloid and tau PET: A report from the Alzheimer's Association and Society for Nuclear Medicine and Molecular Imaging Workgroup. *Alzheimers Dement.* **2025**, *21*, e14338. [CrossRef] [PubMed]
15. Jansen, W.J.; Janssen, O.; Tijms, B.M.; Vos, S.J.B.; Ossenkoppele, R.; Visser, P.J.; Amyloid Biomarker Study Group; Aarsland, D.; Alcolea, D.; Altomare, D.; et al. Prevalence estimates of amyloid abnormality across the Alzheimer disease clinical spectrum. *JAMA Neurol.* **2022**, *79*, 228–243. [CrossRef] [PubMed]
16. Collij, L.E.; Bollack, A.; La Joie, R.; Shekari, M.; Bullich, S.; Roé-Vellvé, N.; Koglin, N.; Jovalekic, A.; Valléz Garciá, D.; Drzezga, A.; et al. Centiloid recommendations for clinical context-of-use from the AMYPAD consortium. *Alzheimers Dement.* **2024**, *20*, 9037–9048. [CrossRef]
17. Farrell, M.E.; Jiang, S.; Schultz, A.P.; Properzi, M.J.; Price, J.C.; Becker, J.A.; Jacobs, H.I.L.; Hanseeuw, B.J.; Rentz, D.M.; Villemagne, V.L.; et al. Defining the Lowest Threshold for Amyloid-PET to Predict Future Cognitive Decline and Amyloid Accumulation. *Neurology* **2021**, *96*, e619–e631. [CrossRef]
18. Villemagne, V.L.; Burnham, S.; Bourgeat, P.; Brown, B.; Ellis, K.A.; Salvado, O.; Szoeke, C.; Macaulay, S.L.; Martins, R.; Maruff, P.; et al. Amyloid β deposition, neurodegeneration, and cognitive decline in sporadic Alzheimer's disease: A prospective cohort study. *Lancet Neurol.* **2013**, *12*, 357–367. [CrossRef]
19. Aizenstein, H.J.; Nebes, R.D.; Saxton, J.A.; Price, J.C.; Mathis, C.A.; Tsopelas, N.D.; Ziolko, S.K.; James, J.A.; Snitz, B.E.; Houck, P.R.; et al. Frequent amyloid deposition without significant cognitive impairment among the elderly. *Arch. Neurol.* **2008**, *65*, 1509–1517. [CrossRef]
20. Marchant, N.L.; Reed, B.R.; Sanossian, N.; Madison, C.M.; Kriger, S.; Dhada, R.; Mack, W.J.; DeCarli, C.; Weiner, M.W.; Mungas, D.M.; et al. The aging brain and cognition: Contribution of vascular injury and Aβ to mild cognitive dysfunction. *JAMA Neurol.* **2013**, *70*, 488–495. [CrossRef]
21. Palmqvist, S.; Janelidze, S.; Quiroz, Y.T.; Zetterberg, H.; Lopera, F.; Stomrud, E.; Su, Y.; Chen, Y.; Serrano, G.E.; Leuzy, A.; et al. Discriminative accuracy of plasma phospho-tau217 for Alzheimer disease vs other neurodegenerative disorders. *JAMA* **2020**, *324*, 772–781. [CrossRef]
22. Milà-Alomà, M.; Salvadó, G.; Shekari, M.; Ashton, N.J.; Grau-Rivera, O.; Benedet, A.L.; Karikari, T.K.; Lantero-Rodriguez, J.; Vanmechelen, E.; Day, T.A.; et al. Plasma p-tau231 and p-tau217 as state markers of amyloid-β pathology in preclinical Alzheimer's disease. *Nat. Med.* **2022**, *28*, 1797–1806. [CrossRef]
23. Xie, L.; Kang, H.; Xu, Q.; Chen, M.J.; Liao, Y.; Thiyagarajan, M.; O'Donnell, J.; Christensen, D.J.; Nicholson, C.; Iliff, J.J.; et al. Sleep drives metabolite clearance from the adult brain. *Science* **2013**, *342*, 373–377. [CrossRef]
24. Ju, Y.S.; Ooms, S.J.; Sutphen, C.; Macauley, S.L.; Zangrilli, M.A.; Jerome, G.; Fagan, A.M.; Mignot, E.; Zempel, J.M.; Claassen, J.A.; et al. Slow wave sleep disruption increases cerebrospinal fluid amyloid-β levels. *Brain* **2017**, *140*, 2104–2111. [CrossRef]
25. Ooms, S.; Overeem, S.; Besse, K.; Rikkert, M.O.; Verbeek, M.; Claassen, J.A.H.R. Effect of 1 night of total sleep deprivation on cerebrospinal fluid β-amyloid 42 in healthy middle-aged men. *JAMA Neurol.* **2014**, *71*, 971–977. [CrossRef]
26. An, S.S.A.; Lee, B.S.; Yu, J.S.; Lim, K.; Kim, G.J.; Lee, R.; Kim, S.; Kang, S.; Park, Y.H.; Wang, M.J.; et al. Dynamic changes of oligomeric amyloid β levels in plasma induced by spiked synthetic Aβ42. *Alzheimers Res. Ther.* **2017**, *9*, 86. [CrossRef] [PubMed]
27. Sciaccaluga, M.; Megaro, A.; Bellomo, G.; Ruffolo, G.; Romoli, M.; Palma, E.; Costa, C. An unbalanced synaptic transmission: Cause or consequence of the amyloid oligomers neurotoxicity? *Int. J. Mol. Sci.* **2021**, *22*, 5991. [CrossRef] [PubMed]
28. Pyun, J.M.; Ryu, J.S.; Lee, R.; Shim, K.H.; Youn, Y.C.; Ryoo, N.; Han, S.W.; Park, Y.H.; Kang, S.; An, S.S.A.; et al. Plasma amyloid-β oligomerization tendency predicts amyloid PET positivity. *Clin. Interv. Aging* **2021**, *16*, 749–755. [CrossRef] [PubMed]
29. Youn, Y.C.; Lee, B.S.; Kim, G.J.; Ryu, J.S.; Lim, K.; Lee, R.; Suh, J.; Park, Y.H.; Pyun, J.-M.; Ryu, N.; et al. Blood amyloid-β oligomerization as a biomarker of Alzheimer's disease: A blinded validation study. *J. Alzheimers Dis.* **2020**, *75*, 493–499. [CrossRef]
30. Wang, S.M.; Kang, D.W.; Um, Y.H.; Kim, S.; Lee, C.U.; Scheltens, P.; Lim, H.K. Plasma oligomer beta-amyloid is associated with disease severity and cerebral amyloid deposition in Alzheimer's disease spectrum. *Alzheimers Res. Ther.* **2024**, *16*, 55. [CrossRef]
31. Wang, M.J.; Yi, S.; Han, J.Y.; Park, S.Y.; Jang, J.W.; Chun, I.K.; Kim, S.E.; Lee, B.S.; Kim, G.J.; Yu, J.S.; et al. Oligomeric forms of amyloid-β protein in plasma as a potential blood-based biomarker. *Alzheimers Res. Ther.* **2017**, *9*, 98. [CrossRef]
32. Tomic, J.L.; Pensalfini, A.; Head, E.; Glabe, C.G. Soluble fibrillar oligomer levels are elevated in Alzheimer's disease brain and correlate with cognitive dysfunction. *Neurobiol. Dis.* **2009**, *35*, 352–358. [CrossRef]

 https://doi.org/10.3390/jpm16030157

33. Blömeke, L.; Rehn, F.; Kraemer-Schulien, V.; Kutzsche, J.; Pils, M.; Bujnicki, T.; Lewczuk, P.; Kornhuber, J.; Freiesleben, S.D.; Schneider, L.; et al. Aβ oligomers peak in early stages of Alzheimer's disease preceding tau pathology. *Alzheimers Dement.* **2024**, *16*, e12589. [CrossRef]
34. Okello, A.; Koivunen, J.; Edison, P.; Archer, H.A.; Turkheimer, F.E.; Någren, K.; Bullock, R.; Walker, Z.; Kennedy, A.; Fox, N.C.; et al. Conversion of amyloid positive and negative MCI to AD over 3 years: An 11C-PIB PET study. *Neurology* **2009**, *73*, 754–760. [CrossRef]
35. Fong, T.G.; Inouye, S.K. The inter-relationship between delirium and dementia. *Lancet Neurol.* **2015**, *14*, 823–832. [CrossRef]
36. Goldberg, T.E.; Chen, C.; Wang, Y.; Jung, E.; Swanson, A.; Ing, C.; Garcia, P.S.; Whittington, R.A.; Moitra, V. Association of delirium with long-term cognitive decline: A meta-analysis. *JAMA Neurol.* **2020**, *77*, 1373–1381. [CrossRef]
37. Wilson, J.E.; Mart, M.F.; Cunningham, C.; Shehabi, Y.; Girard, T.D.; MacLullich, A.M.J.; Slooter, A.J.C.; Ely, E.W. Delirium. *Nat. Rev. Dis. Primers* **2020**, *6*, 90. [CrossRef]
38. Devinney, M.J.; Wong, M.K.; Wright, M.C.; Marcantonio, E.R.; Terrando, N.; Browndyke, J.N.; Whitson, H.E.; Cohen, H.J.; Nackley, A.G.; Klein, M.E.; et al. Role of blood-brain barrier dysfunction in delirium following non-cardiac surgery in older adults. *Ann. Neurol.* **2023**, *94*, 1024–1035. [CrossRef]
39. Taylor, J.; Parker, M.; Casey, C.P.; Tanabe, S.; Kunkel, D.; Rivera, C.; Zetterberg, H.; Blennow, K.; Pearce, R.A.; Lennertz, R.C.; et al. Postoperative delirium and changes in the blood–brain barrier, neuroinflammation, and cerebrospinal fluid lactate: A prospective cohort study. *Br. J. Anaesth.* **2022**, *129*, 219–230. [CrossRef]
40. Xie, Z.; Swain, C.A.; Ward, S.A.; Zheng, H.; Dong, Y.; Sunder, N.; Burke, D.W.; Escobar, D.; Zhang, Y.; Marcantonio, E.R. Preoperative cerebrospinal fluid β-Amyloid/Tau ratio and postoperative delirium. *Ann. Clin. Transl. Neurol.* **2014**, *1*, 319–328. [CrossRef]
41. Payne, T.; Taylor, J.; Casey, C.; Kunkel, D.; Parker, M.; Blennow, K.; Zetterberg, H.; Pearce, R.A.; Lennertz, R.C.; Sanders, R.D. Prospective analysis of plasma amyloid beta and postoperative delirium in the Interventions for Postoperative Delirium: Biomarker-3 study. *Br. J. Anaesth.* **2023**, *130*, 546–556. [CrossRef]
42. van Dyck, C.H.; Swanson, C.J.; Aisen, P.; Bateman, R.J.; Chen, C.; Gee, M.; Kanekiyo, M.; Li, D.; Reyderman, L.; Cohen, S.; et al. Lecanemab in early Alzheimer's disease. *N. Engl. J. Med.* **2023**, *388*, 9–21. [CrossRef]
43. Sims, J.R.; Zimmer, J.A.; Evans, C.D.; Lu, M.; Ardayfio, P.; Sparks, J.; Wessels, A.M.; Shcherbinin, S.; Wang, H.; Monkul Nery, E.S.; et al. Donanemab in early symptomatic Alzheimer disease: The TRAILBLAZER-ALZ 2 randomized clinical trial. *JAMA* **2023**, *330*, 512–527. [CrossRef]
44. Avitan, I.; Halperin, Y.; Saha, T.; Bloch, N.; Atrahimovich, D.; Polis, B.; Samson, A.O.; Braitbard, O. Towards a Consensus on Alzheimer's Disease Comorbidity? *J. Clin. Med.* **2021**, *10*, 4360. [CrossRef]
45. Weinmann, S.; Roll, S.; Schwarzbach, C.; Vauth, C.; Willich, S.N. Effects of Ginkgo biloba in dementia: Systematic review and meta-analysis. *BMC Geriatr.* **2010**, *10*, 14. [CrossRef]
46. Gauthier, S.; Schlaefke, S. Efficacy and tolerability of Ginkgo biloba extract EGb 761® in dementia: A systematic review and meta-analysis. *Clin. Interv. Aging* **2014**, *9*, 2065–2077. [CrossRef]
47. DeKosky, S.T.; Williamson, J.D.; Fitzpatrick, A.L.; Kronmal, R.A.; Ives, D.G.; Saxton, J.A.; Lopez, O.L.; Burke, G.; Carlson, M.C.; Fried, L.P.; et al. Ginkgo biloba for prevention of dementia: A randomized controlled trial. *JAMA* **2008**, *300*, 2253–2262. [CrossRef] [PubMed]
48. Vellas, B.; Coley, N.; Ousset, P.J.; Berr, C.; Dartigues, J.F.; Dubois, B.; Grandjean, H.; Pasquier, F.; Piette, F.; Robert, P.; et al. Long-term use of standardised Ginkgo biloba extract for the prevention of Alzheimer's disease (GuidAge). *Lancet Neurol.* **2012**, *11*, 851–859. [CrossRef] [PubMed]

https://doi.org/10.3390/jpm16030157

Journal of
Personalized Medicine

MDPI

Review

Coronary Microvascular Dysfunction and Lipid Molecules: Pathophysiological Mechanisms, Clinical Assessment, and Therapeutic Implications

Abdelrahman Hafez, Juan M. Farina, Kamal Awad, Milagros Pereyra Pietri, Isabel G. Scalia, Hesham Sheashaa, Fatmaelzahraa E. Abdelfattah, Mahshad Razaghi, Sherif Ahmed, Ramzi Ibrahim, David Simper, Steven J. Lester, Balaji Tamarappoo, Chadi Ayoub and Reza Arsanjani *

Department of Cardiovascular Medicine, Mayo Clinic, Phoenix, AZ 85054, USA;
hafez.abdelrahman@mayo.edu (A.H.); farina.juanmaria@mayo.edu (J.M.F.);
awad.kamal@mayo.edu (K.A.); pereyra.milagros@mayo.edu (M.P.P.); scalia.isabel@mayo.edu (I.G.S.);
abdelfattah.fatmaelzahraa@mayo.edu (F.E.A.); razaghi.mahshad@mayo.edu (M.R.);
ahmed.sherif@mayo.edu (S.A.); ibrahim.ramzi@mayo.edu (R.I.); simper.david@mayo.edu (D.S.);
lester.steven@mayo.edu (S.J.L.); tamarappoo.balaji@mayo.edu (B.T.); ayoub.chadi@mayo.edu (C.A.)
* Correspondence: arsanjani.reza@mayo.edu; Tel.: +1-480-342-2000

Abstract

Coronary microvascular dysfunction (CMD) has emerged as a crucial contributor to cardiovascular morbidity and mortality, particularly in patients with ischemia and non-obstructive coronary arteries (INOCA). The condition arises from a complex interplay of structural and functional abnormalities within the small coronary vessels, driven by underlying molecular mechanisms including endothelial nitric oxide synthase (eNOS) uncoupling, oxidative stress, and chronic inflammation. Lipid metabolism plays a central role in this pathology, especially in the setting of elevated low-density lipoprotein cholesterol (LDL-C). Furthermore, the protective capacity of high-density lipoprotein (HDL) is increasingly understood to depend on its functionality rather than absolute levels, as it can become dysfunctional and pro-inflammatory in pathological states. Emerging evidence has identified lipoprotein(a) [Lp(a)] and triglyceride-rich lipoproteins as significant, independent contributors to microvascular injury. Comprehensive clinical assessment of microvascular dysfunction therefore requires integration of advanced lipid profiling, including apolipoprotein B (ApoB), [Lp(a)], and the triglyceride-glucose (TyG) index with invasive and non-invasive measures of coronary flow reserve to more precisely stratify risk. In this narrative review, we synthesize current observational, mechanistic, and early interventional data linking diverse lipid phenotypes to coronary microvascular dysfunction. We propose a concept of lipid-driven CMD endotypes, such as ApoB-/particle overload, dysfunctional HDL, Lp(a)-mediated risk, and metabolic/TyG-high states, and map these to a practical, mechanism-informed management framework. While intensive LDL-C lowering with high-intensity statins and combination therapy remains guideline-directed care for high-risk patients, evidence for dedicated microvascular benefit from newer lipid and cardiometabolic agents is still largely hypothesis-generating. A personalized approach that aligns lipid phenotyping, CMD endotyping, and existing guideline-based therapies may help refine risk assessment and inform future trials.

Keywords: coronary microvascular dysfunction (CMD); ischemia with non-obstructive coronary arteries (INOCA); lipid metabolism; low-density lipoprotein (LDL); lipoprotein(a); triglycerides; endothelial dysfunction; oxidative stress; statins; apolipoprotein B (ApoB); coronary flow reserve (CFR)

https://doi.org/10.3390/jpm16050254

1. Introduction

Coronary microvascular dysfunction (CMD) affects the coronary vessels with diameters less than 500 μm and has emerged as a significant contributor to cardiovascular morbidity and mortality [1,2]. Unlike epicardial coronary artery disease, microvascular dysfunction often presents with normal or non-obstructive coronary angiography, leading to the clinical syndrome of ischemia with non-obstructive coronary arteries (INOCA) [3]. Recent studies demonstrate that CMD is associated with a threefold increased risk of major adverse cardiovascular events and represents the primary mechanism responsible for angina and ischemia in patients with non-obstructive coronary artery disease [4,5].

The relationship between lipid metabolism and microvascular function is multifaceted, involving complex interactions between different lipoprotein particles, endothelial function, oxidative stress, and inflammatory pathways [6,7]. Understanding these associations is crucial for developing targeted therapeutic strategies and improving clinical outcomes in patients with microvascular disease. While prior authoritative reviews have expertly detailed the broad pathophysiology of CMD across various cardiac conditions [8] and summarized key clinical takeaways for practitioners [9], a dedicated, concept-driven review that centers specifically on lipid and lipoprotein metabolism from mechanism to management is currently lacking. In this narrative review, we do not attempt a formal, systematic or quantitative synthesis. Instead, we performed focused searches of major biomedical databases, including PubMed, Embase, Cochrane, and Web of Science, emphasizing studies on coronary microvascular dysfunction, lipid biology, diagnostic assessment, and therapeutic strategies. Priority was given to recent, clinically relevant studies, while seminal earlier reports were included when foundational. Based on this approach, we integrate observational and mechanistic evidence to propose a lipid-focused CMD framework, highlighting how distinct lipid phenotypes, including dysfunctional HDL, Lp(a), triglyceride-rich lipoproteins, and TyG-defined metabolic dysfunction, may define testable CMD endotypes and inform hypothesis-generating, phenotype-guided management strategies.

2. Core Mechanisms of Microvascular Injury: Structural and Molecular Alterations

Microvascular dysfunction encompasses both structural and functional abnormalities of the coronary microcirculation [2,5]. Structural remodeling involves changes in vessel architecture, including increased media-to-lumen ratio, reduced capillary density, and alterations in perivascular fibrosis. These changes are primarily driven by chronic inflammation, oxidative stress, and neurohormonal activation [3,10].

Functional abnormalities include impaired endothelium-dependent and independent vasodilation, altered vascular reactivity, and increased microvascular resistance [5,11]. The endothelial glycocalyx, a crucial component of vascular homeostasis, undergoes degradation in response to cardiovascular risk factors, leading to disrupted laminar flow and enhanced platelet-endothelial interactions [5,11].

The pathophysiology of microvascular dysfunction involves several interconnected molecular pathways. Endothelial nitric oxide synthase (eNOS) uncoupling represents a central mechanism, where eNOS produces superoxide anion instead of nitric oxide, exacerbating oxidative stress [8,12]. This process is mediated by oxidative depletion of tetrahydrobiopterin (BH4), substrate deficiency, and accumulation of asymmetric dimethylarginine (ADMA) [12].

Inflammatory pathways, including activation of nuclear factor-κB (NF-κB) and production of pro-inflammatory cytokines, contribute to endothelial dysfunction and microvas-

https://doi.org/10.3390/jpm16050254

cular impairment [6,7]. The complement system, neutrophil extracellular traps, and NLRP3 inflammasome activation have been identified as additional inflammatory mechanisms contributing to microvascular dysfunction [7].

2.1. Low-Density Lipoprotein (LDL) Cholesterol and Endothelial Damage

Low-density lipoprotein cholesterol (LDL-C) exerts profound effects on microvascular function through multiple mechanisms. LDL particles can penetrate the endothelial barrier and accumulate in the vessel wall, where they undergo oxidative modification [6,13]. Oxidized LDL (oxLDL) directly impairs endothelial function by reducing nitric oxide bioavailability, increasing oxidative stress, and promoting inflammatory responses [7,14].

Previous clinical studies have demonstrated a strong association between elevated LDL-C levels and coronary microvascular dysfunction. Mayala et al. conducted a single-center, hospital-based observational study with 40 patients (20 with CMD and 20 with obstructive CAD), comparing clinical characteristics and biomarkers between these groups. They identified LDL-C as an independent predictor for the development of CMD with an odds ratio of 5.24 [15]. Importantly, the association between high LDL-C and impaired microvascular function has been observed across different patient populations, including those with and without obstructive CAD [16]. For instance, Mangiacapra et al. reported in a cohort of 95 patients that elevated total cholesterol—especially LDL cholesterol—correlated strongly with worse coronary microvascular function. In that study, higher LDL-C levels were significantly associated with increased index of microvascular resistance (IMR), indicating poorer microvascular perfusion despite angiographically unobstructed or minimally obstructed arteries [16].

2.2. HDL Cholesterol: Protective Mechanisms and Dysfunction

High-density lipoprotein cholesterol (HDL-C) has traditionally been considered protective against cardiovascular disease, but recent research emphasizes HDL functionality over absolute cholesterol levels [17,18]. HDL particles possess multiple cardioprotective functions, including reverse cholesterol transport, antioxidant effects, anti-inflammatory properties, and direct endothelial protection [17,18].

HDL promotes nitric oxide production by endothelial cells through lysophospholipid-mediated pathways and supports endothelial barrier function [19]. The particle also carries paraoxonase-1 (PON1), an enzyme that protects against LDL oxidation and reduces oxidative stress [19]. Additionally, HDL modulates inflammatory responses by inhibiting nuclear factor-κB activation and reducing the expression of adhesion molecules [20].

Patients with CMD were found to have markedly reduced HDL-C levels compared with those without CMD, underscoring the pivotal role of HDL-C in maintaining coronary microvascular integrity [21]. When HDL-C levels are diminished, these protective mechanisms are compromised—cholesterol clearance from peripheral tissues is reduced, oxidative stress is amplified, and nitric oxide bioavailability is impaired—culminating in endothelial dysfunction, a central mechanism in CMD pathogenesis [22]. Low HDL-C further promotes lipid peroxidation and accelerates vascular injury, setting the stage for microcirculatory disturbances [23]. In clinical evaluation, HDL-C serves as a core indicator of lipid metabolism, and its interplay with triglyceride levels, reflected in the triglyceride-to-HDL-C (TG/HDL-C) ratio, offers a more integrated assessment of metabolic and vascular risk [24]. Elevated TG/HDL-C ratios, driven in part by reduced HDL-C, are strongly associated with insulin resistance, atherosclerotic progression, and adverse cardiovascular outcomes, including myocardial infarction, coronary death, and vascular remodeling following ischemic events [21,24]. This relationship highlights the mechanistic and prognostic significance of HDL-C reduction in the context of CMD.

 https://doi.org/10.3390/jpm16050254

2.3. Lipoprotein(a): An Emerging Risk Factor

Lipoprotein(a) [Lp(a)] is a low-density lipoprotein-like particle consisting of apolipoprotein B-100 covalently bound to apolipoprotein(a) [25,26]. Lp(a) levels are primarily genetically determined and serve as an independent, heritable risk factor for atherosclerotic cardiovascular disease [25,26]. The particle is the preferential carrier for oxidized phospholipids and contributes to vascular inflammation, endothelial dysfunction, and thrombogenicity [25,26].

Emerging evidence suggests that elevated Lp(a) levels are associated with increased prevalence of CMD, even in asymptomatic individuals [27]. The mechanisms underlying this association include enhanced oxidative stress, pro-inflammatory effects, and interference with fibrinolysis due to structural homology with plasminogen [28,29]. Lp(a) is more prone to oxidation than LDL-C and can more readily penetrate endothelial barriers to promote foam cell formation [28,29].

2.4. Triglycerides and Metabolic Dysfunction

Elevated triglycerides and triglyceride-rich lipoproteins (TRLs) contribute significantly to microvascular dysfunction through multiple pathogenic mechanisms [30]. The triglyceride-glucose (TyG) index has emerged as a reliable marker of insulin resistance and shows strong associations with coronary microvascular dysfunction [31,32]. In patients with chronic coronary syndrome, the TyG index was identified as an independent predictor of CMD with an odds ratio of 1.436 [32].

Hypertriglyceridemia promotes microvascular dysfunction through several pathways. Elevated triglycerides are associated with insulin resistance, which impairs endothelial function and reduces nitric oxide bioavailability [33]. Free fatty acids released from triglyceride-rich lipoproteins can directly impair myocardial microcirculation, as demonstrated by studies showing reduced myocardial blood flow during lipid infusion [34–36].

3. Novel Lipid Molecules and Coronary Microvascular Dysfunction

3.1. Apolipoprotein B and Particle Number

Apolipoprotein B (ApoB) represents the number of atherogenic particles and may provide superior risk assessment compared to cholesterol concentrations alone [37]. Based on a recent retrospective analysis of 145 CAD patients who underwent rest/dipyridamole-stress dynamic SPECT, higher ApoB levels (>1.28 g/L) were independently associated with reduced MFR and greater CMD severity, with an adjusted odds ratio of 11.78 for MFR < 2.5 compared to patients with ApoB < 1.0 g/L, and demonstrated strong predictive performance for CMD (AUC = 0.87) [38]. ApoB measurement is particularly valuable in patients with metabolic syndrome, diabetes, and hypertriglyceridemia, where discordance between LDL-C and particle number is common [39].

Apolipoprotein B (ApoB) offers an additional layer of lipid-related risk stratification. Elevated ApoB levels, even in patients who have achieved target LDL-C levels, signal underlying particle overload. High ApoB correlates with increased microvascular resistance and is predictive of five-year MACE after adjusting for lipid profiles [40].

3.2. Oxidized LDL and Advanced Glycation End Products

Oxidized LDL represents a pathophysiologically relevant biomarker directly involved in microvascular injury [41]. The lectin-like oxidized LDL receptor-1 (LOX-1) mediates cellular uptake of oxLDL and contributes to endothelial dysfunction through activation of inflammatory and oxidative stress pathways [42]. Advanced glycation end products (AGEs) accumulate in diabetes and contribute to microvascular complications through receptor for AGE (RAGE)-mediated inflammation [43].

https://doi.org/10.3390/jpm16050254

4. Special Populations

In diabetes mellitus, hyperglycemia accelerates advanced glycation end-product (AGE) formation and small-vessel fibrosis. TyG-guided lipid therapy intensification has been shown to reduce microvascular complications, including nephropathy and neuropathy [44,45]. In women and those with myocardial infarction and non-obstructive coronary arteries (MINOCA), CMD is often a key underlying factor. A female predominance in low CFR cases highlights the necessity for sex-specific therapeutic strategies [46,47]. Among patients with autoimmune diseases, tumor necrosis factor-alpha (TNF-α) antagonists in rheumatoid arthritis improve capillary density and nailfold microvascular metrics, reinforcing the link between inflammation and lipid dysregulation [48,49].

5. Clinical Assessment of Lipid-Mediated Coronary Microvascular Dysfunction

CMD is prevalent among individuals at intermediate to high cardiovascular risk, with a rate of 78.6% observed in patients with an ASCVD risk score above 7.5% [50]. Importantly, CMD is independently associated with an elevated risk of cardiac mortality, even after adjustment for traditional cardiovascular risk factors in the general population [50–52]. These observations underscore the importance of careful risk stratification and phenotype-oriented evaluation in patients with suspected microvascular disease.

Clinical assessment of lipid-mediated CMD should integrate functional evaluation of the coronary microcirculation with both standard and advanced lipid profiling. Invasive coronary function testing, including coronary flow reserve (CFR), index of microcirculatory resistance (IMR), and acetylcholine-based vasoreactivity testing, remains central to the identification and phenotyping of CMD. Non-invasive imaging, particularly quantitative PET-derived myocardial flow reserve (MFR), also provides valuable diagnostic and prognostic information [53,54].

Beyond the standard lipid panel, several biomarkers may refine CMD risk assessment. While HDL-C levels have long been considered protective, contemporary evidence emphasizes HDL functionality over quantity. Multiple meta-analyses have shown that HDL cholesterol efflux capacity (HDL-CEC) is inversely associated with major adverse cardiovascular events, independent of HDL-C levels [55,56]. In addition, patients with endothelial dysfunction exhibit reduced HDL particle concentrations and a loss of large HDL subspecies [57], supporting the concept that qualitative HDL abnormalities may contribute to microvascular risk.

Lipoprotein(a) [Lp(a)] also represents an important component of CMD-oriented lipid assessment. Despite affecting approximately 20% of the global population, Lp(a) testing remains underutilized in clinical practice [58]. Elevated Lp(a) levels ($\geq$125 nmol/L) have been associated with a twofold increase in CMD prevalence [28,29], suggesting that Lp(a) measurement may help identify a genetically mediated high-risk phenotype not captured by the standard lipid panel.

Metabolic biomarkers provide additional insight into CMD risk. The triglyceride-glucose (TyG) index, calculated as Ln[fasting triglycerides $\times$ fasting glucose/2], reflects insulin resistance and metabolic dysfunction [59]. A TyG index of $\geq$9.2 independently predicts vulnerable plaques and coronary slow flow, and meta-analyses suggest that each unit increase in TyG index is associated with a 42% higher risk of in-stent restenosis [60–62]. The interaction between TyG and visceral adiposity further highlights the complex metabolic contribution to coronary microvascular disease [63]. The TG/HDL-C ratio may also serve as a practical marker of atherogenic dyslipidemia and insulin resistance in this setting.

Taken together, the assessment of lipid-mediated CMD should move beyond conventional cholesterol measurements alone and incorporate advanced lipid biomark-

 https://doi.org/10.3390/jpm16050254

ers, metabolic indices, and physiologic measures of coronary microvascular function. Figure 1 and Table 1 summarize the principal lipid-related mechanisms involved in CMD pathophysiology and the corresponding approaches to clinical assessment and monitoring.

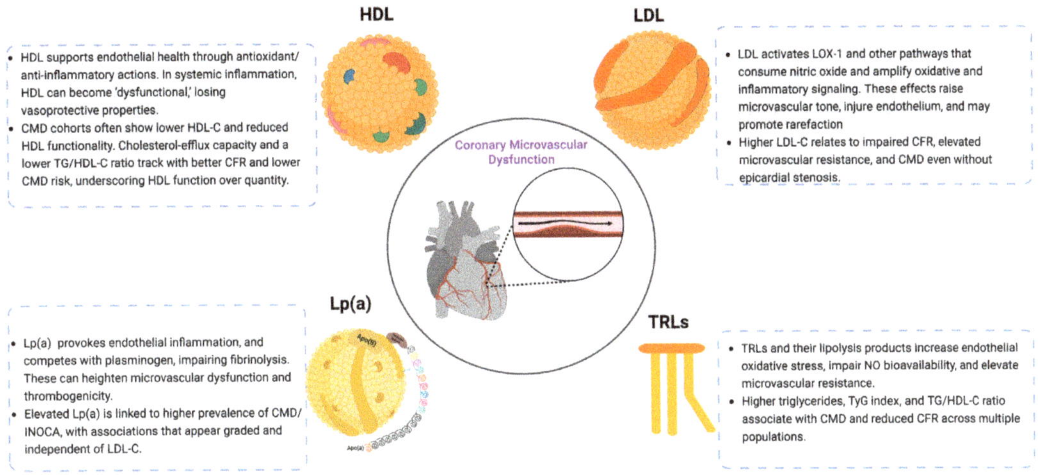

Figure 1. Lipid pathways converging on coronary microvascular dysfunction (CMD).

Table 1. Clinical Assessment and Monitoring of Coronary Microvascular Dysfunction.

Assessment Category	Method/Biomarker	Purpose and What It Measures	Clinical Utility in CMD
Invasive Functional Testing [54]	Coronary Function Testing (e.g., with Acetylcholine)	Directly assesses endothelium-dependent and independent vasodilation and measures coronary flow reserve (CFR) and index of microcirculatory resistance (IMR).	Gold standard for diagnosing and phenotyping CMD (e.g., high- vs. low-resistance subtypes).
Non-Invasive Imaging [53]	Quantitative PET Perfusion	Ratio that normalizes methodological variability; integrates resting and stress flow to reflect coronary vasodilator reserve.	Universal diagnostic cutoff Myocardial Flow Reserve (MFR) < 2.0 for CMD; <1.7 or <1.5 identifies markedly elevated risk of MACE.
Standard Lipid Panel	LDL-C, HDL-C, Triglycerides	Measures cholesterol and triglyceride concentrations within lipoproteins.	Foundational for cardiovascular risk assessment; high LDL-C and TG are associated with CMD.
Advanced Lipid Biomarkers [38]	Apolipoprotein B (ApoB)	Measures the total number of atherogenic lipoprotein particles (LDL, VLDL, Lp(a)).	Superior risk predictor than LDL-C, especially in metabolic syndrome; correlates with microvascular resistance.
	Lipoprotein(a) [Lp(a)]	Measures the concentration of a distinct, highly atherogenic particle.	Identifies a significant genetic risk factor for CMD, independent of other lipids. Recommended for screening.
Metabolic Biomarkers	Triglyceride-Glucose (TyG) Index	A surrogate marker for insulin resistance.	A simple, accessible tool that independently predicts CMD and vulnerable plaques.
	TG/HDL-C Ratio	A marker of atherogenic dyslipidemia and insulin resistance.	Strong association with reduced CFR and is an independent predictor of microvascular dysfunction.

Abbreviations: CMD = Coronary Microvascular Dysfunction; CFR = Coronary Flow Reserve; IMR = Index of Microcirculatory Resistance; PET = Positron Emission Tomography; MFR = Myocardial Flow Reserve; LDL-C = Low-Density Lipoprotein Cholesterol; HDL-C = High-Density Lipoprotein Cholesterol; TG = Triglycerides; ApoB = Apolipoprotein B; VLDL = Very-Low-Density Lipoprotein; Lp(a) = Lipoprotein(a); TyG = Triglyceride-Glucose Index; TG/HDL-C = Triglyceride-to-HDL Cholesterol Ratio; MACE = Major Adverse Cardiovascular Events.

 https://doi.org/10.3390/jpm16050254

6. Therapeutic Strategies

Although several lipid-lowering and cardiometabolic therapies may influence mechanisms relevant to coronary microvascular dysfunction, direct evidence for CMD-specific clinical benefit remains limited, and much of the available literature is based on observational data, mechanistic studies, or surrogate physiological endpoints.

6.1. Lipid-Lowering Therapies

High-intensity statin therapy represents the cornerstone of lipid management in patients at high atherosclerotic risk who may also harbor CMD [64]. Beyond LDL-C reduction, statins exert pleiotropic effects, including improved endothelial function, anti-inflammatory actions, and enhanced nitric oxide bioavailability, that are plausibly beneficial for the coronary microcirculation [65]. Small mechanistic studies suggest that statins may improve CFR and reduce microvascular resistance in selected populations [66], but these data remain limited, and CMD-specific outcome benefits have not been definitively established.

PCSK9 inhibitors provide potent LDL-C lowering and modest reductions in Lp(a), with robust evidence for macrovascular risk reduction in very-high-risk patients [67]. Preliminary data from trials such as EVOCATION and FITTER suggest possible favorable effects on CFR in selected subgroups, although evolocumab pretreatment did not consistently prevent periprocedural microvascular dysfunction, and residual CMD remained common [68]. Thus, PCSK9 inhibitors should currently be viewed as guideline-directed agents for LDL-C and Lp(a) risk reduction, with any putative microvascular benefits considered exploratory. Ezetimibe offers incremental LDL-C lowering and is well tolerated in combination with statins, and its role in CMD is similarly inferred from its impact on overall cardiovascular risk rather than from dedicated CMD trials [69,70].

6.2. Targeted Microvascular Therapies

Calcium channel blockers, particularly those with long half-lives, provide effective symptom relief and improved exercise tolerance in patients with microvascular dysfunction [60]. Ranolazine offers anti-ischemic effects through improved diastolic function and has demonstrated symptom improvement and quality of life benefits [60]. Nebivolol, a beta-blocker with nitric oxide-mediated vasodilatory properties, may provide specific benefits for microvascular function without compromising heart rate response [60]. Renin-angiotensin system inhibitors prevent free fatty acid-induced microvascular dysfunction and provide long-term endothelial protection [60].

6.3. Metabolic and Lifestyle Interventions

For patients with type 2 diabetes or cardiometabolic disease, SGLT2 inhibitors and GLP-1 receptor agonists confer substantial cardiovascular and renal benefits that extend beyond glucose control [61,62]. Experimental data and small clinical studies suggest that these agents may favorably influence endothelial function, inflammation, and myocardial energetics, raising the possibility of beneficial effects on the coronary microcirculation [61,62,71]. However, microvascular endpoints have rarely been prespecified, and available CMD data are hypothesis-generating rather than definitive. Accordingly, SGLT2 inhibitors and GLP-1 receptor agonists should be prescribed based on established indications (heart failure, ASCVD, diabetes with high risk), with any potential CMD benefit considered an attractive but as yet unproven advantage. Metformin remains foundational therapy for type 2 diabetes and has been associated with improved endothelial function, but its impact on CMD-specific outcomes also requires further study [71].

Exercise training represents a powerful intervention for improving microvascular function through enhanced nitric oxide bioavailability, angiogenesis, and reduced oxidative

https://doi.org/10.3390/jpm16050254

stress [72]. Structured exercise programs demonstrate improvements in coronary flow reserve and quality of life measures [73]. Therapeutic strategies and management approaches for coronary microvascular dysfunction are summarized in Table 2.

Table 2. Therapeutic Strategies and Management of Coronary Microvascular Dysfunction.

Therapeutic Class	Specific Agent(s)	Primary Mechanism of Action in CMD	Key Clinical Benefit
Lipid-Lowering Therapies	Statins	↓ LDL-C; Pleiotropic effects: improves endothelial function, ↓ inflammation, ↑ nitric oxide bioavailability.	First-line therapy for risk reduction, with possible benefit on CFR.
	Ezetimibe	Inhibits cholesterol absorption, providing incremental LDL-C reduction.	Used in combination with statins to achieve LDL-C goals.
	PCSK9 Inhibitors	Potently ↓ LDL-C and Lp(a) by increasing LDL receptor recycling.	Significant LDL-C reduction, with possible benefit on CFR.
	Lp(a)-Targeted Therapies	Antisense Oligonucleotides (e.g., Zerlasiran)	Specifically inhibits the production of apolipoprotein(a).
Targeted Microvascular Therapies	Calcium Channel Blockers	Causes coronary vasodilation and reduces microvascular spasm.	Symptom relief (angina) and improved exercise tolerance.
	Ranolazine	Anti-ischemic effects through inhibition of the late sodium current, improving diastolic function.	Symptom improvement and enhanced quality of life.
	Nebivolol	Beta-blockade with added nitric oxide-mediated vasodilation.	Reduces heart rate while potentially improving endothelial function.
	RAS Inhibitors (ACEi/ARBs)	Prevent angiotensin II-mediated vasoconstriction and inflammation; protect against free fatty acid-induced dysfunction.	Long-term endothelial protection and blood pressure control.
Metabolic and Lifestyle Interventions	SGLT2 Inhibitors/GLP-1 RAs	Glucose-lowering with added anti-inflammatory, anti-fibrotic, and direct cardiovascular benefits.	Reduce cardiovascular events and may improve microvascular function in diabetes.
	Metformin	Enhances insulin sensitivity and improves endothelial function.	Foundational therapy for type 2 diabetes with microvascular benefits.
	Structured Exercise Training	↑ Nitric oxide bioavailability, promotes angiogenesis, ↓ oxidative stress.	Powerful non-pharmacological tool to improve CFR and quality of life.

Abbreviations: ↑, increased/higher than baseline; ↓, decreased/lower than baseline; CMD = Coronary Microvascular Dysfunction; LDL-C = Low-Density Lipoprotein Cholesterol; Lp(a) = Lipoprotein(a); CFR = Coronary Flow Reserve; PCSK9 = Proprotein Convertase Subtilisin/Kexin Type 9; ACEi = Angiotensin-Converting Enzyme Inhibitor; ARB = Angiotensin II Receptor Blocker; RAS = Renin–Angiotensin System; SGLT2 = Sodium–Glucose Cotransporter 2; GLP-1 RA = Glucagon-Like Peptide-1 Receptor Agonist.

7. Current Guidelines and Clinical Recommendations

7.1. 2024. ESC Guidelines Updates

CMD is prevalent among people with moderate to high cardiovascular risk and is independently associated with an increased likelihood of cardiac mortality, even after accounting for traditional cardiovascular risk factors [50–52]. The 2024 European Society of Cardiology guidelines introduce new blood pressure categories and emphasize comprehensive cardiovascular risk assessment, especially for high-risk patients [74]. The guidelines maintain aggressive LDL-C targets below 1.4 mmol/L for very high-risk patients while recognizing the importance of non-HDL cholesterol and apolipoprotein B as secondary targets [75,76].

Recent updates emphasize the role of combination therapy for achieving lipid targets, with increased utilization of ezetimibe and PCSK9 inhibitors in appropriate patients [75,77]. The guidelines acknowledge the emerging role of lipoprotein(a) as an independent risk factor and recommend screening in intermediate-risk patients [75,77].

https://doi.org/10.3390/jpm16050254

7.2. Personalized Medicine Approaches

Current evidence supports consideration of phenotype-informed management approaches based on individual patient characteristics and microvascular dysfunction patterns, although prospective validation remains limited [78]. The identification of different CMD endotypes using invasive functional testing allows for targeted therapy selection [79]. High-hyperemic-resistance and low-hyperemic-resistance subtypes require different therapeutic approaches based on underlying pathophysiological mechanisms [2].

7.2.1. Genetic Insights and Pharmacogenomics

Recent genetic studies have begun to uncover single-nucleotide polymorphisms (SNPs) associated with an increased risk of CMD. Variants in genes such as eNOS and CDKN2B-AS1, as well as those regulating endothelin-1, have been implicated in the pathogenesis of microvascular dysfunction [80,81]. Notably, some of these genetic loci are also involved in pathways governing lipid metabolism, suggesting a potential genetic link between dyslipidemia and a predisposition to CMD [80]. The identification of these and other genetic markers may help inform future risk stratification and targeted preventive strategies in susceptible individuals.

Furthermore, the field of pharmacogenomics offers the potential to tailor lipid-lowering therapies to maximize efficacy and minimize adverse effects. It is well-established that there is significant inter-individual variability in the response to statins, the cornerstone of lipid-lowering therapy [82]. Genetic polymorphisms can influence the pharmacokinetics and pharmacodynamics of statins, affecting both the degree of LDL-C reduction and the risk of statin-associated muscle symptoms [82]. For patients with CMD and concomitant dyslipidemia, genotype-guided statin therapy may eventually help optimize treatment outcomes, although this approach is not yet established. For instance, individuals with certain genetic variants may respond differently to lipid-lowering agents or require alternative dosing strategies, though further validation is needed before routine clinical application [83].

7.2.2. Deep Phenotyping with Advanced Lipid and Inflammatory Biomarkers

Moving beyond standard lipid panels towards "deep phenotyping" is crucial for a personalized assessment of CMD. Advanced lipid profiling, or lipidomics, can identify specific lipid signatures associated with microvascular dysfunction that are not captured by routine cholesterol measurements [84,85]. For example, the previous literature has shown that distinct profiles of ceramides and other sphingolipids, which play a role in inflammation and endothelial dysfunction, are associated with an increased risk of cardiovascular events [84,85]. Assessing these novel lipid biomarkers can provide a more granular understanding of an individual's pathological state and guide more targeted therapeutic interventions [84,85].

In addition to advanced lipid profiling, a comprehensive assessment of inflammatory biomarkers is critical. Given the central role of inflammation in both dyslipidemia and CMD, measuring markers such as high-sensitivity C-reactive protein (hs-CRP), interleukin-6 (IL-6), and lipoprotein-associated phospholipase A2 (Lp-PLA2) can help to stratify risk and monitor response to therapy [86,87].

7.3. Clinical Implications and Practice Points

7.3.1. Personalized Therapeutic Mapping of Coronary Microvascular Dysfunction

Clinicians should maintain high clinical suspicion for microvascular dysfunction in patients presenting with angina and non-obstructive coronary arteries, particularly women and patients with diabetes [88]. The triglyceride-glucose index and LDL/HDL

https://doi.org/10.3390/jpm16050254

ratio provide accessible tools for metabolic risk assessment and early identification of microvascular dysfunction risk [89,90]. Comprehensive lipid assessment should include non-HDL cholesterol, apolipoprotein B, and lipoprotein(a) measurement in appropriate patients [91].

Building on these insights, emerging evidence emphasizes that not all coronary microvascular dysfunction is the same; distinct endotypes, such as endothelial dysfunction with vasospasm, impaired microvascular dilation, structural high-resistance remodeling, metabolic CMD, and Lp(a)-driven disease, carry different pathophysiological mechanisms and therapeutic implications. Recognizing these subtypes may help clinicians move beyond a 'one-size-fits-all' approach and support a mechanism-informed, individualized management framework. The following table (Table 3) summarizes how diagnostic phenotyping, biomarker profiles, and lipid metrics may be aligned with potential therapeutic considerations, offering a hypothesis-generating framework for precision-oriented management.

Table 3. Precision Medicine Approach: Matching CMD Phenotypes with Biomarker and Suggested Treatment Strategies.

CMD Endotype (Phenotyping Anchor)	Typical Testing Modality [53,54,78,92]	Biomarker [53,54,78,92]	Potential First-Line Management Consideration	Possible Add-On Strategies
Endothelial dysfunction/microvascular spasm [9,54,60]	ACh: spasm or impaired dilation; variable CFR; symptoms at low ACh dose	Often Lp(a) ↑, ApoB ↑; inflammation signal	Long-acting CCBs; RAS inhibition for endothelial support	Ranolazine for symptoms; consider statin + ezetimibe/PCSK9 to hit LDL-C/ApoB targets; address Lp(a) where high (PCSK9 now; ASO/siRNA emerging)
Impaired microvascular dilation [64–66]	CFR ↓, MFR < 2.0; IMR elevated or normal	ApoB ↑, sdLDL burden, TG/HDL-C ↑	High-intensity statin ± ezetimibe; ACEi/ARB; exercise prescription	PCSK9 inhibitor if targets unmet; SGLT2i/GLP-1RA in diabetes/metabolic syndrome; Ranolazine for persistent angina
High-resistance/structural remodeling [16,53,54]	IMR ↑, minimal vasodilator reserve; PET MFR often <1.7	ApoB ↑; may see TyG ↑	Aggressive LDL/ApoB lowering (statin ± ezetimibe ± PCSK9) and BP control; exercise	Consider cardiac rehab; evaluate for lipidomics/inflammation panel if refractory
Metabolic CMD (insulin resistance dominant) [31,32]	Flow depression under stress; slow flow phenomenon	TyG ≥ 9.2, TG/HDL-C ↑, HDL-CEC often low	SGLT2 inhibitor or GLP-1RA (if T2D), statin per risk, weight loss interventions	Intensify statin; add fibrate only for severe hypertriglyceridemia; focus on lifestyle and CRF gains
Lp(a)-driven risk [26,27,93–95]	May have discordant risk vs. LDL-C; structural/functional changes	Lp(a) ≥ 125 nmol/L	PCSK9 inhibitor (modest Lp(a) lowering) + strict LDL-C/ApoB targets	Consider ongoing trials for ASO/siRNA (e.g., zerlasiran) when available; apheresis in extreme cases

Abbreviations: ↑, increased; ↓, decreased. CMD = Coronary Microvascular Dysfunction; ACh = Acetylcholine; CFR = Coronary Flow Reserve; MFR = Myocardial Flow Reserve; IMR = Index of Microcirculatory Resistance; Lp(a) = Lipoprotein(a); ApoB = Apolipoprotein B; sdLDL = Small Dense Low-Density Lipoprotein; TG/HDL-C = Triglyceride-to-HDL Cholesterol Ratio; TyG = Triglyceride-Glucose Index; HDL-CEC = HDL Cholesterol Efflux Capacity; CCB = Calcium Channel Blocker; RAS = Renin–Angiotensin System; ACEi = Angiotensin-Converting Enzyme Inhibitor; ARB = Angiotensin II Receptor Blocker; PCSK9 = Proprotein Convertase Subtilisin/Kexin Type 9; SGLT2i = Sodium–Glucose Cotransporter 2 Inhibitor; ASO = Antisense Oligonucleotide; siRNA = Small Interfering RNA; CRF = Cardiorespiratory Fitness; T2D = Type 2 Diabetes.

7.3.2. Monitoring and Follow-Up

Regular assessment of symptoms, functional capacity, and lipid parameters is essential for optimizing long-term outcomes [9]. Non-invasive imaging modalities can be used for monitoring treatment response and disease progression [9]. Patient education regarding the

https://doi.org/10.3390/jpm16050254

chronic nature of microvascular dysfunction and the importance of long-term adherence to medical therapy is crucial for successful management [96].

8. Knowledge Gap and Critical Appraisal

The available evidence linking lipid abnormalities to coronary microvascular dysfunction remains heterogeneous and largely observational. Most studies in this review rely on cross-sectional imaging, single-center cohorts, or small mechanistic interventions, with limited adjustment for confounders and substantial variation in how CMD is defined and measured [24,31,32,61,62,71]. As a result, associations between ApoB, triglyceride-rich lipoproteins, TG/HDL-C, TyG, Lp(a), and impaired CFR or elevated IMR should be interpreted as signals of potential mechanistic relevance rather than proof that modifying any single lipid parameter will reverse CMD. Likewise, data on therapeutic interventions (statins, PCSK9 inhibitors, GLP-1 receptor agonists, SGLT2 inhibitors, and lifestyle/exercise programs) are strongest for macrovascular outcomes, whereas microvascular benefits are inferred from surrogate endpoints or small substudies [55–57,75–83].

From a clinical standpoint, these limitations argue against overextending the current evidence and instead support a cautious, phenotype-informed approach. Advanced lipid profiling (ApoB, non-HDL-C, TG/HDL-C, TyG, and Lp(a)) can help identify patients with high atherogenic and metabolic burden who are already candidates for intensive guideline-directed therapy under contemporary guidelines recommendations [70,87]. In such patients, the recognition of CMD, particularly in women with INOCA/MINOCA, individuals with diabetes or insulin resistance, and those with autoimmune disease, may serve as an additional "red flag" that justifies stricter LDL-C and ApoB targets, combination lipid-lowering strategies, and aggressive cardiometabolic risk modification, without claiming CMD-specific benefit beyond established outcome data.

Practically, clinicians can integrate these insights into three critical steps: (1) maintain a high index of suspicion for CMD in symptomatic patients with non-obstructive CAD or discordant ischemia–anatomy findings, especially in high-risk phenotypes highlighted in this review; (2) use advanced lipid and cardiometabolic indices to refine global risk assessment and to guide intensity of guideline-directed therapy, rather than to drive off-label or unproven CMD-specific interventions; and (3) monitor symptoms, functional capacity, lipid profile, and non-invasive CMD surrogates over time to ensure that treatment decisions remain anchored in both patient-reported outcomes and evolving evidence [96]. In this way, a lipid-centric CMD framework can support thoughtful, individualized care while explicitly acknowledging that definitive microvascular outcome data are still needed and that many of the proposed endotypes and therapeutic links remain hypothesis-generating.

9. Conclusions

Coronary microvascular dysfunction represents a pivotal, yet heterogeneous, cardiovascular pathology in which lipid disturbances play a central but not uniform role. Rather than a single entity, CMD appears to comprise multiple lipid-linked endotypes, including ApoB-/particle overload, dysfunctional HDL, Lp(a)-mediated risk, and metabolic/TyG-driven phenotypes, that intersect with sex, diabetes, and inflammatory states. In this narrative review, we synthesize observational, mechanistic, and early interventional evidence to propose a lipid-centric CMD framework that connects these endotypes to practical, phenotype-informed management strategies. Optimal care currently relies on guideline-directed risk factor modification, including intensive LDL-C lowering, blood pressure control, cardiometabolic therapies, and targeted microvascular-directed agents, while recognizing that definitive CMD-specific outcome data for many lipid and cardiometabolic drugs are still lacking. Moving forward, integrating advanced lipid and inflammatory

https://doi.org/10.3390/jpm16050254

profiling with invasive and PET-based CMD phenotyping, and designing prospective trials that prespecify microvascular endpoints, will be essential to test whether targeting specific lipid phenotypes can truly modify CMD and its clinical consequences. Until such data are available, lipid-focused personalization of CMD management should be viewed as a rigorous, hypothesis-generating paradigm, not as established causal proof.

Author Contributions: Conceptualization, A.H. and R.A.; investigation, A.H., J.M.F., K.A., M.P.P., I.G.S., H.S., R.I., F.E.A., M.R. and D.S.; writing—original draft preparation, A.H.; writing—review and editing, J.M.F., K.A., M.P.P., I.G.S., H.S., S.A., F.E.A., M.R., D.S., S.J.L., B.T., C.A. and R.A.; supervision, S.J.L., B.T., C.A. and R.A.; project administration, R.A. All authors have read and agreed to the published version of the manuscript.

Funding: This research received no external funding.

Institutional Review Board Statement: Not applicable.

Informed Consent Statement: Not applicable.

Data Availability Statement: No new data were created or analyzed in this study. Data sharing is not applicable to this article.

Conflicts of Interest: The authors declare no conflicts of interest.

Abbreviations

The following abbreviations are used in this manuscript:

CMD	Coronary Microvascular Dysfunction
INOCA	Ischemia with Non-Obstructive Coronary Arteries
eNOS	Endothelial Nitric Oxide Synthase
LDL-C	Low-Density Lipoprotein Cholesterol
HDL-C	High-Density Lipoprotein Cholesterol
Lp(a)	Lipoprotein(a)
ApoB	Apolipoprotein B
TyG	Triglyceride-Glucose Index
IMR	Index of Microvascular Resistance
CFR	Coronary Flow Reserve
PET	Positron Emission Tomography
MFR	Myocardial Flow Reserve
MACE	Major Adverse Cardiovascular Events
HDL-CEC	HDL Cholesterol Efflux Capacity
oxLDL	Oxidized Low-Density Lipoprotein
BH4	Tetrahydrobiopterin
ADMA	Asymmetric Dimethylarginine
NF-κB	Nuclear Factor Kappa-B
NLRP3	NOD-Like Receptor Pyrin Domain-Containing 3 (Inflammasome)
PON1	Paraoxonase-1
TRL	Triglyceride-Rich Lipoproteins
sdLDL	Small Dense Low-Density Lipoprotein
EVOCATION	Evolocumab for the Prevention of Coronary Microvascular Dysfunction Trial
FITTER	Evolocumab Clinical Trial (Future Investigation Targeting Triglycerides and Endothelial Reserve)
LOX-1	Lectin-Like Oxidized LDL Receptor-1
AGE	Advanced Glycation End Product
RAGE	Receptor for Advanced Glycation End Products
MINOCA	Myocardial Infarction with Non-Obstructive Coronary Arteries
TNF-α	Tumor Necrosis Factor-Alpha

https://doi.org/10.3390/jpm16050254

PCSK9	Proprotein Convertase Subtilisin/Kexin Type 9
ACEi	Angiotensin-Converting Enzyme Inhibitor
ARB	Angiotensin Receptor Blocker
SGLT2	Sodium-Glucose Cotransporter-2
GLP-1 RA	Glucagon-Like Peptide-1 Receptor Agonist
ESC	European Society of Cardiology
ASCVD	Atherosclerotic Cardiovascular Disease

References

1. Yin, J.; Wang, S.; Liu, Y.; Chen, J.; Li, D.; Xu, T. Coronary microvascular dysfunction pathophysiology in COVID-19. *Microcirculation* **2021**, *28*, e12718. [CrossRef]
2. Scarica, V.; Rinaldi, R.; Animati, F.M.; Manzato, M.; Montone, R.A. Coronary microvascular dysfunction: Pathophysiology, diagnosis, and therapeutic strategies across cardiovascular diseases. *EXCLI J.* **2025**, *24*, 454–478. [CrossRef]
3. La Vecchia, G.; Fumarulo, I.; Caffè, A.; Chiatto, M.; Montone, R.A.; Aspromonte, N. Microvascular Dysfunction across the Spectrum of Heart Failure Pathology: Pathophysiology, Clinical Features and Therapeutic Implications. *Int. J. Mol. Sci.* **2024**, *25*, 7628. [CrossRef]
4. Cook, J. Fundamentals of coronary interventional complications. *Interv. Cardiol.* **2024**, *16*, 573–587. [CrossRef]
5. Jan, Y.-K.; Kelhofer, N.; Tu, T.; Mansuri, O.; Onyemere, K.; Dave, S.; Pappu, S. Diagnosis, Pathophysiology and Management of Microvascular Dysfunction in Diabetes Mellitus. *Diagnostics* **2024**, *14*, 2830. [CrossRef]
6. Kei, C.Y.; Singh, K.; Dautov, R.F.; Nguyen, T.H.; Chirkov, Y.Y.; Horowitz, J.D. Coronary "Microvascular Dysfunction": Evolving Understanding of Pathophysiology, Clinical Implications, and Potential Therapeutics. *Int. J. Mol. Sci.* **2023**, *24*, 11287. [CrossRef]
7. Jan, Y.-K. Advances in Diagnosis and Pathophysiology of Microvascular Dysfunction. *Diagnostics* **2022**, *12*, 620. [CrossRef] [PubMed]
8. Crea, F.; Montone, R.A. Pathophysiology of coronary microvascular dysfunction. *Vasc. Pharmacol.* **2023**, *153*, 107239. [CrossRef] [PubMed]
9. Marano, P.; Wei, J.; Merz, C.N.B. Coronary Microvascular Dysfunction: What Clinicians and Investigators Should Know. *Curr. Atheroscler. Rep.* **2023**, *25*, 435–446. [CrossRef]
10. Okada, T.; Kurihara, O.; Takano, M. Takotsubo syndrome during percutaneous coronary intervention: The role of myocardial ischaemia and microvascular dysfunction in pathophysiology. *Eur. Heart J.* **2025**, *46*, 1078. [CrossRef] [PubMed]
11. Alatta, A.; Das, R.; Mohammed, A.; Spray, L.; Purcell, I.; Spyridopoulos, I. The role of arginine vasopressin in the patho-physiology of microvascular dysfunction after ST-elevation myocardial infarction. *Eur. Heart J.* **2023**, *44*. [CrossRef]
12. Bilak, J.M.; Alam, U.; Miller, C.A.; McCann, G.P.; Arnold, J.R.; Kanagala, P. Microvascular Dysfunction in Heart Failure with Preserved Ejection Fraction: Pathophysiology, Assessment, Prevalence and Prognosis. *Card. Fail. Rev.* **2022**, *8*, e24. [CrossRef] [PubMed]
13. Masi, S.; Rizzoni, D.; Taddei, S.; Widmer, R.J.; Montezano, A.C.; Lüscher, T.F.; Schiffrin, E.L.; Touyz, R.M.; Paneni, F.; Lerman, A.; et al. Assessment and pathophysiology of microvascular disease: Recent progress and clinical implications. *Eur. Heart J.* **2020**, *42*, 2590–2604. [CrossRef] [PubMed]
14. La, S.; Tavella, R.; Pasupathy, S.; Beltrame, J.F. Clinico-pathophysiological considerations in coronary microvascular disorders. *Vessel Plus* **2022**, *6*. [CrossRef]
15. Mayala, H.A.; Yan, W.; Jing, H.; Shuang-Ye, L.; Gui-Wen, Y.; Chun-Xia, Q.; Xiao-Li, L.; Zhao-Hui, W. Clinical characteristics and biomarkers of coronary microvascular dysfunction and obstructive coronary artery disease. *J. Int. Med. Res.* **2019**, *47*, 6149–6159. [CrossRef]
16. Mangiacapra, F.; De Bruyne, B.; Peace, A.J.; Melikian, N.; Wijns, W.; Barbato, E. High cholesterol levels are associated with coronary microvascular dysfunction. *J. Cardiovasc. Med.* **2012**, *13*, 439. [CrossRef]
17. E Kosmas, C.; Martinez, I.; Sourlas, A.; Bouza, K.V.; Campos, F.N.; Torres, V.; Montan, P.D.; Guzman, E. High-density lipoprotein (HDL) functionality and its relevance to atherosclerotic cardiovascular disease. *Drugs Context* **2018**, *7*, 212525. [CrossRef]
18. Franczyk, B.; Rysz, J.; Ławiński, J.; Rysz-Górzyńska, M.; Gluba-Brzózka, A. Is a High HDL-Cholesterol Level Always Beneficial? *Biomedicines* **2021**, *9*, 1083. [CrossRef]
19. Tran-Dinh, A.; Diallo, D.; Delbosc, S.; Varela-Perez, L.M.; Dang, Q.B.; Lapergue, B.; Burillo, E.; Michel, J.B.; Levoye, A.; Martin-Ventura, J.L.; et al. HDL and endothelial protection. *Br. J. Pharmacol.* **2013**, *169*, 493–511. [CrossRef]
20. Bonacina, F.; Pirillo, A.; Catapano, A.L.; Norata, G.D. HDL in Immune-Inflammatory Responses: Implications beyond Cardiovascular Diseases. *Cells* **2021**, *10*, 1061. [CrossRef] [PubMed]
21. Liao, L.P.; Wu, L.; Yang, Y. The relationship between triglyceride/high-density lipoprotein cholesterol ratio and coronary microvascular disease. *BMC Cardiovasc. Disord.* **2023**, *23*, 228. [CrossRef] [PubMed]

https://doi.org/10.3390/jpm16050254

22. Zanatta, E.; Colombo, C.; D'amico, G.; D'humières, T.; Lin, C.D.; Tona, F. Inflammation and Coronary Microvascular Dysfunction in Autoimmune Rheumatic Diseases. *Int. J. Mol. Sci.* **2019**, *20*, 5563. [CrossRef]
23. Maldonado, C.; Nguyen, M.-D.; Bauer, P.; Nakamura, S.; Khundmiri, S.J.; Perez-Abadia, G.; Stowers, H.L.; Wu, W.-J.; Tang, X.-L. Rapid Lipid Modification of Endothelial Cell Membranes in Cardiac Ischemia/Reperfusion Injury: A Novel Therapeutic Strategy to Reduce Infarct Size. *Cardiovasc. Drugs Ther.* **2020**, *35*, 113–123. [CrossRef] [PubMed]
24. Prasad, M.; Sara, J.; Widmer, R.J.; Lennon, R.; Lerman, L.O.; Lerman, A. Triglyceride and Triglyceride/HDL (High Density Lipoprotein) Ratio Predict Major Adverse Cardiovascular Outcomes in Women with Non-Obstructive Coronary Artery Disease. *J. Am. Heart Assoc.* **2019**, *8*, e009442. [CrossRef] [PubMed]
25. Khovidhunkit, W. Lipoprotein(a). In *Endotext [Internet]*; MDText.com, Inc.: South Dartmouth, MA, USA, 2023.
26. Reyes-Soffer, G.; Ginsberg, H.N.; Berglund, L.; Duell, P.B.; Heffron, S.P.; Kamstrup, P.R.; Lloyd-Jones, D.M.; Marcovina, S.M.; Yeang, C.; Koschinsky, M.L.; et al. Lipoprotein(a): A Genetically Determined, Causal, and Prevalent Risk Factor for Atherosclerotic Cardiovascular Disease: A Scientific Statement from the American Heart Association. *Arterioscler. Thromb. Vasc. Biol.* **2022**, *42*, e48–e60. [CrossRef]
27. Wodaje, T.; Mahdi, A.; Venkateshvaran, A.; Häbel, H.; Zenlander, R.; Gaylard, B.; Angelin, B.; Pernow, J.; Brinck, J. Higher prevalence of coronary microvascular dysfunction in asymptomatic individuals with high levels of lipoprotein(a) with and without heterozygous familial hypercholesterolaemia. *Atherosclerosis* **2024**, *389*, 117439. [CrossRef]
28. Yao, M.; Dickeson, S.K.; Dhanabalan, K.; Solomevich, S.; Dennewitz, C.; Gailani, D.; Song, W.-L. Investigation of the Influence of Lipoprotein(a) and Oxidized Lipoprotein(a) on Plasminogen Activation and Fibrinolysis. *J. Lipid Atheroscler.* **2025**, *14*, 229–235. [CrossRef]
29. Xu, R.; Wang, Z.; Dong, J.; Yu, M.; Zhou, Y. Lipoprotein(a) and panvascular disease. *Lipids Health Dis.* **2025**, *24*, 186. [CrossRef]
30. Budoff, M. Triglycerides and Triglyceride-Rich Lipoproteins in the Causal Pathway of Cardiovascular Disease. *Am. J. Cardiol.* **2016**, *118*, 138–145. [CrossRef]
31. Tao, L.-C.; Xu, J.-N.; Wang, T.-T.; Hua, F.; Li, J.-J. Triglyceride-glucose index as a marker in cardiovascular diseases: Landscape and limitations. *Cardiovasc. Diabetol.* **2022**, *21*, 68. [CrossRef]
32. Zhang, W.; Liu, L.; Chen, H.; Li, S.; Wan, M.; Mohammed, A.-Q.; Xu, B.; Yin, G.; Lv, X.; Shi, T.; et al. Association between the triglyceride-glucose index and the presence and prognosis of coronary microvascular dysfunction in patients with chronic coronary syndrome. *Cardiovasc. Diabetol.* **2023**, *22*, 113. [CrossRef] [PubMed]
33. Ormazabal, V.; Nair, S.; Elfeky, O.; Aguayo, C.; Salomon, C.; Zuñiga, F.A. Association between insulin resistance and the development of cardiovascular disease. *Cardiovasc. Diabetol.* **2018**, *17*, 122. [CrossRef]
34. Hexeberg, S.; Hessevik, I.; Hexeberg, E. Intravenous lipid infusion results in myocardial lipid droplet accumulation combined with reduced myocardial performance in heparinized rabbits. *Acta Physiol. Scand.* **1995**, *153*, 159–168. [CrossRef] [PubMed]
35. Xu, D.; Xie, L.; Cheng, C.; Xue, F.; Sun, C. Triglyceride-rich lipoproteins and cardiovascular diseases. *Front. Endocrinol.* **2024**, *15*, 1409653. [CrossRef] [PubMed]
36. Stehr, S.N.; Ziegeler, J.C.; Pexa, A.; Oertel, R.; Deussen, A.; Koch, T.; Hübler, M. The Effects of Lipid Infusion on Myocardial Function and Bioenergetics in l-Bupivacaine Toxicity in the Isolated Rat Heart. *Anesth. Analg.* **2007**, *104*, 186–192. [CrossRef]
37. De Oliveira-Gomes, D.; Joshi, P.H.; Peterson, E.D.; Rohatgi, A.; Khera, A.; Navar, A.M. Apolipoprotein B: Bridging the Gap Between Evidence and Clinical Practice. *Circulation* **2024**, *150*, 62–79. [CrossRef]
38. Yang, L.; Zhang, J.; Han, J.; Jiang, X. Relationship between lipoprotein B and the severity of coronary microvascular dys-function. *Clin. Exp. Hypertens.* **2025**, *41*, 2477651. [CrossRef]
39. Witt, C.; Renfroe, L.G.; Lyons, T.S. Discordance between serum cholesterol concentration and atherogenic lipoprotein particle number in people with metabolic disease: A systematic review. *Diabetes Obes. Metab.* **2025**, *27*, 2940–2954. [CrossRef]
40. Hukportie, D.N.; Li, F.; Zhou, R.; Zheng, J.; Wu, X.; Zou, M.; Wu, X. Lipid variability and risk of microvascular complications in Action to Control Cardiovascular Risk in Diabetes (ACCORD) trial: A post hoc analysis. *J. Diabetes* **2022**, *14*, 365–376. [CrossRef]
41. Xu, L.; Wang, S.; Li, B.; Sun, A.; Zou, Y.; Ge, J. A protective role of ciglitazone in ox- LDL -induced rat microvascular endothelial cells via modulating PPAR γ-dependent AMPK/eNOS pathway. *J. Cell. Mol. Med.* **2014**, *19*, 92–102. [CrossRef]
42. Chen, M.; Masaki, T.; Sawamura, T. LOX-1, the receptor for oxidized low-density lipoprotein identified from endothelial cells: Implications in endothelial dysfunction and atherosclerosis. *Pharmacol. Ther.* **2002**, *95*, 89–100. [CrossRef]
43. Lee, J.; Yun, J.-S.; Ko, S.-H. Advanced Glycation End Products and Their Effect on Vascular Complications in Type 2 Diabetes Mellitus. *Nutrients* **2022**, *14*, 3086. [CrossRef]
44. Vithian, K.; Hurel, S. Microvascular complications: Pathophysiology and management. *Clin. Med.* **2010**, *10*, 505–509. [CrossRef] [PubMed]
45. Jha, R.; Lopez-Trevino, S.; Kankanamalage, H.R.; Jha, J.C. Diabetes and Renal Complications: An Overview on Pathophysiology, Biomarkers and Therapeutic Interventions. *Biomedicines* **2024**, *12*, 1098. [CrossRef]

https://doi.org/10.3390/jpm16050254

46. Namkoong, J.; McCarthy, M.; Toleva, O.; Nield, L.; Rinfret, S.; Miner, S. Abstract 4138528: Clinical Characteristics of Five Different Endotypes from Coronary Reactivity Testing, and the Emergence of Sex Patterns in Coronary Microvascular Dys-function. *Circulation* **2024**, *150*. [CrossRef]
47. Mohan, A.; Rajotia, A.; Bagheri, S.; Bhattar, K.; Reddy, S.; Reddy, K.T.; Ho, A. Abstract 4140648: Wake up call for the need of standardized medical management for Myocardial Infarction with non-obstructive coronary arteries (MINOCA): A Meta-analysis. *Circulation* **2024**, *150*. [CrossRef]
48. Weber, B.; Weisenfeld, D.; Massarotti, E.; Seyok, T.; Cremone, G.; Lam, E.; Golnik, C.; Brownmiller, S.; Liu, F.; Huang, S.; et al. Interplay Between Systemic Inflammation, Myocardial Injury, and Coronary Microvascular Dysfunction in Rheumatoid Arthritis: Results from the LiiRA Study. *J. Am. Hear. Assoc.* **2024**, *13*, e030387. [CrossRef] [PubMed]
49. Caraba, A.; Stancu, O.; Crișan, V.; Georgescu, D. Anti TNF-Alpha Treatment Improves Microvascular Endothelial Dysfunction in Rheumatoid Arthritis Patients. *Int. J. Mol. Sci.* **2024**, *25*, 9925. [CrossRef]
50. Weber, B.; Weisenfeld, D.; Seyok, T.; Huang, S.; Massarotti, E.; Barrett, L.; Bibbo, C.; Solomon, D.H.; Plutzky, J.; Bolster, M.; et al. Relationship Between Risk of Atherosclerotic Cardiovascular Disease, Inflammation, and Coronary Microvascular Dysfunction in Rheumatoid Arthritis. *J. Am. Hear. Assoc.* **2022**, *11*, e025467. [CrossRef]
51. Liao, K.P.; Huang, J.; He, Z.; Cremone, G.; Lam, E.; Hainer, J.M.; Morgan, V.; Bibbo, C.; Di Carli, M. Coronary Microvascular Dysfunction in Rheumatoid Arthritis Compared to Diabetes Mellitus and Association with All-Cause Mortality. *Arthritis Care Res.* **2021**, *73*, 159–165. [CrossRef]
52. Weber, B.N.; Stevens, E.; Perez-Chada, L.M.; Brown, J.M.; Divakaran, S.; Bay, C.; Bibbo, C.; Hainer, J.; Dorbala, S.; Blankstein, R.; et al. Impaired Coronary Vasodilator Reserve and Adverse Prognosis in Patients with Systemic Inflammatory Disorders. *Cardiovasc. Imaging* **2021**, *14*, 2212–2220. [CrossRef] [PubMed]
53. Schindler, T.H.; Fearon, W.F.; Pelletier-Galarneau, M.; Ambrosio, G.; Sechtem, U.; Ruddy, T.D.; Patel, K.K.; Bhatt, D.L.; Bateman, T.M.; Gewirtz, H.; et al. Myocardial Perfusion PET for the Detection and Reporting of Coronary Microvascular Dysfunction. *Cardiovasc. Imaging* **2023**, *16*, 536–548. [CrossRef]
54. Gurgoglione, F.L.; Vignali, L.; Montone, R.A.; Rinaldi, R.; Benatti, G.; Solinas, E.; Leone, A.M.; Galante, D.; Campo, G.; Biscaglia, S.; et al. Coronary Spasm Testing with Acetylcholine: A Powerful Tool for a Personalized Therapy of Coronary Vasomotor Disorders. *Life* **2024**, *14*, 292. [CrossRef]
55. Lee, J.J.; Chi, G.; Fitzgerald, C.; Kazmi, S.H.A.; Kalayci, A.; Korjian, S.; Duffy, D.; Shaunik, A.; Kingwell, B.; Yeh, R.W.; et al. Cholesterol Efflux Capacity and Its Association with Adverse Cardiovascular Events: A Systematic Review and Meta-Analysis. *Front. Cardiovasc. Med.* **2021**, *8*, 774418. [CrossRef]
56. Hisauchi, I.; Ishikawa, T.; Yamada, K.; Ukaji, T.; Shimura, M.; Tamura, Y.; Kondo, Y.; Takeyama, T.; Mori, K.; Arai, M.; et al. Association between the High-density Lipoprotein Cholesterol Efflux Capacity and the Long-term Prognosis in Patients with Coronary Artery Disease: A Meta-analysis. *J. Atheroscler. Thromb.* **2025**, *32*, 491–501. [CrossRef] [PubMed]
57. Monette, J.S.; Hutchins, P.M.; Ronsein, G.E.; Wimberger, J.; Irwin, A.D.; Tang, C.; Sara, J.D.; Shao, B.; Vaisar, T.; Lerman, A.; et al. Patients with Coronary Endothelial Dysfunction Have Impaired Cholesterol Efflux Capacity and Reduced HDL Particle Concentration. *Circ. Res.* **2016**, *119*, 83–90. [CrossRef]
58. Tsimikas, S.; Fazio, S.; Ferdinand, K.C.; Ginsberg, H.N.; Koschinsky, M.L.; Marcovina, S.M.; Moriarty, P.M.; Rader, D.J.; Remaley, A.T.; Reyes-Soffer, G.; et al. NHLBI Working Group Recommendations to Reduce Lipoprotein(a)-Mediated Risk of Cardiovascular Disease and Aortic Stenosis. *J. Am. Coll. Cardiol.* **2018**, *71*, 177–192. [CrossRef]
59. Kurniawan, L.B. Triglyceride-Glucose Index As A Biomarker Of Insulin Resistance, Diabetes Mellitus, Metabolic Syndrome, And Cardiovascular Disease: A Review. *EJIFCC* **2024**, *35*, 44–51.
60. Soleymani, M.; Masoudkabir, F.; Shabani, M.; Vasheghani-Farahani, A.; Behnoush, A.H.; Khalaji, A. Updates on Pharmacologic Management of Microvascular Angina. *Cardiovasc. Ther.* **2022**, *2022*, 6080258. [CrossRef]
61. Fatima, A.; Rasool, S.; Devi, S.; Talha, M.; Waqar, F.; Nasir, M.; Khan, M.R.; Jaffari, S.M.I.A.; Haider, A.; Shah, S.U.; et al. Exploring the Cardiovascular Benefits of Sodium-Glucose Cotransporter-2 (SGLT2) Inhibitors: Expanding Horizons Beyond Diabetes Management. *Cureus* **2023**, *15*, e46243. [CrossRef] [PubMed]
62. Luna-Marco, C.; Iannantuoni, F.; Hermo-Argibay, A.; Devos, D.; Salazar, J.D.; Víctor, V.M.; Rovira-Llopis, S. Cardiovascular benefits of SGLT2 inhibitors and GLP-1 receptor agonists through effects on mitochondrial function and oxidative stress. *Free. Radic. Biol. Med.* **2024**, *213*, 19–35. [CrossRef]
63. Yang, Y.; Li, S.; Ren, Q.; Qiu, Y.; Pan, M.; Liu, G.; Zheng, R.; An, Z.; Li, S. The interaction between triglyceride-glucose index and visceral adiposity in cardiovascular disease risk: Findings from a nationwide Chinese cohort. *Cardiovasc. Diabetol.* **2024**, *23*, 427. [CrossRef] [PubMed]
64. Huang, B.; Han, X.; Pan, Y.; Chen, D. A systematic review and meta-analysis of the effect of high-intensity statin on coronary microvascular dysfunction. *BMC Cardiovasc. Disord.* **2023**, *23*, 370. [CrossRef]
65. Oesterle, A.; Laufs, U.; Liao, J.K. Pleiotropic Effects of Statins on the Cardiovascular System. *Circ. Res.* **2017**, *120*, 229–243. [CrossRef]

https://doi.org/10.3390/jpm16050254

66. Baller, D.; Notohamiprodjo, G.; Gleichmann, U.; Holzinger, J.; Weise, R.; Lehmann, J. Improvement in Coronary Flow Reserve Determined by Positron Emission Tomography After 6 Months of Cholesterol-Lowering Therapy in Patients with Early Stages of Coronary Atherosclerosis. *Circulation* **1999**, *99*, 2871–2875. [CrossRef]
67. Chen, H.; Chen, X. PCSK9 inhibitors for acute coronary syndrome: The era of early implementation. *Front. Cardiovasc. Med.* **2023**, *10*, 1138787. [CrossRef]
68. Ishihara, M.; Asakura, M.; Hibi, K.; Okada, K.; Shimizu, W.; Takano, H.; Suwa, S.; Fujii, K.; Okumura, Y.; Mano, T.; et al. Evolocumab for prevention of microvascular dysfunction in patients undergoing percutaneous coronary intervention: The randomised, open-label EVOCATION trial. *EuroIntervention* **2022**, *18*, e647–e655. [CrossRef]
69. Ballantyne, C.M.; Houri, J.; Notarbartolo, A.; Melani, L.; Lipka, L.J.; Suresh, R.; Sun, S.; LeBeaut, A.P.; Sager, P.T.; Veltri, E.P. Effect of Ezetimibe Coadministered with Atorvastatin in 628 Patients with Primary Hypercholesterolemia. *Circulation* **2003**, *107*, 2409–2415. [CrossRef] [PubMed]
70. Banach, M.; Reiner, Ž.; Surma, S.; Bajraktari, G.; Bielecka-Dabrowa, A.; Bunc, M.; Bytyçi, I.; Ceska, R.; Cicero, A.F.G.; Dudek, D.; et al. 2024 Recommendations on the Optimal Use of Lipid-Lowering Therapy in Established Atherosclerotic Cardiovascular Disease and Following Acute Coronary Syndromes: A Position Paper of the International Lipid Expert Panel (ILEP). *Drugs* **2024**, *84*, 1541–1577. [CrossRef] [PubMed]
71. Mather, K.J.; Verma, S.; Anderson, T.J. Improved endothelial function with metformin in type 2 diabetes mellitus. *J. Am. Coll. Cardiol.* **2001**, *37*, 1344–1350. [CrossRef]
72. Hong, J.; Park, Y. Microvascular Function and Exercise Training: Functional Implication of Nitric Oxide Signaling and Ion Channels. *Pulse* **2024**, *12*, 27–33. [CrossRef] [PubMed]
73. Bruning, R.S.; Sturek, M. Benefits of Exercise Training on Coronary Blood Flow in Coronary Artery Disease Patients. *Prog. Cardiovasc. Dis.* **2015**, *57*, 443–453. [CrossRef]
74. McEvoy, J.W.; McCarthy, C.P.; Bruno, R.M.; Brouwers, S.; Canavan, M.D.; Ceconi, C.; Christodorescu, R.M.; Daskalopoulou, S.S.; Ferro, C.J.; Gerdts, E.; et al. 2024 ESC Guidelines for the management of elevated blood pressure and hypertension. *Eur. Hear. J.* **2024**, *45*, 3912–4018. [CrossRef]
75. Ray, K.K.; Reeskamp, L.F.; Laufs, U.; Banach, M.; Mach, F.; Tokgözoğlu, L.S.; Connolly, D.L.; Gerrits, A.J.; Stroes, E.S.G.; Masana, L.; et al. Combination lipid-lowering therapy as first-line strategy in very high-risk patients. *Eur. Hear. J.* **2022**, *43*, 830–833. [CrossRef]
76. Cannon, C.P.; Blazing, M.A.; Giugliano, R.P.; McCagg, A.; White, J.A.; Théroux, P.; Darius, H.; Lewis, B.S.; Ophuis, T.O.; Jukema, J.W.; et al. Ezetimibe Added to Statin Therapy after Acute Coronary Syndromes. *N. Engl. J. Med.* **2015**, *372*, 2387–2397. [CrossRef]
77. Khan, S.U.; Yedlapati, S.H.; Lone, A.N.; Hao, Q.; Guyatt, G.; Delvaux, N.; Bekkering, G.E.; Vandvik, P.O.; Bin Riaz, I.; Li, S.; et al. PCSK9 inhibitors and ezetimibe with or without statin therapy for cardiovascular risk reduction: A systematic review and network meta-analysis. *BMJ* **2022**, *377*, e069116. [CrossRef] [PubMed]
78. Ang, D.T.Y.; Berry, C.; Kaski, J.-C. Phenotype-based management of coronary microvascular dysfunction. *J. Nucl. Cardiol.* **2022**, *29*, 3332–3340. [CrossRef]
79. Maas, A.M.; Damman, P. Some endotypes of microvascular dysfunction may be more worrisome than others. *EuroIntervention* **2022**, *18*, 703–704. [CrossRef] [PubMed]
80. Wayne, N.; Singamneni, V.S.; Venkatesh, R.; Cherlin, T.; Verma, S.S.; Guerraty, M.A. Genetic Insights Into Coronary Micro-vascular Disease. *Microcirculation* **2025**, *32*, e12896. [CrossRef]
81. Stein, A.P.; Harder, J.; Holmes, H.R.; Merz, C.N.B.; Pepine, C.J.; Keeley, E.C. Single Nucleotide Polymorphisms in Coronary Microvascular Dysfunction. *J. Am. Heart Assoc.* **2024**, *13*, e032137. [CrossRef]
82. Sheikhy, A.; Fallahzadeh, A.; Meybodi, H.R.A.; Hasanzad, M.; Tajdini, M.; Hosseini, K. Personalized medicine in cardiovascular disease: Review of literature. *J. Diabetes Metab. Disord.* **2021**, *20*, 1793–1805. [CrossRef]
83. Yow, H.-Y.; Hamzah, S.; Abdul Rahim, N.; Suppiah, V. Pharmacogenomics of response to statin treatment and susceptibility to statin-induced adverse drug reactions in Asians: A scoping review. *Asian Biomed. Res. Rev. News* **2023**, *17*, 95–114. [CrossRef] [PubMed]
84. Zhu, D.; Vernon, S.T.; D'agostino, Z.; Wu, J.; Giles, C.; Chan, A.S.; Kott, K.A.; Gray, M.P.; Gholipour, A.; Tang, O.; et al. Lipidomics Profiling and Risk of Coronary Artery Disease in the BioHEART-CT Discovery Cohort. *Biomolecules* **2023**, *13*, 917. [CrossRef] [PubMed]
85. Lindner, J.R.; Davidson, B.P.; Song, Z.; Maier, C.S.; Minnier, J.; Stevens, J.F.; Ferencik, M.; Taqui, S.; Belcik, J.T.; Moccetti, F.; et al. Plasma Lipidomic Patterns in Patients with Symptomatic Coronary Microvascular Dysfunction. *Metabolites* **2021**, *11*, 648. [CrossRef]
86. Liu, H.; Yao, Y.; Wang, Y.; Ji, L.; Zhu, K.; Hu, H.; Chen, J.; Yang, J.; Cui, Q.; Geng, B.; et al. Association between high-sensitivity C-reactive protein, lipoprotein-associated phospholipase A2 and carotid atherosclerosis: A cross-sectional study. *J. Cell. Mol. Med.* **2018**, *22*, 5145–5150. [CrossRef]

 https://doi.org/10.3390/jpm16050254

87. Alfaddagh, A.; Martin, S.S.; Leucker, T.M.; Michos, E.D.; Blaha, M.J.; Lowenstein, C.J.; Jones, S.R.; Toth, P.P. Inflammation and cardiovascular disease: From mechanisms to therapeutics. *Am. J. Prev. Cardiol.* **2020**, *4*, 100130. [CrossRef]
88. Kunadian, V.; Chieffo, A.; Camici, P.G.; Berry, C.; Escaned, J.; Maas, A.H.E.M.; Prescott, E.; Karam, N.; Appelman, Y.; Fraccaro, C.; et al. An EAPCI Expert Consensus Document on Ischaemia with Non-Obstructive Coronary Arteries in Collaboration with European Society of Cardiology Working Group on Coronary Pathophysiology & Microcirculation Endorsed by Coronary Vasomotor Disorders International Study Group. *Eur. Hear. J.* **2020**, *41*, 3504–3520. [CrossRef]
89. Araújo, S.P.; Juvanhol, L.L.; Bressan, J.; Hermsdorff, H.H.M. Triglyceride glucose index: A new biomarker in predicting cardiovascular risk. *Prev. Med. Rep.* **2022**, *29*, 101941. [CrossRef] [PubMed]
90. Millán, J.; Pintó, X.; Muñoz, A.; Zúñiga, M.; Rubiés-Prat, J.; Pallardo, L.F.; Masana, L.; Mangas, A.; Hernández-Mijares, A.; González-Santos, P.; et al. Lipoprotein ratios: Physiological significance and clinical usefulness in cardiovascular prevention. *Vasc. Health Risk Manag.* **2009**, *5*, 757–765. [CrossRef]
91. Katsi, V.; Argyriou, N.; Fragoulis, C.; Tsioufis, K. The Role of Non-HDL Cholesterol and Apolipoprotein B in Cardiovascular Disease: A Comprehensive Review. *J. Cardiovasc. Dev. Dis.* **2025**, *12*, 256. [CrossRef]
92. Taqueti, V.R.; Di Carli, M.F. Coronary Microvascular Disease Pathogenic Mechanisms and Therapeutic Options. *J. Am. Coll. Cardiol.* **2018**, *72*, 2625–2641. [CrossRef] [PubMed]
93. Shapiro, M.D.; Minnier, J.; Tavori, H.; Kassahun, H.; Flower, A.; Somaratne, R.; Fazio, S. Relationship Between Low-Density Lipoprotein Cholesterol and Lipoprotein(a) Lowering in Response to PCSK9 Inhibition with Evolocumab. *J. Am. Hear. Assoc.* **2019**, *8*, e010932. [CrossRef] [PubMed]
94. Greco, A.; Finocchiaro, S.; Spagnolo, M.; Faro, D.C.; Mauro, M.S.; Raffo, C.; Sangiorgio, G.; Imbesi, A.; Laudani, C.; Mazzone, P.M.; et al. Lipoprotein(a) as a Pharmacological Target: Premises, Promises, and Prospects. *Circulation* **2025**, *151*, 400–415. [CrossRef] [PubMed]
95. Nissen, S.E.; Wang, Q.; Nicholls, S.J.; Navar, A.M.; Ray, K.K.; Schwartz, G.G.; Szarek, M.; Stroes, E.S.G.; Troquay, R.; Dorresteijn, J.A.N.; et al. Zerlasiran—A Small-Interfering RNA Targeting Lipoprotein(a). *JAMA* **2024**, *332*, 1992. [CrossRef]
96. Mller, A. Adherence to Long-Term Therapy—A Model of Assessment Into Primary Care. In *Primary Care at a Glance—Hot Topics and New Insights*; INTECH Open Access Publisher: London, UK, 2012. [CrossRef]

 https://doi.org/10.3390/jpm16050254

Journal of
Personalized Medicine

MDPI

Review

Prolactin as a Candidate Biomarker in Non-Small Cell Lung Cancer: Implications for Personalized Medicine and Post-Treatment Risk Stratification

Filip Gajewski [1,*], Grzegorz Kurec [1], Aleksandra Litkowska [1], Joanna Pec [1], Jakub Kleinrok [2], Weronika Pająk [1], Oliwia Burdan [1], Paweł Krawczyk [3,*] and Agnieszka Korolczuk [2]

1 Department of Pneumonology, Oncology and Allergology, Medical University of Lublin, Doktora Kazimierza Jaczewskiego 8, 20-090 Lublin, Poland; a_litkowska@interia.pl (A.L.); apec1410@gmail.com (J.P.)
2 Chair and Department of Clinical Pathomorphology at Medical University of Lublin, Kazimierza Jaczewskiego 8b, 20-090 Lublin, Poland
3 Laboratory of Immunology and Genetics, Medical University of Lublin, Doktora Kazimierza Jaczewskiego 8, 20-090 Lublin, Poland
* Correspondence: 63380@umlub.edu.pl (F.G.); pawelkrawczyk@umlub.edu.pl (P.K.)

Abstract

Background/Objectives: Non-small cell lung cancer (NSCLC) remains associated with high mortality, frequent late-stage diagnosis, biological heterogeneity, and recurrence after treatment. Although molecular and immunohistochemical biomarkers have transformed treatment selection, there remains a need for accessible, repeatable, and clinically practical circulating biomarkers that may support prognosis and post-treatment monitoring. This review discusses prolactin (PRL) as a candidate supplementary biomarker in NSCLC, with particular emphasis on its biological rationale, potential prognostic relevance, and possible role in personalized risk stratification after systemic therapy. **Methods:** This narrative review summarizes current evidence on established biomarkers in NSCLC, the physiology and regulation of PRL, PRL/PRLR signaling in cancer biology, mechanisms of PRL dysregulation in lung cancer, and available clinical observations concerning PRL alterations in NSCLC. Particular attention is given to the distinction between prognostic and predictive biomarkers, longitudinal monitoring, pituitary involvement, immune checkpoint inhibitor-related endocrine effects, and biological, pharmacological, and analytical confounders affecting PRL interpretation. **Results:** Current evidence suggests that PRL may be biologically relevant in NSCLC through its involvement in pathways related to cell proliferation, survival, angiogenesis, invasion, epithelial–mesenchymal transition, immune modulation, and possible therapy resistance. Clinical observations indicate that altered PRL levels may occur in advanced disease, pituitary involvement, systemic inflammation, stress, or during anticancer and supportive treatment. However, PRL lacks cancer specificity and is influenced by multiple confounders, including circadian rhythm, stress, endocrine disorders, macroprolactin, cachexia, medications, and assay variability. Available clinical data remain limited and are largely derived from small studies or case-based evidence. **Conclusions:** PRL should not currently be considered a standalone diagnostic, predictive, or treatment-selective biomarker in NSCLC. Its most realistic potential role is as a supplementary circulating marker within multimarker prognostic and monitoring models. Prospective validation with standardized sampling, assay procedures, and confounder adjustment is required before clinical implementation.

Keywords: non-small cell lung cancer; prolactin; biomarker; personalized medicine; circulating biomarkers; risk stratification; prognosis; treatment monitoring; hyperprolactinemia; PRLR signaling

1. Introduction

Global Burden and Clinical Significance of NSCLC

Lung cancer remains one of the most significant challenges in modern oncology, due to its prevalence, high mortality rate, and the rising number of cases among younger patients. Non-small cell lung cancer (NSCLC) is of particular significance, accounting for approximately 85% of lung cancer cases and primarily comprising adenocarcinoma, squamous cell carcinoma and large cell carcinoma [1–3].

Despite significant diagnostic and therapeutic advances, NSCLC continues to be associated with high mortality. This is due to several factors. A significant proportion of cases are diagnosed at a locally advanced or metastatic stage. Clinical symptoms in the early stages are often non-specific, and the disease is characterised by high biological heterogeneity. Furthermore, even after radical treatment, some patients experience recurrence [3].

In oncology, biomarkers are of particular importance because they enable a shift from treatment based solely on histopathological diagnosis to a management approach tailored to the biology of a specific tumour and the patient's characteristics. Their use in personalised medicine stems not only from the possibility of selecting treatment methods, but also from more vigilant, objective monitoring following therapy [4,5].

The characteristics that an ideal clinical biomarker should possess are reliability, reproducibility, easy access, relatively low cost, the ability to be measured in routine practice, and ease of interpretation in the context of prognosis and therapeutic decisions. For this reason, there is growing interest in circulating biomarkers, which can be measured repeatedly and non-invasively [6].

Currently, many key NSCLC biomarkers rely on the analysis of tissue samples. Histopathological and molecular examination of the tumour remains essential, but has significant limitations. Biopsy material may be insufficient in terms of quantity or quality; a single biopsy does not always reflect the full heterogeneity of the tumour, and re-sampling tissue in the event of disease progression is often impossible or burdensome for the patient.

This clinical gap presents an opportunity for potential endocrine markers. The endocrine system influences proliferation, metabolism, inflammation, anti-tumour immunity, and the body's stress response. This means that selected hormones may not only reflect the patient's general condition but also participate in mechanisms promoting tumour progression. With regard to NSCLC, markers that can be measured in serum, which may change in response to treatment and which potentially correlate with clinical outcome following chemotherapy, are of particular interest.

Personalised medicine has significantly transformed the treatment of NSCLC, particularly through molecular and immunohistochemical testing. Nevertheless, there remains a need for markers that are inexpensive, reproducible, easy to measure, and useful for assessing prognosis and monitoring patients following treatment.

2. Scope of the Review

The aim of this review is to evaluate the potential role of prolactin as a supplementary circulating biomarker in patients with NSCLC, with particular emphasis on its prognostic significance following systemic treatment, including chemotherapy. We discuss the biological rationale for PRL involvement in NSCLC, summarize the available clinical evidence,

 https://doi.org/10.3390/jpm16070342

and highlight the methodological challenges and future research directions required before PRL can be considered for routine clinical application. PRL is not currently recognised as a diagnostic marker or a factor determining treatment selection. Therefore, this review primarily analyses it as a potential adjunctive marker.

3. Personalized Medicine in NSCLC: Current Biomarker Landscape and Remaining Gaps

3.1. Molecular Biomarkers Currently Used in NSCLC

Molecular profiling has become a central component of personalized treatment in NSCLC, particularly in patients with advanced non-squamous tumors. The most clinically relevant actionable alterations include mutations in the EGFR gene, rearrangements involving ALK and ROS1 proto-oncogene 1, BRAF p.(Val600Glu) mutations, MET exon 14 skipping alterations, RET proto-oncogene fusions, NTRK fusions, KRAS p.(Gly12Cys) mutations, and selected human epidermal growth factor receptor 2 (HER2/ERBB2) alterations [7–10]. These biomarkers are primarily predictive, as their identification allows the selection of molecularly targeted therapies that may provide substantial clinical benefit compared with non-selective systemic treatment [11,12]. In addition to genomic alterations, PD-L expression remains an important immunohistochemical biomarker used to guide the selection of immune checkpoint inhibitor-based therapy, especially in tumors without actionable driver alterations, although its interpretation may be affected by tumour heterogeneity, assay variability, and the broader immune context of the tumour microenvironment (TME) [11,13].

Broad-panel next-generation sequencing (NGS), performed on tissue and increasingly supported by liquid biopsy when tissue is insufficient, is therefore recommended to identify actionable alterations efficiently and to avoid sequential single-gene testing [9,10]. However, despite the major therapeutic impact of these biomarkers, they do not fully address prognosis, longitudinal treatment monitoring, or risk assessment after systemic therapy.

Although tissue biopsy remains the gold standard for molecular profiling in NSCLC, alternative specimen types have also been explored. In particular, bronchoalveolar lavage fluid (BALF) has emerged as a potential source of tumor-derived material, including cell-free DNA, extracellular vesicles, proteins, and other biomolecules. Several studies have demonstrated the feasibility of detecting actionable genomic alterations, such as EGFR mutations, using BALF, with some reports suggesting higher sensitivity than plasma-based liquid biopsy in selected clinical settings. However, despite these promising findings, BALF-based molecular analyses have not yet been incorporated into routine biomarker testing algorithms because of limited standardization, heterogeneous methodologies, and insufficient prospective validation. Therefore, BALF should currently be regarded as an investigational complementary source of molecular information rather than an established alternative to tissue-based testing in NSCLC [14–16].

3.2. Prognostic Versus Predictive Biomarkers in NSCLC

In NSCLC, the distinction between prognostic and predictive biomarkers is essential for the correct interpretation of biomarker studies. A prognostic biomarker provides information about the likely clinical outcome of the disease, such as overall survival (OS), progression-free survival (PFS), recurrence risk, or disease aggressiveness, independently of a specific therapeutic intervention [12,17]. In contrast, a predictive biomarker indicates the likelihood of response or resistance to a particular treatment and is therefore directly linked to therapeutic decision-making [12,17,18].

This distinction is particularly important during the evaluation of prolactin as a potential biomarker in NSCLC. If elevated prolactin levels are associated with shorter

 https://doi.org/10.3390/jpm16070342

survival or higher risk of progression, prolactin should be interpreted primarily as a prognostic biomarker [13]. However, to define prolactin as a predictive biomarker, studies would need to demonstrate that prolactin levels modify the probability of benefit from a specific treatment, such as chemotherapy, immunotherapy, or targeted therapy.

3.3. Established Blood-Based and Serum Biomarkers

Several blood-based biomarkers have been evaluated in NSCLC, mainly as supportive tools for prognosis and treatment monitoring rather than as independent diagnostic markers. The most frequently studied serum tumour markers include CEA, CYFRA 21-1, SCC antigen, and NSE [19,20]. CEA is more frequently associated with adenocarcinoma, CYFRA 21-1 and SCC antigen with squamous cell carcinoma, whereas NSE is primarily linked to neuroendocrine differentiation and small cell lung cancer, although it may occasionally be assessed in NSCLC [19,20].

Among these markers, CEA and CYFRA 21-1 have the strongest evidence for prognostic and monitoring utility. Elevated baseline levels have been associated with higher tumour burden and poorer outcomes, while decreases during systemic therapy may correlate with treatment response and radiological disease control [21,22]. However, their clinical value remains limited by insufficient sensitivity and specificity, histology-dependent performance, variable cut-off values, and possible elevation in non-malignant diseases or other cancers [19–22].

In parallel, systemic inflammatory and nutritional markers, including the NLR, CRP, albumin, CRP/albumin ratio, and LDH, have been explored as inexpensive prognostic indicators in NSCLC [23]. These parameters reflect host inflammation, immune status, nutritional decline, and disease burden, but they are highly non-specific and lack standardized thresholds. Therefore, although serum and inflammatory biomarkers are clinically attractive because they are inexpensive and repeatable, their limitations support the search for additional circulating markers, such as prolactin, that could complement existing prognostic models rather than replace established biomarkers.

3.4. Limitations of Current Biomarkers and Remaining Gaps in Personalized Monitoring

Despite major progress in molecularly guided treatment, current biomarkers in NSCLC do not fully address all clinical needs. Genomic alterations such as EGFR mutations, ALK and ROS1 rearrangements, BRAF, MET, RET, NTRK, KRAS, and HER2/ERBB2 alterations are highly valuable for treatment selection, but they mainly function as predictive biomarkers and are not always sufficient for continuous assessment of disease dynamics or post-treatment risk [8–10]. Similarly, PD-L1 expression supports immunotherapy selection, but its interpretation is limited by spatial and temporal heterogeneity, assay variability, and imperfect prediction of clinical benefit [11,19].

Classical serum biomarkers, including CEA, CYFRA 21-1, SCC antigen, and NSE, are inexpensive and repeatable, yet their sensitivity, specificity, and clinical interpretability remain limited [19–22]. Inflammatory and nutritional indices, such as NLR, CRP, albumin-based markers, and LDH, may provide additional prognostic information, but they are non-specific and strongly influenced by systemic conditions unrelated to cancer [23].

Therefore, an important gap remains in NSCLC personalized medicine: the need for accessible, low-cost, repeatable biomarkers that could complement molecular, immunohistochemical, and serum tumor markers in risk assessment and longitudinal monitoring. In this context, prolactin should not be viewed as a replacement for established biomarkers, but as a potential supplementary circulating marker that may contribute to broader multimarker prognostic models.

https://doi.org/10.3390/jpm16070342

Given the biological complexity of prolactin regulation discussed in later sections, future research should investigate whether PRL can improve the performance of existing serum biomarker panels through multimarker predictive algorithms.

4. Physiology and Regulation of Prolactin

4.1. Prolactin Synthesis, Secretion and Neuroendocrine Regulation

Prolactin is a peptide hormone with a molecular weight of 23 kDa, consisting of 199 amino acids. In humans, prolactin is encoded by a single gene located on chromosome 6. It has a 3D structure composed of four anti-parallel α-helices, and thus exhibits strong structural homology not only with placental lactogen but also with growth hormone (GH) [23]. It is formed by the proteolytic cleavage of the signal peptide from the prohormone of prolactin, known as proprolactin [24].

The primary source of PRL is the pituitary gland. Lactophores located in the anterior lobe of the pituitary gland are responsible for the synthesis and release of prolactin [25]. PRL secretion is regulated by various factors. The pattern of PRL secretion is linked to the circadian rhythm. In humans, the highest levels are typically observed at night, between 2:00 and 4:00 a.m. During the day, PRL levels decrease [26]. The primary neuroendocrine factor regulating prolactin secretion is dopamine (DA). DA released by tuberoinfundibular dopamine (TIDA) neurons in the hypothalamus binds to D2 receptors on lactophores, thereby inhibiting dopamine synthesis and secretion [27,28].

In contrast, factors such as thyrotropin-releasing hormone (TRH), estrogen, and dopamine antagonists stimulate PRL secretion [24]. TRH has a stimulating effect on PRL secretion. It stimulates the lactotrophic cells of the pituitary gland [27]. Estrogens also play a role in stimulating PRL secretion. They directly stimulate lactophores and weaken the inhibitory effect of DA [27,29]. The secretion of PRL also increases in stressful situations. Stress is one of the physiological stimuli that increases its secretion. Its effects are associated, among other things, with a reduction in the activity of dopaminergic neurons through the action of endogenous opioids via the μ, κ, and δ opioid receptors [30].

Hyperprolactinemia can be physiological, pharmacological, or pathological in nature [26,31]. Physiological causes include pregnancy, lactation, stress, and nipple stimulation [31]. The most common pharmacological causes are antipsychotic medications, as well as certain antidepressants or opioids, which disrupt dopaminergic transmission [26,30]. The most common pathological cause is prolactinoma, but other pathologies are also mentioned, such as hypothyroidism or other tumors of the hypothalamic–pituitary region [31,32].

PRL is also synthesized outside the pituitary gland. Its synthesis is observed in peripheral tissues such as the endometrium, mammary gland, brain, and immune system cells. Extrapituitary prolactin exerts primarily local, autocrine, and paracrine effects. The regulation of its secretion does not depend on the hypothalamic–pituitary axis [33].

Physiological Functions of PRL

One of the main roles of prolactin is its mammogenic effect, that is, stimulating the growth and development of the mammary glands, as well as its lactogenic effect, which induces lactation, and its galactopoietic effect, which helps maintain milk production [34,35]. PRL influences milk production by inducing the enzyme that synthesizes milk components such as casein, lactose, and lipids [24].

PRL also has an effect on the hypothalamic–pituitary–gonadal axis, as it can, with pulsatility, inhibit the release of gonadotropin-releasing hormone (GnRH) by the hypothalamus [34].

Within the immune system, PRL may function similarly to a cytokine. It may play a role in both the innate and adaptive immune responses [36]. This hormone may influence

https://doi.org/10.3390/jpm16070342

the proliferation and survival of immune cells. Its potential role in autoimmunity is also emphasized, where it may disrupt the activity of regulatory T cells (Treg) and B-cell tolerance, lowering their activation threshold in a state of anergy [37].

PRL also influences metabolic processes in the body. Its effects depend, among other factors, on its concentration. Both a significant excess and a deficiency of prolactin can have a negative impact on metabolism, leading to excess body weight and disturbances in lipid and carbohydrate metabolism [38,39].

PRL also plays a role in regulating cell proliferation and differentiation through prolactin receptor (PRLR)-dependent signaling [40]. This is significant in carcinogenesis. Hormone-dependent cancers, such as breast, ovarian, endometrial, or prostate cancer, may be characterized by enhanced prolactin signaling [41].

An additional aspect that should be considered when evaluating prolactin as a potential biomarker is the existence of biologically distinct prolactin isoforms and proteolytic fragments. In addition to the full-length 23 kDa form, prolactin can undergo enzymatic cleavage to generate smaller peptides collectively referred to as vasoinhibins. These fragments exhibit biological activities that differ substantially from those of native prolactin, particularly with regard to vascular regulation. Vasoinhibins have been shown to exert anti-angiogenic, anti-vasopermeability, and pro-apoptotic effects on endothelial cells, partly through interactions with integrin $\alpha5\beta1$ and the modulation of endothelial signaling pathways [42]. More recent evidence has highlighted the importance of the prolactin/vasoinhibin axis in cardiovascular diseases, emphasizing the distinct physiological and pathological roles of these peptide forms [43]. Given that angiogenesis is a fundamental process in NSCLC progression and metastatic dissemination, the relative balance between full-length prolactin and vasoinhibins may have important implications for tumour biology. Therefore, future studies investigating prolactin as a biomarker in NSCLC should consider not only total circulating prolactin concentrations but also the potential contribution of specific prolactin isoforms and their differential biological activities.

4.2. PRLR Isoforms and Intracellular Signaling Pathways

PRLR is linked to the non-receptor tyrosine kinase Janus 2 (JAK2) and is a member of the class I cytokine receptor family. It exists in several isoforms that differ in their functional and structural properties [44]. Three isoforms of the PRLR have been described in humans: long, short, and intermediate. These isoforms arise from alternative splicing of the primary transcript. The differences between the isoforms concern variations in the length of the amino acid chain in the intracellular region. The transmembrane domains and extracellular regions remain the same [45]. This affects their varying ability to activate signaling pathways. PRL signaling seems to be significantly influenced by the long PRLR isoform. Many kinases, including JAK2, mitogen-activated protein kinase (MAPK), and phosphoinositide 3-kinase (PI3K), are activated when PRL binds to this receptor. Cell survival, differentiation, and proliferation are all aided by their activation. A frameshift mutation produces the intermediate isoform, which likewise activates the Janus kinase/signal transducer and activator of transcription (JAK/STAT) pathway but cannot promote cell division [44]. PRL, by binding to PRLR, leads to the activation of several key signaling pathways associated with tumorigenesis, such as JAK/STAT, mitogen-activated protein kinase/extracellular signal-regulated kinase (MAPK/ERK), and phosphoinositide 3-kinase/protein kinase B (PI3K/AKT) [41].

The JAK/STAT pathway is considered the canonical signaling pathway activated upon PRLR activation. It is particularly associated with its long isoform. Following the binding of PRL to PRLR, JAK2 is activated, STAT proteins are phosphorylated, and subsequently translocated to the cell nucleus, where they regulate the expression of target

 https://doi.org/10.3390/jpm16070342

genes. Activation of this pathway promotes cell differentiation, proliferation, and survival. Particular importance is attributed to the STAT5A and STAT5B proteins [41,44].

The RAS/MAPK/ERK pathway is also associated with prolactin signaling. It is linked to neoplastic transformation and cell proliferation [41,46]. Abramicheva et al. indicate that the MAPK/ERK pathway can be activated by both the long and short isoforms of PRLR [44]. More recent data suggest that the intermediate isoform of PRLR may contribute to breast cancer oncogenesis by activating the RAS/MAPK/ERK pathway [47].

Prolactin signaling is also significantly influenced by the PI3K/AKT pathway [45]. Cell growth, proliferation, and survival can all be impacted by PI3K/AKT activation [44]. This pathway may be one of the primary pathways of PRLR signaling in prolactin-dependent tumors and other malignancies [45].

PRLR expression exhibits tissue specificity, which enables tissue-specific responses to PRL that also depend on the organism's physiological state. The presence of the receptor has been described in many tissues and organs involved in the regulation of water and electrolyte balance, growth and development, endocrine and metabolic functions, brain activity and behavior, reproduction, and the immune response [48,49]. Disorders of the PRL/PRLR axis have been described in tumors, particularly hormone-dependent ones. It is worth noting, however, that research indicates this pathway may also play a role in promoting the development of other types of cancer, including liver, colorectal, and pancreatic cancer [41]. Not only the expression levels of individual PRLR isoforms, but also the ratio between them and the dominance of a specific isoform may have biological significance. In Abramicheva's study, the researchers emphasize that the long PRLR isoform may promote cell proliferation and survival, whereas some short isoforms may exhibit antiproliferative and proapoptotic effects [23]. In the study by Standing et al., the researchers suggest that the intermediate PRLR isoform may be of particular importance, as it has been associated with increased proliferation, viability, and transformation of breast cancer cells (Figure 1) [41].

Prolactin in Tumor-Related Processes

As it was mentioned before, PRL is considered a pleiotropic hormone whose effects surpass classic endocrine functions. In the cancer context, PRL regulates multiple key biological processes such as cell proliferation, cell survival, angiogenesis, and migration and modulation of the TME.

PRL has been shown to have an impact on tumor proliferation by the activation of the PRL-PRLR pathway, which leads to phosphorylation of JAK2 and further activation of STAT5 transcriptional factors, which regulate gene expression and cell survival. At the same time, the activated PI3K/AKT pathway promotes cell survival by inhibiting proapoptotic proteins and activating mTOR, favouring cell growth. It has also been reported that PRL may modulate tumor cell response to oxidative stress and DNA impairment, enhancing their capability of survival during treatment. Therefore, it suggests that PRL may have an impact on treatment resistance development, especially chemotherapy and targeted therapies [41,50–52].

What is more, PRL may influence angiogenesis. A full-length PRL plays a proangiogenic role via factors such as VEGF, whereas proteolytic fragments—vasoinhibins—may have an antiangiogenic role. This dual role shows that the PRL effect on tumor angiogenesis may depend on local TME, activity of proteolytic enzymes, and the balance between different isoforms of the hormone [53–56].

https://doi.org/10.3390/jpm16070342

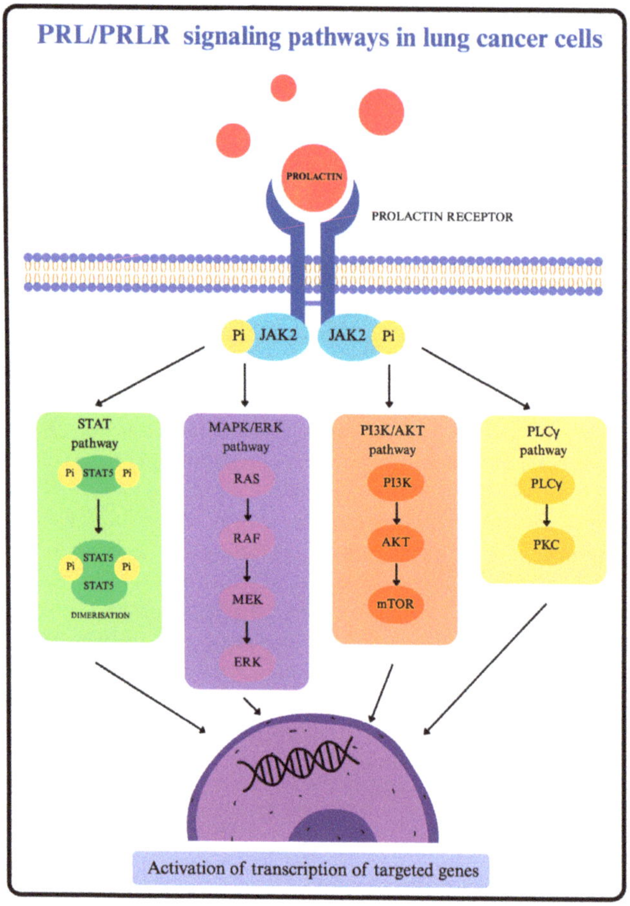

Figure 1. PRL/PRLR signaling pathways implicated in NSCLC biology. Binding of prolactin (PRL) to the prolactin receptor (PRLR) activates JAK2 and downstream signaling cascades, including the JAK/STAT, MAPK/ERK, PI3K/AKT/mTOR, and PLCγ pathways. These pathways regulate transcriptional programs involved in cell proliferation, survival, differentiation, and tumour progression.

Multiple studies report that PRL may influence the ability of tumor cells to migrate and invade by regulating cell adhesion and extracellular matrix degradation. Activation of the MAPK/ERK and PI3K/AKT pathways leads to increased expression of metalloproteinases (MMP-2, MMP-9), which play a key role in tissue invasion [57–59].

Furthermore, evidence suggests that PRL may participate in the regulation of epithelial–mesenchymal transition (EMT). These mechanisms include the modulation of the expression of adhesion proteins and transcription factors associated with EMT. Despite the limited research for NSCLC, observations from other tumors support the hypothesis of a potential role for PRL in promoting a more aggressive phenotype [50,60].

PRL also plays a significant role in shaping the TME through its immunomodulatory abilities. It can influence the function of T cells, NK cells, macrophages, and dendritic cells, modulating both the antitumor response and immunosuppressive mechanisms. Particularly, PRL may promote the differentiation of macrophages toward the M2 phenotype, which favors tumor progression, angiogenesis, and suppression of the immune response. Additionally, PRL may influence the production of cytokines and chemokines, thereby

 https://doi.org/10.3390/jpm16070342

modifying communication between tumor cells and components of the microenvironment [61–63].

NSCLC may influence the hypothalamic–pituitary axis through paraneoplastic mechanisms and chronic activation of the stress axis. Disruptions in the dopaminergic control of PRL secretion can lead to its overproduction in the course of cancer. Moreover, proinflammatory cytokines may stimulate PRL secretion both on the pituitary level and in the peripheral endocrine tissues, highlighting the connection between immune and endocrine systems [62–64]. Secretion of proinflammatory cytokines, such as IL-6, affects neuroendocrine pathways and impairs hormone regulation, leading to high PRL levels. PRL itself presents immunomodulatory effects and may modulate signal pathways such as JAK/STAT, MAPK/ERK or PI3K/AKT, suggesting its potential role not only as a biomarker but also as an active participant of tumor processes [64,65].

In the context of paraneoplastic syndromes, it should be highlighted that despite ectopic hormone production in lung cancer concerning mostly ACTH or ADH, the systemic effects of cytokines and growth factors produced by the tumor can lead to impairments in the hypothalamic–pituitary axis, thereby affecting prolactin secretion [65,66]. What is more, chronic activation of the stress axis (HPA) in patients with advanced NSCLC may lead to hormonal dysregulation. Disruptions of this axis, also observed during immunotherapy, affect the balance between cortisol and the dopaminergic system, which in turn may modulate PRL secretion [66,67].

4.3. Mechanisms of Prolactin Dysregulation in Lung Cancer

PRL dysregulation in patients with NSCLC is an effect of multiple endocrine, inflammatory and iatrogenic mechanisms. In contrast to other hormone-dependent tumors, in NSCLC, changes in the PRL levels mirror a complex response to the disease rather than one pathological process [64,68].

4.3.1. Therapy-Related Effects on Prolactin Levels

Lung cancer treatment is an important element influencing the PRL levels. The effect is complex and dependent on the type of treatment [69,70]. Chemotherapy may indirectly influence PRL secretion through inflammatory response induction and metabolic impairments [71]. Even though the direct impact of chemotherapy on the pituitary gland is not conclusive, the systemic nature of the treatment contributes to hormonal homeostasis disorders [70]. Other treatment methods that may lead to high PRL levels include antipsychotic treatment, which is used in oncological patients. The usage of antipsychotic drugs is reported to raise the PRL levels [72,73]. Opioids, commonly used in the treatment of cancer pain, may contribute to high PRL levels by inhibiting the activity of dopaminergic neurons [74]. Glucocorticoids affect the HPA axis, and their impact on PRL levels remains variable and context-dependent [75]. Recently, attention has been drawn to the potential impact of immunotherapy on hormonal balance. Immune checkpoint inhibitors (ICIs), such as anti-PD-1 and anti-PD-L1 antibodies used in NSCLC, may induce endocrine disorders. Reports have emerged suggesting the possibility of high PRL levels during treatment with nivolumab. The mechanism behind it is not fully understood, but it is believed to result from an interaction between the immune and endocrine systems, in which prolactin acts as a cytokine modulating lymphocyte activity [76–79].

4.3.2. Inflammation, Stress, and Systemic Illness as Mediators

An important role of PRL regulation in NSCLC is played by chronic inflammation, immune response, and the general condition of the patient. NSCLC presents a strong inflammatory component where proinflammatory cytokines, including interleukins and TNF-α, may influence PRL secretion both directly and through modulation of the hypothalamic–

https://doi.org/10.3390/jpm16070342

pituitary axis [80]. Therefore, a stress response may play a crucial role as a PRL-secretion mediator. Activation of the HPA axis in response to chronic cancer-related stress leads to changes in cortisol secretion and neurotransmitter imbalances, including dopamine, which secondarily influence prolactin secretion. What is more, malnutrition and cancer cachexia further enhance endocrine disruptions. Metabolic disturbances affect the functioning of endocrine axes, including PRL regulation (Figure 2) [81–83].

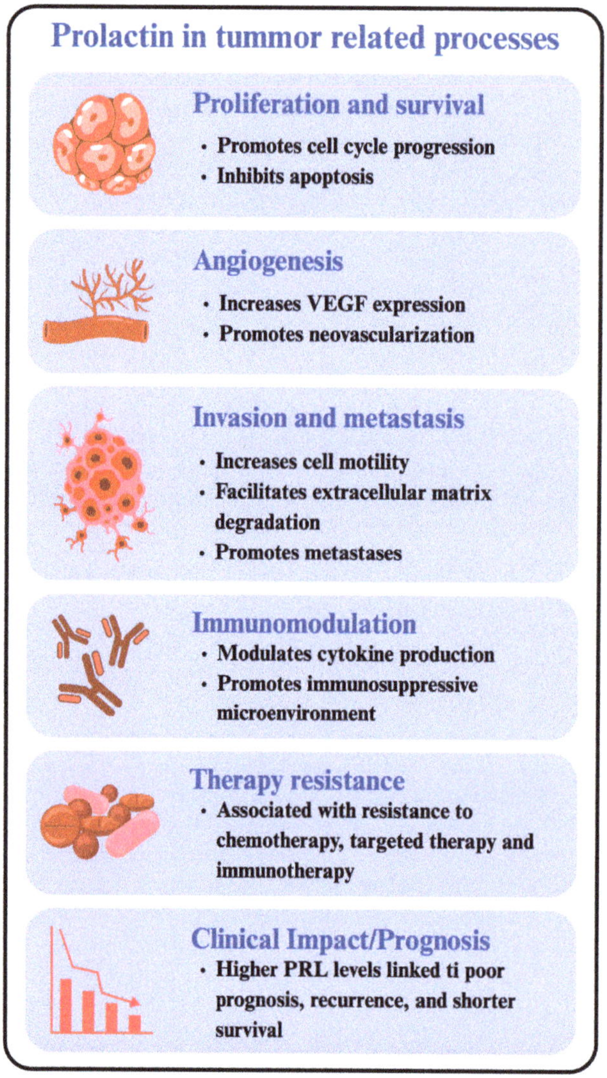

Figure 2. Proposed roles of prolactin in tumour-related processes relevant to NSCLC. Experimental evidence suggests that prolactin signaling contributes to tumour cell proliferation and survival, angiogenesis, invasion and metastatic dissemination, modulation of the tumour microenvironment, therapy resistance, and adverse clinical outcomes. The figure summarizes the potential biological and clinical implications of PRL dysregulation in NSCLC.

https://doi.org/10.3390/jpm16070342

4.4. Integrative Multimarker Predictive Modeling Incorporating Prolactin

Given that prolactin is influenced by systemic inflammation, stress, pharmacotherapy, and comorbid conditions, isolated PRL elevations may introduce substantial biological variability and reduce its interpretative specificity in NSCLC [23,30,80]. For this reason, its clinical utility is likely to be most robust when assessed in combination with other biomarkers rather than in isolation.

A practical approach is the integration of PRL into multimarker predictive models together with established tumor-associated biomarkers such as CEA, CYFRA 21-1, NSE, and SCC antigen [19–22]. In this framework, biomarkers contribute weighted information within a unified predictive score for diagnostic, prognostic, or monitoring purposes.

From a methodological perspective, multivariable regression models (e.g., logistic regression and Cox proportional hazards models) enable estimation of independent biomarker contributions while accounting for clinical covariates [21,23]. In parallel, machine learning approaches, including penalized regression (e.g., LASSO), random forests, and gradient boosting methods, may improve model performance by capturing nonlinear relationships and mitigating the impact of biologically variable markers.

The rationale for such integration is the complementary nature of the included biomarkers: classical tumor markers primarily reflect tumor burden and histological subtype, whereas PRL may provide additional information on systemic endocrine–immune and tumor–host interactions. Their combined assessment may therefore improve discrimination between tumor-associated biological changes and nonspecific fluctuations in PRL levels.

These multimarker strategies require rigorous validation and calibration across independent cohorts but are increasingly applied in oncology to enhance predictive accuracy beyond single-marker approaches [11,21,23].

5. Clinical Evidence on Prolactin in NSCLC

5.1. Clinical Observations and Methodological Challenges in Prolactin Assessment

Current clinical data suggest that prolactin serves a functional role across various malignancies, including lung cancer, rather than acting as a mere physiological bystander. Consequently, its presence in patients with non-small cell lung cancer should not be dismissed as an incidental finding, but rather viewed as a component of a sophisticated oncogenic mechanism. When evaluating the frequency of hyperprolactinemia, we must account for three distinct sources of the hormone identified in the recent literature: classic endocrine secretion from the pituitary gland, autocrine and paracrine production by the neoplastic epithelium itself, and stromal-sourced secretion. This latter factor is particularly noteworthy, as cells within the tumor microenvironment have been shown to synthesize PRL, thereby driving tumor progression. The variability in reported hyperprolactinemia rates likely stems from a fundamental methodological gap: standard assays measure systemic, circulating PRL while overlooking localized production within the tumor. Such a limitation may lead to a significant underestimation of the hormone's biological impact in a substantial subset of patients [60].

Estimates of hyperprolactinemia frequency in lung cancer remain scattered throughout the literature. However, cohort studies consistently reveal significant elevations when compared to healthy populations. While systemic dysregulation is common, direct structural damage to the endocrine axis must also be considered in advanced cases. Autopsy data indicate that pituitary metastases occur in 1% to 4% of patients with terminal malignancies, a factor that may further complicate the interpretation of prolactinemia in the final stages of the disease [84]. These lesions account for approximately 1% of all pituitary tumors and roughly 0.4% of all intracranial metastatic growth. Interestingly, while autopsy findings

https://doi.org/10.3390/jpm16070342

suggest a higher prevalence, the clinical frequency diagnosed during a patient's lifetime remains near 1% [85]. Lung and breast cancers combined account for approximately 50% of all pituitary metastases, with the highest incidence observed in patients aged 60 to 70 years. Recent reports highlight an increasing frequency of anterior hypopituitarism among those with metastatic involvement of the gland. In one clinical case involving a patient with metastatic adenocarcinoma, mild hyperprolactinemia was documented at 110 μIU/mL, significantly exceeding the reference range of 3.5–26 μIU/mL. Following the surgical resection of the tumor mass, prolactin levels plummeted to 20 μIU/mL. This rapid normalization underscores that the hyperprolactinemia was a direct consequence of mechanical compression of the pituitary gland or stalk by the tumor [84].

Clinical symptoms suggesting pituitary axis dysfunction, including those related to PRL, manifest in only about 20% of patients. This suggests that for the vast majority, hyperprolactinemia remains an undiagnosed, subclinical condition. While lung cancer stands as the leading cause of pituitary metastases, the actual prevalence of hyperprolactinemia in NSCLC patients without central nervous system involvement is poorly documented. This gap in the literature underscores a pressing need for broader screening within this population.

Another barrier lies in the phenomenon of macroprolactinemia—the presence of high-molecular-weight hormone isoforms that possess minimal biological activity yet remain detectable by standard immunoassays. As Biagetti et al. (2022) [86] point out, the lack of a universal requirement for polyethylene glycol (PEG) precipitation to eliminate macroprolactin is a primary driver of misdiagnosis and inconsistency in reported hyperprolactinemia rates. Within the oncological literature, it is rare to find clarification on whether results were corrected for the macroprolactin fraction. This oversight suggests that the true prevalence of biologically active hyperprolactinemia may be systematically overestimated across many patient cohorts [86].

The lack of a standardized cutoff for "oncological hyperprolactinemia", particularly in patients dealing with cancer cachexia or chronic stress, creates a diagnostic gray area. A result of 30 ng/mL might be flagged as pathological in one cohort but dismissed as a reactive, normal finding in another. The pharmacological profile of concurrent medications is another critical driver of these reporting discrepancies. Recent analyses indicate that using prolactin-sparing agents, such as aripiprazole, results in significantly lower serum PRL levels compared to standard regimens involving potent dopamine antagonists. Such therapeutic variables must be carefully accounted for when comparing data across different patient cohorts [87].

The discrepancies in reported hyperprolactinemia rates among NSCLC patients stem largely from a lack of standardized research methodology. A primary challenge is the absence of uniform cut-off points. Ken-Dror et al. (2024) [88] demonstrated that even when studies focused on "low prolactin," their definitions varied wildly: for men, "low" was defined as <3.6 ng/mL in one study, yet reached <7.2 ng/mL in another. Among women, this spread was even more pronounced, ranging from <4.5 ng/mL to <8 ng/mL. Laboratory techniques present a further barrier to consistency. Although all studies analyzed by Ken-Dror et al. (2024) [88] utilized chemiluminescence immunoassay technology, significant inconsistencies remained. Even with modern immunoassays, variations in equipment and reagents, such as those between Roche platforms and other manufacturers, mean that identical serum concentrations can lead to divergent clinical interpretations. Finally, the systemic failure to control for confounding variables remains a critical flaw in current data. Many studies overlook the impact of hospitalization-related stress, diurnal secretion fluctuations, and the influence of supportive pharmacotherapy. Without accounting for these external drivers, the true prevalence of tumor-associated hyperprolactinemia remains difficult to isolate [88].

 https://doi.org/10.3390/jpm16070342

The biological complexity of this axis is further deepened by the promiscuity of the prolactin receptor (PRLR), which can be activated by ligands other than PRL itself, such as growth hormone (GH) and placental lactogen. This cross-reactivity introduces a significant diagnostic blind spot: a patient may present with perfectly normal serum prolactin levels, yet their pulmonary PRLRs could be "bombarded" by GH. This alternative signaling pathway can trigger the same deleterious oncogenic effects as hyperprolactinemia, effectively masking the true intensity of the receptor's activation in the tumor microenvironment (Table 1) [60].

Table 1. Summary of clinical evidence, cohort characteristics, and prolactin level dynamics in lung cancer populations.

Study Type	Sample Size	Demographics	Clinical Stage & Histology	Treatment Status	Observations	Ref.
Autopsy Cohorts	In total, 1% to 4% of advanced terminal cancer cases.	Elderly patients (predominantly 60 to 70 years old).	Advanced metastatic disease with direct pituitary involvement; accounts for ~1% of all pituitary tumors.	Post mortem analysis (end-stage disease).	Lung and breast cancers combined account for approximately 50% of all pituitary metastases. Associated with an increasing frequency of anterior hypopituitarism.	[63]
Clinical Cohorts	In total, ~1% clinically diagnosed during lifetime.	Mean age of ~49.5 years; strong male predominance (64% of cases).	Advanced NSCLC (Adenocarcinoma, Squamous Cell Carcinoma); Stage IVB (M1 category).	Active disease, pre-intervention phase, or progression during targeted therapies (e.g., crizotinib resistance).	Markedly elevated PRL (often >110–200 ng/mL) driven by the "stalk effect" (mechanical compression blocking dopamine) or direct tumor tissue invasion. Correlates with secondary mutations (e.g., ALK-I1171S).	[85,89]
Ectopic Neuroendocrine Cohorts	Individual advanced cases (highly metabolic thoracic masses).	Adult patients presenting with exceptionally high tumor burden.	Advanced Pulmonary Neuroendocrine Tumors (NETs); presenting as large thoracic masses (e.g., 75 × 87 × 106 mm).	Pre-operative diagnostic phase vs. Post-radical surgical resection.	Extreme "tumoral range" hyperprolactinemia (330–832 ng/mL) caused by ectopic GHRH hypersecretion (38,088 ng/L) driving secondary lactotroph hyperplasia. Post-op: Rapid drop to 1.9 ng/mL within 5 days, stabilizing at 3.6 ng/mL in the long term.	[90]
Immunotherapy Cohorts	Target populations monitored on immune checkpoint inhibitors.	Adult patients receiving anti-PD-1/PD-L1 checkpoint blockades.	Advanced NSCLC showing partial response (PR) or stable disease.	On-treatment monitoring and post-treatment follow-up (up to 17 months after initial dose).	Stable/Normal PRL levels. The stability of PRL helps differentiate immune-related adverse events (e.g., Isolated ACTH Deficiency/hypophysitis) from mechanical pituitary metastases.	[91]

ACTH, adrenocorticotropic hormone; ALK, anaplastic lymphoma kinase; GHRH, growth hormone-releasing hormone; M1, distant metastasis; NET, neuroendocrine tumor; NSCLC, non-small cell lung cancer; PD-1, programmed cell death protein 1; Post-op, post-operative; Pre-op, pre-operative; PRL, prolactin.

Pre-Analytical Standardization Framework for Longitudinal Prolactin Assessment

To improve comparability of longitudinal prolactin measurements, a minimal standardized protocol is required to reduce pre-analytical variability and ensure clinically meaningful interpretation of temporal trends.

1. Pre-sampling conditions
   Patients should avoid intense physical activity and unnecessary stressors for 24 h prior to sampling. Blood collection should preferably be performed in a stable outpatient setting rather than during acute hospitalization whenever possible.

https://doi.org/10.3390/jpm16070342

2. Medication and confounder control
All concomitant therapies influencing prolactin secretion (e.g., antipsychotics, antidepressants, antiemetics, opioids) should be systematically documented at each time point, including recent dose changes.
3. Sampling procedure
Morning fasting blood samples are recommended. A short rest period (15–30 min) prior to venipuncture should be ensured. For repeated measurements, the use of an indwelling venous catheter is preferred to minimize procedure-related variability.
4. Analytical consistency
The same immunoassay platform should be used throughout follow-up when possible. Reporting should include whether macroprolactin screening (e.g., PEG precipitation) was performed.
5. Longitudinal design and interpretation
Assessment should rely on predefined serial time points rather than isolated measurements. Interpretation should prioritize intra-individual trajectories over fixed population cut-offs, integrating clinical context and treatment status.

5.2. Prolactin Alterations in Advanced NSCLC and Pituitary Involvement

The dynamics of prolactin concentrations in lung cancer patients are intricately linked to both the disease stage and the specific therapeutic interventions employed. Clinical case analyses demonstrate that these hormonal parameters can fluctuate rapidly, positioning them as a sensitive indicator of the patient's current clinical status. Evidence from clinical studies suggests a higher prevalence of elevated PRL levels in patients with advanced-stage NSCLC. In these settings, the hormone may function as more than a passive marker of tumor burden. It appears to act as an active promoter of dissemination. This association is driven by the direct involvement of prolactin in the molecular and cellular processes underlying metastasis [41].

During the diagnostic phase, particularly in metastatic disease, the hormonal profile can become profoundly disrupted. A striking example involves a patient with a pulmonary neuroendocrine tumor (NET) measuring 75 × 87 × 106 mm, whose pre-intervention prolactin levels reached "tumoral" ranges, oscillating between 330 and 832 ng/mL against a reference norm of 25 ng/mL. While such extreme elevations typically point toward a macroprolactinoma, the underlying cause here was an ectopic stimulatory mechanism. The lung tumor secreted massive quantities of GHRH (38,088 ng/L), triggering secondary lactotroph hyperplasia and enlarging the pituitary gland to 22 × 30 × 34 mm. This case demonstrates that in advanced disease, high prolactin can be a direct byproduct of the metabolic activity of the primary thoracic mass [90].

However, while the role of prolactin in late-stage malignancy is increasingly well-documented, the impact of early-stage, small nodules on the hormonal profile remains poorly understood and warrants prioritized clinical investigation. The most dramatic shifts in prolactin levels are observed following radical surgical intervention. Clinical case reports indicate that as early as five days post-resection, PRL levels can plummet from tumoral peaks to as low as 1.9 ng/mL. In the long term, as demonstrated in follow-up observations approximately nine months post-surgery, prolactin concentrations tend to stabilize within the physiological range (around 3.6 ng/mL), while the previously hyperplastic pituitary volume can regress by as much as 70%. The clinical validation of this systemic normalization is often evidenced by the return of spontaneous menstrual cycles in female patients. Such a radical transformation of endocrine parameters following lung surgery provides compelling evidence that the hyperprolactinemia was entirely tumor-dependent, positioning it as a dynamic marker of therapeutic efficacy [90].

https://doi.org/10.3390/jpm16070342

The use of potent analgesics, specifically opioids, represents another significant variable in the hormonal landscape of oncological patients. A 2021 meta-analysis by Diasso et al. confirms that prolonged opioid administration profoundly disrupts the prolactin axis. This pharmacological interference adds a layer of complexity to blood test interpretations, as the resulting shifts in serum PRL levels may reflect drug-induced alterations rather than tumor dynamics alone [92]. In the context of tumor staging according to the 8th edition of the TNM (where T stands for primary tumor, N for regional lymph nodes, and M for distant metastasis) classification, the occurrence of NSCLC metastasis to the pituitary gland (M1 category) is of particular clinical significance. The presence of such a neoplastic mass profoundly alters the hormonal profile, with a rapid surge in prolactin levels—often exceeding 200 ng/mL—serving as a critical red flag. This phenomenon is driven by the "stalk effect," where the tumor compresses the pituitary stalk and obstructs the dopaminergic flow that normally inhibits PRL secretion, compounded by the direct invasion of aggressive adenocarcinoma cells into the surrounding tissues. Clinically, such extreme hyperprolactinemia acts as a clear indicator of heavy systemic tumor burden and rapid disease progression. Unfortunately, these findings are synonymous with a poor prognosis. In such cases, the median survival rarely extends beyond a single year [93].

It is noteworthy that hyperprolactinemia in advanced NSCLC (stage IVB) is not always a baseline finding. It often emerges as a herald of disease progression during active therapy. This is vividly illustrated by a case involving a patient with an ALK gene fusion who, after maintaining a year of stability on crizotinib, experienced a sudden onset of neurological symptoms accompanied by a surge in prolactin to 113.35 ng/mL. Such a spike in a previously stable patient serves as a definitive clinical alarm, suggesting the emergence of new metastases—specifically to the pituitary in this instance, and a resultant increase in systemic tumor burden. In this case, the hyperprolactinemia occurred in tandem with the development of the secondary resistance mutation in the ALK gene (p.(Ile1171Ser). This suggests that hormonal shifts may indirectly mirror the genetic evolution of the tumor as it escapes the control of targeted therapies. The sensitivity of this marker is further evidenced by the immediate normalization of prolactin levels following the surgical resection of the metastatic lesion [89].

In clinical practice, the profile of a patient with pituitary metastasis typically centers around the age of 50, with a statistical mean of 49.5 years. While biological sex might not initially seem like a decisive factor, the data reveal a clear male predominance, with men accounting for 64% of cases. Furthermore, lung cancer is the undisputed "primary culprit," responsible for nearly half of all metastases in this location—a figure that reaches exactly 50% in the male population. The most immediate "red flag" for a clinician is the combination of two critical factors: the patient's oncological history and the rapid expansion of the intracranial mass. While a standard pituitary adenoma is benign and grows slowly over the years, a metastasis can increase in volume by 20% in just a few months, with some cases progressing in as little as 37 days. On MRI, these lesions are typically substantial, averaging 2.7 cm and often occupying the entire sella turcica. When a patient with a prior history of malignancy presents with a pituitary lesion exhibiting such explosive growth, the diagnostic certainty that it is a metastasis reaches 97.9%. Unfortunately, this aggressive biological behavior translates into a very challenging prognosis. From the moment of diagnosis, the median survival typically spans only six months [94].

5.3. Prolactin in Patients Treated with Immune Checkpoint Inhibitors

The etiology of pituitary dysfunction varies significantly depending on the histological subtype, disease dynamics, and the specific therapeutic strategy employed. While aggressive metastatic involvement is characterized by mechanical invasion and high prolactin

https://doi.org/10.3390/jpm16070342

levels, recent data reveal a different pattern in patients responding well to immunotherapy. In both adenocarcinoma and squamous cell carcinoma, treatment with PD-1 inhibitors, such as pembrolizumab or sintilimab, can trigger immune-related hypophysitis, leading to isolated ACTH deficiency. Interestingly, these endocrine complications often manifest while the primary tumor remains stable or in partial remission (PR), suggesting that a robust anti-tumor immune response may "erroneously" target pituitary tissue. A critical diagnostic distinction lies in the hormonal profile: unlike metastatic infiltration, where prolactin surges drastically, patients with immunotherapy-induced complications typically maintain normal prolactin levels. This stability is a vital clinical clue. The absence of a PRL spike in a patient presenting with symptoms of adrenal insufficiency—such as fatigue, nausea, or hyponatremia—allows clinicians to differentiate an autoimmune reaction from physical neoplastic infiltration. Furthermore, in these immunotherapeutic contexts, MRI scans of the pituitary often appear entirely unremarkable, showing no enlargement or stalk thickening despite severe hormonal deficiency. This reinforces the notion that the histological subtype and disease stage dictate whether pituitary damage is the result of mechanical destruction by a tumor or metabolic disruption caused by inflammation [91].

5.4. *Prolactin in Immune-Related Pituitary Dysfunction*

In patients with NSCLC treated with PD-1 inhibitors like pembrolizumab or sintilimab, stable prolactin levels serve as a pivotal tool for differential diagnosis. This stability allows clinicians to distinguish between immune-related complications, such as isolated ACTH deficiency (IAD), and pituitary metastases. While PRL typically remains within the normal range in the former, metastatic involvement usually triggers a rapid hormonal surge. Notably, these endocrine disturbances often coincide with a robust oncological response, including partial remission, which suggests that intense immune activation may inadvertently target the pituitary gland. Post-treatment monitoring requires vigilance for up to 17 months after the initial dose or for at least six months following the complete cessation of immunotherapy, as autoimmune mechanisms can manifest with significant latency.

Despite these promising clinical observations, the utility of prolactin in post-treatment monitoring for NSCLC remains constrained by a lack of large-scale prospective trials. Much of the current evidence is drawn from case reports or small cohorts, which preclude definitive statistical conclusions regarding the sensitivity of PRL when measured against established markers like CEA or CYFRA 21-1.

5.5. *Prolactin, Tumour Progression, Metastatic Potential and Therapy Resistance*

The role of prolactin in the progression of neoplastic diseases extends far beyond the stimulation of primary tumor growth, encompassing key processes that determine progression-free survival and the dynamics of metastatic dissemination. Prolactin contributes to the shortening of PFS by inducing resistance to DNA-damaging chemotherapeutic agents, such as doxorubicin and cisplatin. This mechanism relies on the interaction of the PRL-PRLR-JAK2-STAT5 signaling pathway with heat shock proteins (HSP90) and the DNA damage response system (ATM), which collectively promote cancer cell survival despite active treatment.

High serum PRL levels and the overexpression of its receptor directly correlate with shorter times to disease recurrence. Furthermore, the autocrine secretion of prolactin by tumor cells shifts their phenotype toward a more mesenchymal state, enhancing invasive capacity, facilitating migration, and promoting colony formation, which leads to the earlier emergence of new foci following radical treatment. The time to progression is further modified by external factors within the tumor microenvironment. For instance, the rigidity of the extracellular matrix—such as dense collagen—shifts PRL signaling from the

https://doi.org/10.3390/jpm16070342

JAK2/STAT5 pathway to the more aggressive MAPK/ERK route, intensifying invasiveness and accelerating clinical progression. Prolactin also activates RAS/RAF/MAPK/ERK signaling cascades, which are directly linked to invasiveness and the ability to form distant metastases. In cases of bone metastasis, PRL stimulates the secretion of factors like Sonic Hedgehog (SHH), triggering a "vicious cycle" of bone destruction and growth factor release that drastically hastens disease advancement in these areas. The metastatic potential is primarily driven by the long isoform of the PRLR. Research has shown that reducing the activity of this specific form inhibits the formation of lung and liver metastases, suggesting that the long PRLR isoform is a primary driver of oncological progression. In summary, prolactin shortens both progression-free and disease-free survival not only by fueling cell division but also by actively supporting invasiveness, facilitating the creation of metastatic niches, and building resistance to standard oncological therapies [60].

5.6. Limitations in the Prognostic Interpretation of Prolactin

The interpretation of prolactin's role as a prognostic indicator in oncology demands a high degree of critical scrutiny, as elevated levels are not always a direct consequence of the tumor's autonomous secretory activity. Mistaking oncological signals for an infection leads to critical delays in initiating appropriate therapy. Furthermore, aggressive disease progression accompanied by a sudden surge in prolactin can occur in young, non-smoking individuals harboring EGFR mutations. This supports the thesis that the prognostic value of prolactin is inextricably linked to the patient's genetic profile and interactions within the tumor microenvironment. A prime example is the stiffness of the extracellular matrix, which can "switch" PRL signaling from differentiation pathways to pro-metastatic routes. A final limitation to reliable clinical inference is the inability of currently available diagnostic assays to distinguish between PRLR isoforms, despite evidence that the long PRLR isoform is specifically responsible for enhanced metastatic potential, tumor progression, and therapy resistance [95,96]. A major analytical challenge stems from the limitations of currently available immunoenzymatic and immunohistochemical assays. Most commercially available antibody-based methods are designed to detect conserved receptor domains shared by multiple PRLR isoforms and therefore measure total PRLR expression rather than the abundance of individual receptor variants. Because the long and short PRLR isoforms differ primarily in their intracellular domains and downstream signaling capacities, conventional assays cannot determine which isoform predominates within a given tumor. Consequently, patients with markedly different risks of recurrence and metastatic dissemination may be classified similarly based on overall PRLR positivity. This lack of isoform specificity reduces the prognostic value of PRLR assessment and may obscure clinically relevant differences in disease behavior.

5.7. Hormonal Parameters in Treatment Response Monitoring

The relationship between prolactin levels and therapeutic response is not uniform, as it depends heavily on the specific mechanism of action of the treatment and the genetic profile of the tumor (Table 2).

Data analysis demonstrates that hormonal parameters may serve as a potential tool for monitoring NSCLC treatment outcomes. Elevated levels of prolactin and an excess of activin A function as early warning signals, heralding potential resistance to both immunotherapy (specifically nivolumab and atezolizumab) and platinum-based chemotherapy. Gender is a critical variable in this monitoring process. In female patients, superior immunotherapy outcomes may correlate with higher leptin levels, even though estrogens tend to impair PD-L1 expression. Furthermore, a specific clinical paradox is observed during the administration of PD-1 inhibitors: a decline in ACTH levels coupled with nor-

https://doi.org/10.3390/jpm16070342

mal prolactin concentrations often confirms therapeutic efficacy and tumor destruction, despite the induction of hormonal complications. Additionally, because PRL, FSH, and LH promote tumor invasiveness by blocking the HO-1 molecule, achieving the stabilization of these hormonal levels is essential for securing sustained clinical improvement [91] (Table 3).

Table 2. Morphological and biological tumor characteristics vs. hormonal profiles in NSCLC [90,93]. Abbreviations: ACTH—adrenocorticotropic hormone; IHC—immunohistochemistry; Ki-67—proliferation marker; M1—distant metastasis; PRL—prolactin.

Tumor Characteristic	Description and Clinical Significance	Impact on Hormone Levels (PRL/ACTH)
Location and size	Strong correlation with high tumor burden and M1 stage. Tumor mass occupying the sella turcica physically affects pituitary structures.	Induces the so-called stalk effect; mechanical compression blocks dopamine delivery, resulting in a rapid surge of prolactin.
Grading and aggressiveness	High histological grade and significant proliferative activity (Ki-67 index at 5–10% of cells).	Promotes aggressive and rapid infiltration of intracranial structures, leading to sudden manifestation of hormonal symptoms.
Receptor and marker expression	Expression of neuroendocrine markers in metastatic cells confirmed by immunohistochemical (IHC) studies.	Suggests that hormonal disturbances may result from the tumor biology itself and its ability to secrete biologically active substances, rather than solely from mechanical compression.

Table 3. Predictive value of hormonal parameters in monitoring NSCLC treatment response [50,64,67,76].

Parameter/Molecule	Predictive Value and Treatment Monitoring	Impact on Therapeutic Response and Mechanism
Prolactin ↑	Early indicator of poor response to nivolumab immunotherapy.	Induces chemotherapy resistance (cisplatin, doxorubicin) via activation of DNA repair systems (ATM) and interaction with heat shock proteins (HSP90).
Leptin ↑	Favorable prognostic factor, particularly in women with NSCLC.	Correlates with improved OS following the administration of PD-1/PD-L1 checkpoint inhibitors.
Activin A ↑	Marker of resistance to selected forms of immunotherapy.	Associated with a lack of durable clinical benefit following atezolizumab treatment and the risk of developing cancer-related sarcopenia.
FSH/LH ↑	Indicator of increased tumor invasiveness, particularly significant in patients over 50 years of age.	Stimulates tumor aggressiveness and metastatic potential by inhibiting the expression of HO-1.
ACTH ↓ (with normal prolactine)	Signal of isolated ACTH deficiency (IAD) occurrence as an immune-related adverse event.	Often correlates with good disease control and achievement of PR to PD-1 inhibitor therapy.

Abbreviations: ↑—Increase; ↓—Decrease; PR—Partial Remission; OS—Overall Survival; ATM—Ataxia-Telangiectasia Mutated Kinase; HSP90—Heat Shock Protein 90; IAD—Isolated ACTH Deficiency; HO-1—Heme Oxygenase-1.

6. Potential Clinical Utility of Prolactin in Personalized Medicine

Although molecular profiling has substantially improved treatment selection in NSCLC, current biomarkers do not fully address the need for accessible, repeatable, and clinically practical tools for prognostic assessment and longitudinal monitoring [18,97]. In

https://doi.org/10.3390/jpm16070342

this context, PRL should not be interpreted as an independent diagnostic or therapeutic decision-making marker but rather as a potential supplementary circulating biomarker that may add biological and clinical information to existing models [18,50]. Its possible value results from the combination of several features: low-cost serum measurement, biological links with cell proliferation and survival pathways in NSCLC, and preliminary clinical observations suggesting associations between PRL alterations and disease course during systemic therapy [50,76]. Therefore, the potential clinical utility of PRL in personalized medicine should be considered mainly in three areas: risk stratification, longitudinal monitoring, and identification of patient subgroups in whom hormonal or inflammatory dysregulation may reflect more aggressive disease biology [18,21,50,76].

6.1. Risk Stratification

PRL may be considered a potential supplementary marker for risk stratification in NSCLC, particularly when interpreted together with established clinical and laboratory variables. Its value should not be assessed independently from TNM stage, histological subtype, performance status, treatment response, systemic inflammation, and standard serum biomarkers such as CEA or CYFRA 21-1 [18,21,22]. In this setting, elevated or persistently increased PRL could hypothetically indicate a subgroup of patients with more pronounced tumor-related endocrine and inflammatory dysregulation, especially if it coexists with radiological progression, poor clinical status, or increasing conventional biomarkers.

The most clinically realistic approach would be to include PRL in multivariable prognostic models rather than to define a single universal cut-off value. This is in line with current trends in NSCLC in which blood-based risk models are increasingly incorporating tumour markers, inflammatory indices and nutritional parameters to improve prognostic accuracy [22,98]. Experimental data showing that PRL may support cell proliferation and survival through the GHR/JAK2/STAT3 pathway provide a biological rationale for its possible association with aggressive tumor behavior [50]. However, before PRL can be used for risk stratification, future studies must confirm whether it provides independent prognostic information beyond standard clinical, molecular, inflammatory, and serum tumor markers.

6.2. Longitudinal Monitoring

The greatest potential clinical value of PRL in NSCLC may lie in longitudinal monitoring rather than in a single baseline measurement. Serial PRL assessment could theoretically help capture changes in disease activity during and after systemic therapy, especially when interpreted together with imaging, symptoms, performance status, and established serum markers such as CEA, CYFRA 21-1, NSE, or SCC antigen [21,99,100]. In this context, the direction of change may be more informative than an isolated value. Persistent elevation, lack of normalization, or secondary increase during follow-up could suggest disease progression, treatment-related endocrine disturbance, systemic stress, or a combination of these mechanisms.

This idea is supported by studies showing that dynamic changes in serum tumor markers may correlate with treatment response and survival outcomes in advanced NSCLC treated with immunotherapy [99,100]. In addition, preliminary observations in metastatic NSCLC patients treated with nivolumab reported hyperprolactinemia during therapy and suggested its association with disease progression [76]. PRL dynamics might be interesting to investigate as an additional monitoring parameter, particularly in patients receiving systemic treatment. However, its use would require standardized sampling time, repeated measurements at predefined clinical points, control of pharmacological confounders, and validation against radiological response, progression-free survival, and overall survival.

 https://doi.org/10.3390/jpm16070342

6.3. Patient Subgrouping

The clinical value of PRL in NSCLC is unlikely to be uniform across all patients. Its interpretation may differ according to sex, age, menopausal status, histological subtype, disease stage, systemic inflammation, and type of anticancer therapy. These variables are important because PRL is strongly influenced by endocrine and inflammatory regulation, while NSCLC itself represents a biologically heterogeneous disease [18,22]. Therefore, future studies should assess PRL separately in clinically defined subgroups rather than only in unselected NSCLC populations.

Particular attention should be paid to patients receiving systemic therapy, especially immunotherapy or chemotherapy, because treatment may modify endocrine and immune responses. Preliminary data in metastatic NSCLC treated with nivolumab suggest that hyperprolactinemia may occur during therapy and may be associated with disease progression [76]. Another potentially relevant subgroup includes patients with advanced disease, cachexia, high inflammatory burden, or poor performance status, in whom elevated PRL may reflect both tumor biology and systemic deterioration. In contrast, patients using opioids, dopamine antagonists, antipsychotics, or metoclopramide should be analyzed separately or excluded from biomarker validation studies because these drugs may independently increase PRL levels.

6.4. Comparison with Established Biomarkers

Compared with established serum biomarkers such as CEA, CYFRA 21-1, SCC antigen, and NSE, PRL has several practical advantages, including low cost, easy availability, and the possibility of repeated measurement. However, its main weakness is limited cancer specificity. Classical serum markers are more directly associated with tumor burden or histological subtype, whereas PRL may reflect a broader mixture of tumor-related signaling, systemic inflammation, stress response, endocrine dysregulation, and treatment effects [13,21,99,100].

Therefore, PRL should not be presented as an alternative to CEA, CYFRA 21-1, NSE, SCC antigen, molecular testing, or PD-L1 assessment. Its potential role is more realistic as an additional biomarker used in combination with existing tools. This approach is supported by studies showing that multimarker serum panels, including PRL together with markers such as CEA or CYFRA 21-1, may perform better than single-marker assessment in lung cancer-related analyses [101]. In personalized medicine, the most promising application of PRL would therefore be its integration into broader prognostic or monitoring models, where it could provide complementary information on endocrine-inflammatory tumor-host interactions rather than direct tumor specificity.

Overall, the potential clinical utility of PRL in personalized NSCLC management appears to be most realistic when it is treated as a supplementary biomarker rather than an independent clinical tool. Its main value may lie in supporting risk stratification, longitudinal monitoring, and subgroup-specific interpretation, especially when combined with established clinical, molecular, serum, and inflammatory parameters. However, due to its limited specificity and susceptibility to multiple biological, pharmacological, and analytical confounders, PRL requires prospective validation before it can be incorporated into routine clinical decision-making (Figure 3).

https://doi.org/10.3390/jpm16070342

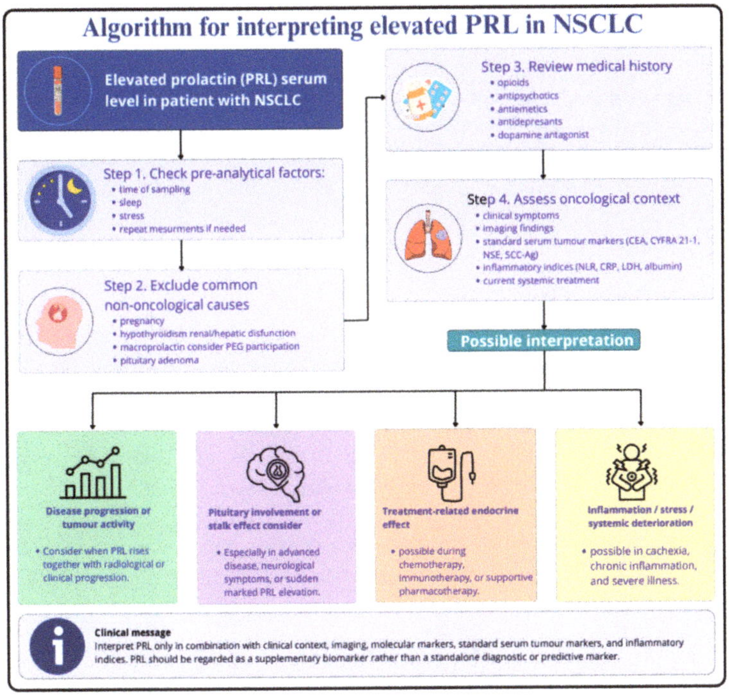

Figure 3. Suggested framework for interpreting prolactin levels in NSCLC.

7. Confounders, Analytical Limitations, and Barriers to Clinical Translation of Prolactin in NSCLC

The interpretation of prolactin as a prognostic biomarker in NSCLC faces significant challenges due to multiple confounding factors and methodological issues, as demonstrated by both clinical and experimental studies [102,103]. Although available data suggest a role for prolactin in NSCLC biology, its clinical significance remains ambiguous [50,76].

7.1. Biological Confounders

The physiological variability of prolactin levels, including the impact of stress, circadian rhythm, and sleep disturbances, as well as the lack of standardization in sample collection, has been extensively discussed in previous sections. These factors collectively limit the reliability of PRL as a prognostic biomarker in NSCLC and must be carefully considered in both research and clinical practice (see, Sections 4.3.1 and 4.3.2) [103–106].

Metabolic factors and the general condition of the patient are also relevant. Cancer cachexia and metabolic disorders affect the regulation of the hypothalamic–pituitary axis, as observed in advanced cancer stages [106]. Importantly, experimental studies have shown that NSCLC cells can produce prolactin, further complicating the interpretation of its systemic levels as a biomarker [50]. Both in vitro and in vivo models have confirmed the presence of prolactin within tumor tissue and its involvement in regulating cancer cell proliferation [50].

7.2. Clinical Confounders

In the NSCLC patient population, comorbidities can significantly influence prolactin levels and lead to erroneous prognostic conclusions [103]. Hypothyroidism is one of the most common causes of secondary hyperprolactinemia via stimulation of thyrotropin-

 https://doi.org/10.3390/jpm16070342

releasing hormone [102]. Renal and hepatic insufficiency, whether as comorbidities or as complications of cancer therapy, result in decreased prolactin clearance and its accumulation [103,107].

Chronic inflammation, characteristic of NSCLC, may affect prolactin secretion through pro-inflammatory cytokines, consistent with its role as an immunomodulatory factor [105]. Notably, prolactin may be directly associated with cancer progression—elevated levels have been correlated with poorer prognosis in lung cancer patients [108]. Rare cases of ectopic prolactin production by lung tumors have also been reported, further complicating differential diagnosis [108].

7.3. Pharmacological Confounders

Pharmacotherapy in NSCLC patients is a major source of prolactin disturbances [107]. Metoclopramide and other antiemetics, routinely used during chemotherapy, induce hyperprolactinemia by blocking dopamine receptors [107]. Antipsychotic and antidepressant medications, frequently prescribed in this patient group, also affect the dopaminergic system and may increase prolactin levels [109]. Opioids, commonly administered for cancer pain, also modulate prolactin secretion via the hypothalamic axis [104].

Additionally, as highlighted in previous sections, immunotherapy (e.g., nivolumab) has been associated with a high incidence of hyperprolactinemia, which may correlate with disease progression [76]. This indicates that changes in prolactin levels may result from both tumor biology and anticancer treatment effects.

7.4. Analytical and Pre-Analytical Limitations

Methodological limitations are a persistent obstacle in evaluating prolactin as a biomarker in NSCLC [110]. Variability in assay techniques, lack of standardized oncology-specific cut-off values, and the infrequent exclusion of macroprolactin all contribute to inconsistent results and hinder direct comparison between studies [102,103]. While prolactin levels tend to be higher in NSCLC patients than in healthy controls, its clinical utility emerges primarily when interpreted alongside established markers such as CEA or CYFRA21, rather than as an isolated parameter [4]. The timing of sample collection and storage conditions remains critical for assay reliability [102,105].

An important analytical limitation identified in the current literature concerns the assessment of prolactin receptor isoforms. Experimental evidence indicates that the long PRLR isoform is the principal mediator of prolactin-driven oncogenic signaling, promoting tumor progression, metastatic dissemination, and resistance to therapy. However, most routinely used clinical immunoassays, including enzyme-linked immunosorbent assays (ELISA), chemiluminescent immunoassays, and standard immunohistochemical protocols, are unable to differentiate between the long and short PRLR variants. This limitation arises because the antibodies employed in these assays typically recognize epitopes located within receptor regions shared by multiple isoforms, resulting in the measurement of total PRLR expression rather than isoform-specific expression patterns. As a consequence, biologically significant differences in receptor signaling may remain undetected, potentially limiting prognostic accuracy and patient stratification.

Bridging this bench-to-bedside gap will require the development and clinical validation of isoform-specific diagnostic methodologies. Potential approaches include monoclonal antibodies directed against unique domains of the long PRLR isoform, isoform-specific immunohistochemical panels, and transcript-based molecular techniques such as quantitative RT-PCR, digital PCR, and RNA sequencing capable of distinguishing alternatively spliced PRLR transcripts. The implementation of these technologies could improve prognostic

 https://doi.org/10.3390/jpm16070342

assessment, facilitate more precise risk stratification, and support the development of personalized therapeutic strategies targeting prolactin-dependent signaling pathways.

7.5. Barriers to Clinical Implementation

Despite the growing body of experimental and clinical data, the use of prolactin as a prognostic biomarker in NSCLC remains limited [50]. As previously discussed, molecular studies indicate that prolactin can promote NSCLC cell proliferation through activation of the GHR/JAK2/STAT3/VEGF pathway, supporting its potential involvement in disease progression [50]. Furthermore, genetic (Mendelian randomization) studies have shown that higher prolactin levels are associated with an increased risk of lung cancer, further supporting its potential role in carcinogenesis [68].

However, it should be emphasized that available clinical studies are few and involve small patient cohorts, limiting their statistical power and generalizability [103]. There is also a lack of external validation and unequivocal evidence that prolactin measurement influences therapeutic decisions or improves patient outcomes [4]. Ultimately, the greatest challenge remains the integration of biological data into clinical practice, as even statistically significant associations do not always translate into clinical utility [111].

8. Conclusions

Prolactin is not yet an established biomarker in NSCLC, but current evidence suggests that it may have potential as a supplementary circulating marker, particularly for prognosis and post-treatment monitoring. Its biological relevance is supported by its involvement in pathways related to tumour proliferation, survival, invasion, angiogenesis, immune modulation and possible therapy resistance.

In clinical practice, PRL should not be interpreted as a standalone diagnostic or predictive marker. Its levels may be influenced by many confounders, including stress, circadian rhythm, inflammation, endocrine disorders, cachexia, pituitary metastases, macroprolactin and medications such as opioids, antipsychotics or antiemetics. Therefore, PRL should be assessed only in combination with clinical data, imaging, molecular markers, standard serum tumour markers and inflammatory indices.

The most realistic future role of PRL in NSCLC lies in multimarker prognostic models and longitudinal monitoring after systemic treatment, including chemotherapy. Serial changes in PRL may potentially help identify patients at higher risk of progression, but this requires confirmation in large prospective studies with standardized sampling, assay methods and adjustment for confounding factors.

In conclusion, prolactin is a promising but still unvalidated candidate biomarker in NSCLC. Its clinical use should remain investigational until robust evidence confirms its independent prognostic value and practical utility in personalised patient management.

Author Contributions: Conceptualization, P.K., F.G., and O.B.; validation, P.K. and A.K.; formal analysis, P.K. and A.K.; investigation, F.G., J.P., J.K., W.P., G.K., and A.L.; writing—original draft preparation, F.G., J.P., J.K., W.P., G.K., and A.L.; writing—review and editing, F.G. and J.P.; visualization, F.G.; supervision, P.K. and A.K.; project administration, P.K. and F.G. All authors have read and agreed to the published version of the manuscript.

Funding: This research received no external funding.

Institutional Review Board Statement: Not applicable.

Informed Consent Statement: Not applicable.

Data Availability Statement: No new data were created or analyzed in this study. Data sharing is not applicable to this article.

https://doi.org/10.3390/jpm16070342

Conflicts of Interest: The authors declare no conflicts of interest.

Abbreviations

The following abbreviations are used in this manuscript:

ACTH	adrenocorticotropic hormone
ADH	antidiuretic hormone
ALK	anaplastic lymphoma kinase
ATM	ataxia-telangiectasia mutated kinase
CEA	carcinoembryonic antigen
CRP	C-reactive protein
CYFRA 21-1	cytokeratin 19 fragment antigen 21-1
DA	dopamine
DFS	disease-free survival
EGFR	epidermal growth factor receptor
EMT	epithelial–mesenchymal transition
ERBB2	erb-b2 receptor tyrosine kinase 2
ERK	extracellular signal-regulated kinase
FSH	follicle-stimulating hormone
GH	growth hormone
GHR	growth hormone receptor
GHRH	growth hormone-releasing hormone
GnRH	gonadotropin-releasing hormone
HER2	human epidermal growth factor receptor 2
HO-1	heme oxygenase-1
HPA axis	hypothalamic–pituitary–adrenal axis
HSP90	heat shock protein 90
IAD	isolated ACTH deficiency
ICI	immune checkpoint inhibitor
IHC	immunohistochemistry
IL-6	interleukin-6
JAK	Janus kinase
JAK2	Janus kinase 2
JAK/STAT	Janus kinase/signal transducer and activator of transcription
Ki-67	marker of cellular proliferation
KRAS	Kirsten rat sarcoma viral oncogene homolog
LDH	lactate dehydrogenase
LH	luteinizing hormone
MAPK	mitogen-activated protein kinase
MAPK/ERK	mitogen-activated protein kinase/extracellular signal-regulated kinase
MET	mesenchymal–epithelial transition factor
MMP	matrix metalloproteinase
MMP-2	matrix metalloproteinase-2
MMP-9	matrix metalloproteinase-9
mTOR	mechanistic target of rapamycin
N	regional lymph node status in TNM classification
NET	neuroendocrine tumor
NGS	next-generation sequencing
NLR	neutrophil-to-lymphocyte ratio
NSE	neuron-specific enolase
NSCLC	non-small cell lung cancer
NTRK	neurotrophic tyrosine receptor kinase
OS	overall survival

 https://doi.org/10.3390/jpm16070342

PD-1	programmed cell death protein 1
PD-L1	programmed death-ligand 1
PEG	polyethylene glycol
PFS	progression-free survival
PI3K	phosphoinositide 3-kinase
PI3K/AKT	phosphoinositide 3-kinase/protein kinase B
PR	partial response/partial remission
PRL	prolactin
PRLR	prolactin receptor
RET	rearranged during transfection proto-oncogene
ROS1	ROS proto-oncogene 1, receptor tyrosine kinase
SCC-Ag	squamous cell carcinoma antigen
SHH	Sonic Hedgehog
STAT	signal transducer and activator of transcription
STAT3	signal transducer and activator of transcription 3
STAT5	signal transducer and activator of transcription 5
STAT5A	signal transducer and activator of transcription 5A
STAT5B	signal transducer and activator of transcription 5B
T	primary tumor status in TNM classification
TIDA neurons	tuberoinfundibular dopamine neurons
TME	tumor microenvironment
TNF-α	tumor necrosis factor alpha
TNM	tumor, node, metastasis classification
TRH	thyrotropin-releasing hormone
Treg	regulatory T cells
VEGF	vascular endothelial growth factor

References

1. Siegel, R.L.; Kratzer, T.B.; Wagle, N.S.; Sung, H.; Jemal, A. Cancer statistics, 2026. *CA Cancer J. Clin.* **2026**, *76*, e70043. [CrossRef] [PubMed]
2. Shong, L.Y.-W.; Lam, D.C.-L. Emerging trends in global lung cancer burden. *Semin. Respir. Crit. Care Med.* **2025**, *46*, 409–418. [CrossRef] [PubMed]
3. Jovanoski, N.; Bowes, K.; Brown, A.; Belleli, R.; Di Maio, D.; Chadda, S.; Abogunrin, S. Survival and quality-of-life outcomes in early-stage NSCLC patients: A literature review of real-world evidence. *Lung Cancer Manag.* **2023**, *12*, LMT60. [CrossRef] [PubMed]
4. Šutić, M.; Vukić, A.; Baranašić, J.; Försti, A.; Džubur, F.; Samaržija, M.; Jakopović, M.; Brčić, L.; Knežević, J. Diagnostic, predictive, and prognostic biomarkers in non-small cell lung cancer (NSCLC) management. *J. Pers. Med.* **2021**, *11*, 1102. [CrossRef] [PubMed]
5. Califf, R.M. Biomarker definitions and their applications. *Exp. Biol. Med.* **2018**, *243*, 213–221. [CrossRef] [PubMed]
6. Nalejska, E.; Mączyńska, E.; Lewandowska, M.A. Prognostic and predictive biomarkers: Tools in personalized oncology. *Mol. Diagn. Ther.* **2014**, *18*, 273–284. [CrossRef] [PubMed]
7. Hendriks, L.; Kerr, K.; Menis, J.; Mok, T.; Nestle, U.; Passaro, A.; Peters, S.; Planchard, D.; Smit, E.; Solomon, B.; et al. Oncogene-addicted metastatic non-small-cell lung cancer: ESMO Clinical Practice Guideline for diagnosis, treatment and follow-up. *Ann. Oncol.* **2023**, *34*, 339–357. [CrossRef] [PubMed]
8. Lindeman, N.I.; Cagle, P.T.; Aisner, D.L.; Arcila, M.E.; Beasley, M.B.; Bernicker, E.H.; Colasacco, C.; Dacic, S.; Hirsch, F.R.; Kerr, K.; et al. Updated molecular testing guideline for the selection of lung cancer patients for treatment with targeted tyrosine kinase inhibitors. *Arch. Pathol. Lab. Med.* **2018**, *142*, 321–346. [CrossRef] [PubMed]
9. Sholl, L.M.; Cooper, W.A.; Kerr, K.M.; Tan, D.S.W.; Tsao, M.-S.; Yang, J.C.-H. (Eds.) *IASLC Atlas of Molecular Testing for Targeted Therapy in Lung Cancer*; International Association for the Study of Lung Cancer: Denver, CO, USA, 2023.
10. Hendriks, L.E.L.; Cortiula, F.; Martins-Branco, D.; Mariamidze, E.; Popat, S.; Reck, M.; ESMO Guidelines Committee. Updated treatment recommendations for systemic treatment: From the ESMO non-oncogene-addicted metastatic NSCLC Living Guideline. *Ann. Oncol.* **2025**, *36*, 1223–1227. [CrossRef] [PubMed]
11. FDA-NIH Biomarker Working Group. *BEST (Biomarkers, EndpointS, and Other Tools) Resource*; Food and Drug Administration: Silver Spring, MD, USA; National Institutes of Health: Bethesda, MD, USA, 2016.

 https://doi.org/10.3390/jpm16070342

12. Oldenhuis, C.N.; Oosting, S.F.; Gietema, J.A.; de Vries, E.G. Prognostic versus predictive value of biomarkers in oncology. *Eur. J. Cancer* **2008**, *44*, 946–953. [CrossRef] [PubMed]
13. Molina, R.; Filella, X.; Augé, J.; Fuentes, R.; Bover, I.; Rifa, J.; Moreno, V.; Canals, E.; Viñolas, N.; Marquez, A.; et al. Tumor markers (CEA, CA 125, CYFRA 21-1, SCC and NSE) in patients with non-small cell lung cancer as an aid in histological diagnosis and prognosis. *Tumor Biol.* **2003**, *24*, 209–218. [CrossRef] [PubMed]
14. Yanev, N.; Mekov, E.; Valev, D.; Yankov, G.; Milanov, V.; Bichev, S.; Gabrovska, N.; Kostadinov, D. EGFR mutation status yield from bronchoalveolar lavage in patients with primary pulmonary adenocarcinoma compared to a venous blood sample and tissue biopsy. *PeerJ* **2021**, *9*, e11448. [CrossRef] [PubMed]
15. Kalkanis, A.; Papadopoulos, D.; Testelmans, D.; Kopitopoulou, A.; Boeykens, E.; Wauters, E. Bronchoalveolar lavage fluid-isolated biomarkers for the diagnostic and prognostic assessment of lung cancer. *Diagnostics* **2022**, *12*, 2949. [CrossRef] [PubMed]
16. Nair, V.S.; Hui, A.B.-Y.; Chabon, J.J.; Esfahani, M.S.; Stehr, H.; Nabet, B.Y.; Zhou, L.; Chaudhuri, A.A.; Benson, J.; Ayers, K.; et al. Genomic profiling of bronchoalveolar lavage fluid in lung cancer. *Cancer Res.* **2022**, *82*, 2838–2847. [CrossRef] [PubMed]
17. Ballman, K.V. Biomarker: Predictive or Prognostic? *J. Clin. Oncol.* **2015**, *33*, 3968–3971. [CrossRef] [PubMed]
18. Odintsov, I.; Sholl, L.M. Prognostic and predictive biomarkers in non-small cell lung carcinoma. *Pathology* **2024**, *56*, 192–204. [CrossRef] [PubMed]
19. Wang, L.; Wang, D.; Zheng, G.; Yang, Y.; Du, L.; Dong, Z.; Zhang, X.; Wang, C. Clinical evaluation and therapeutic monitoring value of serum tumor markers in lung cancer. *Int. J. Biol. Markers* **2016**, *31*, 80–87. [CrossRef] [PubMed]
20. Holdenrieder, S.; Wehnl, B.; Hettwer, K.; Simon, K.; Uhlig, S.; Dayyani, F. Carcinoembryonic antigen and cytokeratin-19 fragments for assessment of therapy response in non-small cell lung cancer: A systematic review and meta-analysis. *Br. J. Cancer* **2017**, *116*, 1037–1045. [CrossRef] [PubMed]
21. Dall'oLio, F.G.; Abbati, F.; Facchinetti, F.; Massucci, M.; Melotti, B.; Squadrilli, A.; Buti, S.; Formica, F.; Tiseo, M.; Ardizzoni, A. CEA and CYFRA 21-1 as prognostic biomarker and as a tool for treatment monitoring in advanced NSCLC treated with immune checkpoint inhibitors. *Ther. Adv. Med. Oncol.* **2020**, *12*, 1758835920952994. [CrossRef] [PubMed]
22. Stares, M.; Brown, L.R.; Abhi, D.; Phillips, I. Prognostic biomarkers of systemic inflammation in non-small cell lung cancer: A narrative review of challenges and opportunities. *Cancers* **2024**, *16*, 1508. [CrossRef] [PubMed]
23. Saleem, M.; Martin, H.; Coates, P. Prolactin biology and laboratory measurement: An update on physiology and current analytical issues. *Clin. Biochem. Rev.* **2018**, *39*, 3–16. [PubMed]
24. Sadiq, N.M.; Tadi, P. *Physiology, Pituitary Hormones*; StatPearls Publishing: Treasure Island, FL, USA, 2023. Available online: https://www.ncbi.nlm.nih.gov/books/NBK557556/ (accessed on 1 May 2023).
25. Thapa, S.; Bhusal, K. *Hyperprolactinemia*; StatPearls Publishing: Treasure Island, FL, USA, 2023. Available online: https://www.ncbi.nlm.nih.gov/books/NBK537331/ (accessed on 30 November 2025).
26. Mendoza, R.A.; Grandner, M.A.; Elali, L.S.; Fernandez, F.-X. Concerning the circadian rhythms of prolactin, its secretion timing, and regulation of the affiliative mind. *Neurosci. Biobehav. Rev.* **2025**, *179*, 106403. [CrossRef] [PubMed]
27. Al-Chalabi, M.; Bass, A.N.; Alsalman, I. *Physiology, Prolactin*; StatPearls Publishing: Treasure Island, FL, USA, 2023. Available online: https://www.ncbi.nlm.nih.gov/books/NBK507829/ (accessed on 30 November 2025).
28. Qi-Lytle, X.; Sayers, S.; Wagner, E.J. Current review of the function and regulation of tuberoinfundibular dopamine neurons. *Int. J. Mol. Sci.* **2023**, *25*, 110. [CrossRef] [PubMed]
29. Faron-Górecka, A.; Latocha, K.; Pabian, P.; Kolasa, M.; Sobczyk-Krupiarz, I.; Dziedzicka-Wasylewska, M.; Maćkowiak, M. The involvement of prolactin in stress-related disorders. *Int. J. Environ. Res. Public Health* **2023**, *20*, 3257. [CrossRef] [PubMed]
30. Kolnikaj, T.S.; Musat, M.; Salehidoost, R.; Korbonits, M. *Pharmacological Causes of Hyperprolactinemia*; MDText.com, Inc.: Portland, OR, USA, 2024. Available online: https://www.ncbi.nlm.nih.gov/books/NBK599196/ (accessed on 30 November 2025).
31. Petersenn, S.; Fleseriu, M.; Casanueva, F.F.; Honegger, J.; Gadelha, M.R.; Vila, G.; Chanson, P.; Persani, L.; Luger, A.; Ansorge, O.; et al. Diagnosis and management of prolactin-secreting pituitary adenomas: A Pituitary Society international consensus statement. *Nat. Rev. Endocrinol.* **2023**, *19*, 722–740. [CrossRef] [PubMed]
32. Monteiro, A.L.S.; Glezer, A. *Hyperprolactinemia*; MDText.com, Inc.: Portland, OR, USA, 2025. Available online: https://www.ncbi.nlm.nih.gov/books/NBK278984/ (accessed on 30 November 2025).
33. Marano, R.J.; Ben-Jonathan, N. Minireview: Extrapituitary prolactin: An update on the distribution, regulation, and functions. *Mol. Endocrinol.* **2014**, *28*, 622–633. [CrossRef] [PubMed]
34. Kamel-ElSayed, S.A.; Schwartz, J. *Physiology, Pituitary Gland*; StatPearls Publishing: Treasure Island, FL, USA, 2023. Available online: https://www.ncbi.nlm.nih.gov/books/NBK459247/ (accessed on 1 May 2023).
35. Ni, Y.; Chen, Q.; Cai, J.; Xiao, L.; Zhang, J. Three lactation-related hormones: Regulation of hypothalamus-pituitary axis and function on lactation. *Mol. Cell. Endocrinol.* **2021**, *520*, 111084. [CrossRef] [PubMed]
36. Borba, V.V.; Bonfá, E. Prolactin as an inflammatory cytokine in systemic autoimmune diseases. *Front. Immunol.* **2019**, *10*, 1823.
37. Legorreta-Haquet, M.V.; Chávez-Rueda, K.; Montoya-Díaz, E.; Arriaga-Pizano, L.; Silva-García, R.; López-Casillas, F. The effect of prolactin on immune cell subsets involved in SLE and other autoimmune diseases. *Clin. Rheumatol.* **2022**, *42*, 1007–1019.

https://doi.org/10.3390/jpm16070342

38. Pirchio, R.; Graziadio, C.; Colao, A.; Pivonello, R.; Auriemma, R.S. Metabolic effects of prolactin. *Front. Endocrinol.* **2022**, *13*, 1015520. [CrossRef] [PubMed]
39. Macotela, Y.; Ruiz-Herrera, X.; Vázquez-Carrillo, D.I.; Ramírez-Hernandez, G.; Martínez de la Escalera, G.; Clapp, C. The beneficial metabolic actions of prolactin. *Front. Endocrinol.* **2022**, *13*, 1001703. [CrossRef] [PubMed]
40. Shams, A.; Binothman, N.; Boudreault, J.; Wang, N.; Shams, F.; Hamam, D.; Tian, J.; Moamer, A.; Dai, M.; Lebrun, J.-J.; et al. Prolactin receptor-driven combined luminal and epithelial differentiation in breast cancer restricts plasticity, stemness, tumorigenesis and metastasis. *Oncogenesis* **2021**, *10*, 10. [CrossRef] [PubMed]
41. Standing, D.; Dandawate, P.; Anant, S. Prolactin receptor signaling: A novel target for cancer treatment—Exploring anti-PRLR signaling strategies. *Front. Endocrinol.* **2023**, *13*, 1112987. [CrossRef] [PubMed]
42. Morohoshi, K.; Mochinaga, R.; Watanabe, T.; Nakajima, R.; Harigaya, T. 16 kDa vasoinhibin binds to integrin alpha5 beta1 on endothelial cells to induce apoptosis. *Endocr. Connect.* **2018**, *7*, 630–636. [CrossRef] [PubMed]
43. Zhao, H.; Gong, S.; Shi, Y.; Luo, C.; Qiu, H.; He, J.; Sun, Y.; Huang, Y.; Wang, S.; Miao, Y.; et al. The role of prolactin/vasoinhibins in cardiovascular diseases. *Anim. Model. Exp. Med.* **2023**, *6*, 81–91. [CrossRef]
44. Abramicheva, P.A.; Smirnova, O.V. Prolactin receptor isoforms as the basis of tissue-specific action of prolactin in the norm and pathology. *Biochemistry* **2019**, *84*, 329–345. [CrossRef] [PubMed]
45. Ferraris, J. Is prolactin receptor signaling a target in dopamine-resistant prolactinomas? *Front. Endocrinol.* **2023**, *13*, 1057749. [CrossRef] [PubMed]
46. Shen, S.; Radhakrishnan, S.K.; Harrell, J.C.; Puchalapalli, M.; Koblinski, J.; Clevenger, C. The human intermediate prolactin receptor I-tail contributes breast oncogenesis by targeting Ras/MAPK pathway. *Endocrinology* **2024**, *165*, bqae039. [CrossRef] [PubMed]
47. Clevenger, C.V.; Rui, H. Breast cancer and prolactin—New mechanisms and models. *Endocrinol. Endocrinol.* **2022**, *163*, bqac122. [CrossRef] [PubMed]
48. Banks, C.M.; Trott, J.F.; Hovey, R.C. The prolactin receptor: A cross-species comparison of gene structure, transcriptional regulation, tissue-specificity, and genetic variation. *J. Neuroendocr.* **2024**, *36*, e13385. [CrossRef] [PubMed]
49. Grible, J.M.; Zot, P.; Olex, A.L.; Hedrick, S.E.; Harrell, J.C.; Woock, A.E.; Idowu, M.O.; Clevenger, C.V. The human intermediate prolactin receptor is a mammary proto-oncogene. *npj Breast Cancer* **2021**, *7*, 37. [CrossRef] [PubMed]
50. Chou, J.-C.; Lieu, F.-K.; Ho, D.M.-T.; Shen, H.-Y.; Lin, P.-H.; Hu, S.; Wang, S.-W.; Lin, H.; Wang, P.S. Regulation of extracellular and intracellular prolactin on cell proliferation and survival rate through GHR/JAK2/STAT3 pathway in NSCLC. *Chemosphere* **2021**, *264*, 128604. [CrossRef] [PubMed]
51. Alkharusi, A.; Yu, S.; Landázuri, N.; Zadjali, F.; Davodi, B.; Nyström, T.; Gräslund, T.; Rahbar, A.; Norstedt, G. Stimulation of prolactin receptor induces STAT-5 phosphorylation and cellular invasion in glioblastoma multiforme. *Oncotarget* **2016**, *7*, 79572–79583. [CrossRef] [PubMed]
52. Biagetti, B.; Simò, R. Molecular pathways in prolactinomas: Translational and therapeutic implications. *Int. J. Mol. Sci.* **2021**, *22*, 11247. [CrossRef] [PubMed]
53. Lenke, L.; Martínez de la Escalera, G.; Clapp, C.; Bertsch, T.; Triebel, J. A Dysregulation of the Prolactin/Vasoinhibin Axis Appears to Contribute to Preeclampsia. *Front. Endocrinol.* **2020**, *10*, 893. [CrossRef] [PubMed]
54. Triebel, J.; Bertsch, T.; Bollheimer, C.; Rios-Barrera, D.; Pearce, C.F.; Hüfner, M.; de la Escalera, G.M.; Clapp, C. Principles of the prolactin/vasoinhibin axis. *Am. J. Physiol. Integr. Comp. Physiol.* **2015**, *309*, R1193–R1203. [CrossRef] [PubMed]
55. Clapp, C.; Thebault, S.; Macotela, Y.; Moreno-Carranza, B.; Triebel, J.; Martínez de la Escalera, G. Regulation of blood vessels by prolactin and vasoinhibins. *Adv. Exp. Med. Biol.* **2015**, *846*, 83–95. [CrossRef] [PubMed]
56. Reuwer, A.Q.; Nowak-Sliwinska, P.; Mans, L.A.; van der Loos, C.M.; von der Thüsen, J.H.; Twickler, M.T.B.; Spek, C.A.; Goffin, V.; Griffioen, A.W.; Borensztajn, K.S. Functional consequences of prolactin signalling in endothelial cells: A potential link with angiogenesis in pathophysiology? *J. Cell. Mol. Med.* **2012**, *16*, 2035–2048. [CrossRef] [PubMed]
57. Rider, L.; Oladimeji, P.; Diakonova, M. PAK1 regulates breast cancer cell invasion through secretion of matrix metalloproteinases in response to prolactin and three-dimensional collagen IV. *Mol. Endocrinol.* **2013**, *27*, 1048–1064. [CrossRef] [PubMed]
58. Cepeda, M.A.; Evered, C.L.; Pelling, J.J.H.; Damjanovski, S. Inhibition of MT1-MMP proteolytic function and ERK1/2 signalling influences cell migration and invasion through changes in MMP-2 and MMP-9 levels. *J. Cell Commun. Signal.* **2017**, *11*, 167–179. [CrossRef] [PubMed]
59. da Silva, P.L.; do Amaral, V.C.; Gabrielli, V.; Montt Guevara, M.M.; Mannella, P.; Baracat, E.C.; Soares, J.M., Jr.; Simoncini, T. Prolactin promotes breast cancer cell migration through actin cytoskeleton remodeling. *Front. Endocrinol.* **2015**, *6*, 186. [CrossRef] [PubMed]
60. Karayazi Atıcı, Ö.; Govindrajan, N.; Lopetegui-González, I.; Shemanko, C.S. Prolactin: A hormone with diverse functions from mammary gland development to cancer metastasis. *Semin. Cell Dev. Biol.* **2021**, *114*, 159–170. [CrossRef] [PubMed]

https://doi.org/10.3390/jpm16070342

61. Lahmar, Q.; Keirsse, J.; Laoui, D.; Movahedi, K.; Van Overmeire, E.; Van Ginderachter, J.A. Tissue-resident versus monocyte-derived macrophages in the tumor microenvironment. *Biochim. Biophys. Acta Rev. Cancer* **2016**, *1865*, 23–34. [CrossRef] [PubMed]
62. Gorvin, C.M. The prolactin receptor: Diverse and emerging roles in pathophysiology. *J. Clin. Transl. Endocrinol.* **2015**, *2*, 85–91. [CrossRef] [PubMed]
63. Costanza, M.; Binart, N.; Steinman, L.; Pedotti, R. Prolactin: A versatile regulator of inflammation and autoimmune pathology. *Autoimmun. Rev.* **2015**, *14*, 223–230. [CrossRef] [PubMed]
64. Safdari, S.; Safdari, S.; Noorabadi, P. Prolactin as a novel biomarker in malignancy. *Clin. Chim. Acta* **2025**, *572*, 120277. [CrossRef] [PubMed]
65. Rahal, Z.; El Darzi, R.; Moghaddam, S.J.; Cascone, T.; Kadara, H. Tumour and microenvironment crosstalk in NSCLC progression and response to therapy. *Nat. Rev. Clin. Oncol.* **2025**, *22*, 463–482. [CrossRef] [PubMed]
66. Wen, J.; Yu, J.-Z.; Liu, C.; Ould Ismail, A.A.O.; Ma, W. Exploring the molecular tumor microenvironment and translational biomarkers in brain metastases of non-small-cell lung cancer. *Int. J. Mol. Sci.* **2024**, *25*, 2044. [CrossRef] [PubMed]
67. Wang, J.; Lan, H.; Mao, X.; Chen, Y. Pituitary-adrenal axis dysfunction induced by tislelizumab immunotherapy for non-small cell lung cancer: A case series and literature review. *BMC Pulm. Med.* **2024**, *24*, 327. [CrossRef] [PubMed]
68. Feng, Z.; Fu, J.; Wang, K.; Yang, J.; Jiang, X.; Wu, Q. Causal relationship between hormone levels and lung cancer: A Mendelian randomization study. *Front. Endocrinol.* **2025**, *16*, 1462531. [CrossRef] [PubMed]
69. Partyńska, A.; Jabłońska, K.; Nowińska, K.; Dzięgiel, P. The role of prolactin and its receptor in cancer development. *Postep. Hig. Med. Dosw.* **2019**, *73*, 232–244. [CrossRef]
70. Schuler, L.A.; O'Leary, K.A. Prolactin: The third hormone in breast cancer. *Front. Endocrinol.* **2022**, *13*, 910978. [CrossRef] [PubMed]
71. Cisoń-Jurek, S.; Czajka-Francuz, P.; Francuz, T.; Owczarek, A.J.; Szymczak, B.; Wojnar, J.; Chudek, J. The value of prolactin, a panel of cytokines, and the soluble human epidermal growth factor receptor 2 in the prediction of rapid progression and shorter survival during palliative chemotherapy of colorectal cancer patients. *Biomedicines* **2023**, *11*, 2014. [CrossRef] [PubMed]
72. Peuskens, J.; Pani, L.; Detraux, J.; De Hert, M. The effects of novel and newly approved antipsychotics on serum prolactin levels: A comprehensive review. *CNS Drugs* **2014**, *28*, 421–453. [CrossRef] [PubMed]
73. Haddad, P.M.; Wieck, A. Antipsychotic-induced hyperprolactinaemia. *Drugs* **2004**, *64*, 2291–2314. [CrossRef] [PubMed]
74. Vuong, C.; Van Uum, S.H.M.; O'Dell, L.E.; Lutfy, K.; Friedman, T.C. The effects of opioids and opioid analogs on animal and human endocrine systems. *Endocr. Rev.* **2010**, *31*, 98–132. [CrossRef] [PubMed]
75. Herman, J.P.; McKlveen, J.M.; Ghosal, S.; Kopp, B.; Wulsin, A.; Makinson, R.; Scheimann, J.; Myers, B. Regulation of the hypothalamic-pituitary-adrenocortical stress response. *Compr. Physiol.* **2016**, *6*, 603–621. [CrossRef]
76. Caponnetto, S.; Iannantuono, G.M.; Barchiesi, G.; Magri, V.; Gelibter, A.; Cortesi, E. Prolactin as a potential early predictive factor in metastatic non-small cell lung cancer patients treated with nivolumab. *Oncology* **2017**, *93*, 62–66. [CrossRef] [PubMed]
77. Barroso-Sousa, R.; Barry, W.T.; Garrido-Castro, A.C.; Hodi, F.S.; Min, L.; Krop, I.E.; Tolaney, S.M. Incidence of endocrine dysfunction following the use of different immune checkpoint inhibitor regimens: A systematic review and meta-analysis. *JAMA Oncol.* **2018**, *4*, 173–182. [CrossRef] [PubMed]
78. Bole-Feysot, C.; Goffin, V.; Edery, M.; Binart, N.; Kelly, P.A. Prolactin and its receptor: Actions, signal transduction pathways and phenotypes observed in PRL receptor knockout mice. *Endocr. Rev.* **1998**, *19*, 225–268. [CrossRef] [PubMed]
79. Liu, Q.; Shaibu, Z.; Xu, A.; Yang, F.; Cao, R.; Yang, F. Predictive value of serum cytokines in patients with non-small-cell lung cancer receiving anti-PD-1 blockade therapy: A meta-analysis. *Clin. Exp. Med.* **2025**, *25*, 59. [CrossRef] [PubMed]
80. Patel, H.J.; Patel, B.M. TNF-α and cancer cachexia: Molecular insights and clinical implications. *Life Sci.* **2017**, *170*, 56–63. [CrossRef] [PubMed]
81. Olson, B.; Diba, P.; Korzun, T.; Marks, D.L. Neural mechanisms of cancer cachexia. *Cancers* **2021**, *13*, 3990. [CrossRef] [PubMed]
82. Wu, Q.; Liu, Z.; Li, B.; Liu, Y.-E.; Wang, P. Immunoregulation in cancer-associated cachexia. *J. Adv. Res.* **2024**, *58*, 45–62. [CrossRef] [PubMed]
83. van Norren, K.; Dwarkasing, J.T.; Witkamp, R.F. The role of hypothalamic inflammation, the hypothalamic–pituitary–adrenal axis and serotonin in the cancer anorexia–cachexia syndrome. *Curr. Opin. Clin. Nutr. Metab. Care* **2017**, *20*, 396–401. [CrossRef] [PubMed]
84. Costanza, F.; Giampietro, A.; Mattogno, P.P.; Chiloiro, S. Colon cancer presenting as pituitary mass and hypopituitarism: Recognition and multidisciplinary approach of a rare case. *JCEM Case Rep.* **2023**, *1*, luad031. [CrossRef] [PubMed]
85. Giuffrida, G.; Ferraù, F.; Alessi, Y.; Cannavò, S. Shrinkage of a pituitary metastasis of melanoma induced by pembrolizumab: A case report. *J. Med. Case Rep.* **2021**, *15*, 555. [CrossRef] [PubMed]
86. Biagetti, B.; Ferrer Costa, R.; Alfayate Guerra, R.; Álvarez García, E.; Berlanga Escalera, E.; Casals, G.; Esteban Salán, M.; Granada Ibern, M.L.; Gorrín Ramos, J.; López Lazareno, N.; et al. Macroprolactin: From laboratory to clinical practice. *Endocrinol. Diabetes Y Nutr.* **2022**, *69*, 63–69. [CrossRef] [PubMed]

 https://doi.org/10.3390/jpm16070342

87. O'Callaghan, L.A.; Blum, C.B.; Powell, K.; Chess-Williams, R.; McDermott, C. From psychiatry to oncology: Exploring the anti-neoplastic mechanisms of aripiprazole and its potential use in cancer treatment. *Pharmacol. Res. Perspect.* **2025**, *13*, e70076. [CrossRef] [PubMed]
88. Ken-Dror, G.; Fluck, D.; Lean, M.E.J.; Casanueva, F.F.; Han, T.S. The relationship between low prolactin and type 2 diabetes. *Rev. Endocr. Metab. Disord.* **2024**, *25*, 1087–1095. [CrossRef] [PubMed]
89. Han, D.; Zhao, K.; Yang, Q.; Zhang, L.; Fei, S. Secondary mutant ALK-I1171s in pituitary metastases from a patient with ALK fusion-positive advanced lung adenocarcinoma: A case report and literature review. *Front. Oncol.* **2022**, *12*, 1016320. [CrossRef] [PubMed]
90. Gupta, A.; Kasaliwal, R.; Das, L.; Sharma, S.K.; Kaur, V.; Vasiljevic, A.; Raverot, V.; Korbonits, M.; Dutta, P. Ectopic acromegaly with tumoral range hyperprolactinemia and apoplexy with a dramatic regression of pituitary hyperplasia. *Front. Endocrinol.* **2024**, *15*, 1473167. [CrossRef] [PubMed]
91. Gu, Y.C.; Liu, Y.; Xie, C.; Cao, B.S. Pituitary immune-related adverse events induced by programmed cell death protein 1 inhibitors in advanced lung cancer patients: A report of 3 cases. *Beijing Da Xue Xue Bao Yi Xue Ban* **2022**, *54*, 369–375. [CrossRef] [PubMed]
92. Diasso, P.D.K.; Frederiksen, B.S.; Nielsen, S.D.; Main, K.M.; Sjøgren, P.; Kurita, G.P. Long-term opioid treatment and endocrine measures in chronic non-cancer pain patients: A systematic review and meta-analysis. *Eur. J. Pain* **2021**, *25*, 1859–1875. [CrossRef] [PubMed]
93. Wang, Q.; Liu, X.-W.; Chen, K.-Y. Pituitary metastasis from lung adenocarcinoma: A case report. *World J. Clin. Cases* **2024**, *12*, 2597–2605. [CrossRef] [PubMed]
94. Yuzkan, S.; Erkan, B.; Dogukan, F.M.; Ozkiziltan, U.; Balsak, S.; Arslan, F.Z.; Tutuncuoglu, B.; Arikan, C.C.; Karatay, H.; Akpinar, E.; et al. Distinguishing pituitary metastasis and pituitary neuroendocrine tumors through conventional MR imaging and clinical features. *Am. J. Neuroradiol.* **2024**, *45*, 1063–1069. [CrossRef] [PubMed]
95. Arafsha, L.; Samargandy, S.A.; Alyazidi, A.S. Endocrine manifestations of lung adenocarcinoma with epidermal growth factor receptor mutation mimicking tuberculosis: A case report and literature review. *Qatar Med. J.* **2025**, *2025*, 64. [CrossRef] [PubMed]
96. Puglisi, M.; May, L.; Gardiyehewa, T.; Landry, J.W. Sex differences in the response to lung cancer and its relation to programmed cell death protein-1/programmed death-ligand-1 checkpoint therapies. *Cancers* **2025**, *17*, 3953. [CrossRef] [PubMed]
97. Wang, M.; Herbst, R.S.; Boshoff, C. Toward personalized treatment approaches for non-small-cell lung cancer. *Nat. Med.* **2021**, *27*, 1345–1356. [CrossRef] [PubMed]
98. Feng, Y.; Qiao, H.; Han, X.; Tang, H. A prognostic nomogram of non-small cell lung cancer based on tumor marker inflammatory nutrition score. *Transl. Lung Cancer Res.* **2024**, *13*, 3392–3406. [CrossRef] [PubMed]
99. Dal Bello, M.G.; Filiberti, R.A.; Alama, A.; Orengo, A.M.; Mussap, M.; Coco, S.; Vanni, I.; Boccardo, S.; Rijavec, E.; Genova, C.; et al. The role of CEA, CYFRA21-1 and NSE in monitoring tumor response to Nivolumab in advanced non-small cell lung cancer patients. *J. Transl. Med.* **2019**, *17*, 74. [CrossRef] [PubMed]
100. Yang, X.; Xiao, Y.; Zhou, Y.; Deng, H.; Yuan, Z.; Dong, L.; Lan, J.; Hu, H.; Huang, J.; Huang, S. Dynamic monitoring of serum tumor markers as prognostic factors in patients with advanced non-small-cell lung cancer treated with first-line immunotherapy: A multicenter retrospective study. *Ther. Adv. Med. Oncol.* **2023**, *15*, 17588359231206282. [CrossRef] [PubMed]
101. Fang, R.; Zhu, Y.; Khadka, V.S.; Zhang, F.; Jiang, B.; Deng, Y. The evaluation of serum biomarkers for non-small cell lung cancer (NSCLC) diagnosis. *Front. Physiol.* **2018**, *9*, 1710. [CrossRef] [PubMed]
102. Melmed, S.; Casanueva, F.F.; Hoffman, A.R.; Kleinberg, D.L.; Montori, V.M.; Schlechte, J.A.; Wass, J.A.H.; Endocrine Society. Diagnosis and treatment of hyperprolactinemia: An Endocrine Society clinical practice guideline. *J. Clin. Endocrinol. Metab.* **2011**, *96*, 273–288. [CrossRef] [PubMed]
103. Vilar, L.; Vilar, C.F.; Lyra, R.; Freitas, M.C. Pitfalls in the diagnostic evaluation of hyperprolactinemia. *Neuroendocrinology* **2019**, *109*, 7–19. [CrossRef] [PubMed]
104. Ben-Jonathan, N.; Hugo, E. Prolactin in adipose tissue: Regulation and functions. *Adv. Exp. Med. Biol.* **2015**, *846*, 1–35. [CrossRef] [PubMed]
105. Touitou, Y.; Haus, E. Alterations with aging of the endocrine and neuroendocrine circadian system in humans. *Chronobiol. Int. Chronobiol. Int.* **2000**, *17*, 369–390. [CrossRef] [PubMed]
106. Argilés, J.M.; Busquets, S.; Stemmler, B.; López-Soriano, F.J. Cancer cachexia: Understanding the molecular basis. *Nat. Rev. Cancer* **2014**, *14*, 754–762. [CrossRef] [PubMed]
107. Molitch, M.E. Medication-Induced Hyperprolactinemia. *Mayo Clin. Proc.* **2005**, *80*, 1050–1057. [CrossRef] [PubMed]
108. Yao, H.; Rui, W.; Zhang, Y.; Liu, Y.; Lin, S.; Tang, H.; Zhao, W.; Wu, Z. Prolactin-secreting lung adenocarcinoma metastatic to the pituitary mimicking a prolactinoma: A case report. *Neurosurgery* **2019**, *85*, E773–E778. [CrossRef] [PubMed]
109. Peveler, R.C.; Branford, D.; Citrome, L.; Fitzgerald, P.; Harvey, P.W.; Holt, R.I.; Howard, L.; Kohen, D.; Jones, I.; O'Keane, V.; et al. Antipsychotics and hyperprolactinaemia: Clinical recommendations. *J. Psychopharmacol.* **2008**, *22*, 98–103. [CrossRef] [PubMed]

110. Fahie-Wilson, M.N.; Soule, S.G. Macroprolactinaemia: Contribution to hyperprolactinaemia in a district general hospital and evaluation of a screening test based on precipitation with polyethylene glycol. *Ann. Clin. Biochem. Int.* **1997**, *34*, 252–258. [CrossRef] [PubMed]
111. Ioannidis, J.P.A. Why most clinical research is not useful. *PLoS Med.* **2016**, *13*, e1002049. [CrossRef] [PubMed]

 https://doi.org/10.3390/jpm16070342

MDPI AG
Grosspeteranlage 5
4052 Basel
Switzerland
Tel.: +41 61 683 77 34

Journal of Personalized Medicine Editorial Office
E-mail: jpm@mdpi.com
www.mdpi.com/journal/jpm

www.ingramcontent.com/pod-product-compliance
Lightning Source LLC
LaVergne TN
LVHW070449061126
851858LV00011B/196